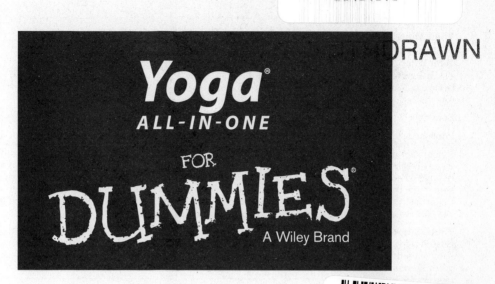

Yoga® ALL-IN-ONE FOR DUMMIES®

A Wiley Brand

by Larry Payne, PhD,
Georg Feuerstein, PhD,
Sherri Baptiste, Doug Swenson,
Stephan Bodian, Therese Iknoian,
LaReine Chabut

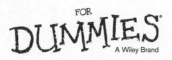

FOR DUMMIES®

A Wiley Brand

Contents at a Glance

Table of Contents

Book II: Basic Yoga Techniques and Postures 41

Chapter 1: The Fundamentals of Yogic Breathing 43

Chapter 2: Please Be Seated 57

Chapter 3: Standing Tall 67

Book VII: Meditation, Mindfulness, and Letting Go of Stress 435

Chapter 1: How Your Mind Stresses You Out and What You Can Do about It................................437

Chapter 2: Relaxed Like a Noodle: The Fine Art of Letting Go of Stress...................................457

Introduction

Yoga is the ultimate mind-body practice. By its very nature, it leads practitioners around the globe toward greater balance and relaxation. Each yoga pose balances alertness and relaxation. By integrating physical movements, breath, and mindfulness, yoga produces both bodily and mental relaxation. The result? A welcome dose of enhanced well-being, which is one reason why yoga has never been more important. In today's hectic schedules, seemingly loaded with constant stimulation and stress, yoga can bring balance and even serenity.

Consider *Yoga All-in-One For Dummies* your complete guide to finding the health and peace of mind that yoga can bring. Whether you're looking for classic poses and routines, more-modern takes on this ancient practice, or ways to incorporate yoga into your life, this book can get you started and well on your way. After all, at its core, yoga is a timeless answer for anyone seeking deeper meaning in life and that elusive treasure called abiding peacefulness.

About This Book

Yoga — and its many schools and philosophies — offers a number of mental and physical benefits to those who practice it. Whether you're interested in becoming more flexible, more fit, less stressed, or more peaceful and joyful, this book contains the guidance you need and the routines that can help you achieve your goals. It takes you step by step into the treasure house of yoga, where you'll find out how to strengthen your mind and enlist it to unlock your body's extraordinary potential. A sound body requires a sound mind, and this book shows you how to improve or regain the health and wholeness of both.

To help you fit yoga into your busy schedule, this book is organized in a way that lets you easily find the information you're looking for. You can read the book from cover to cover, or you can jump in at any section or chapter that interests you. Feel free to skip over the material marked with a Technical Stuff icon and the content in the sidebars; although these bits are interesting, they're not essential to your being able to practice yoga — or to do so safely. But if you see a Warning icon, take note — these tidbits offer suggestions to keep your yoga practice a safe one.

Within this book, you may note that some web addresses break across two lines of text. If you're reading this book in print and want to visit one of these web pages, simply key in the web address exactly as it's noted in the text, pretending as though the line break doesn't exist. If you're reading this as an e-book, you've got it easy — just click the web address to be taken directly to the web page.

Foolish Assumptions

The first assumption that guided the creation of *Yoga All-in-One For Dummies* was that you're looking for sound information about yoga in a no-nonsense presentation. Beyond that, here are a few other assumptions about you and the kind of information you want:

- ✔ If you're new to yoga, you want to start with the basics. No prior exposure to the many aspects of yoga is necessary for you to benefit from this book. In fact, this book is the perfect first step in your exploration. The Additional Yoga Resources section online at www.dummies.com/extras/yogaaio and www.dummies.com/go/yogaaiofd can help you with that, but you get more on that later in this introduction.

- ✔ If you already have some experience with yoga, you want to understand the fundamentals more deeply or go beyond the traditional types of yoga to experience something new. For you, this book provides detail and a fair amount of depth across the yoga spectrum — all in plain English. It also includes some hot trends in yoga, like Partner Yoga and Hot Yoga.

- ✔ If you're looking for yoga workouts that will make you stronger, healthier, more balanced, and more flexible, you'll find information and step-by-step instructions on Power Yoga and Yoga with Weights, both designed to enhance physical fitness.

- ✔ If you're interested in mind-body connection of yoga, you want a more in-depth look at mindfulness and meditation, easy-to-follow meditation instructions, and info on how to use relaxation techniques to let go of stress.

Icons Used in This Book

Throughout this book, you'll see icons in the margins. These icons are intended to draw your attention to particular kinds of information. Here's a key to what those icons mean:

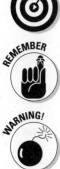

Tips point you toward helpful information that can make your yogic journey a little smoother.

Information you'll want to remember is marked with this icon. Making a mental note of this information can help you down the road in your understanding and practice.

Please take note of all warnings. Yoga is safe, but yoga injuries can and do happen, and you can avoid them by heeding the recommendations highlighted with this icon.

Consider this material "nice to know" information. It's interesting and can add to your experience, but feel free to skip it if you want to breeze through.

When you see this icon, prepare to stop what you're doing, take a few deep breaths, and start meditating. It's your chance to savor the real thing!

At www.dummies.com/go/yogaaiofd, you can find a series of videos that show you how to prepare for and move into several yoga postures. This icon highlights these postures.

Beyond the Book

In addition to the material in the print or e-book you're reading right now, this product also comes with some access-anywhere goodies on the web. You can access a Cheat Sheet that offers suggestions and information you can use to enhance your yoga workout: Discover how stretching can alleviate common aches and pains, find out why warming up before a yoga workout is vital, and be inspired by ways that yoga can improve your physical health. To access this material, go to www.dummies.com/cheatsheet/yogaallinone.

You also have access to additional articles at www.dummies.com/extras/ yogaallinone. There you can find ways to avoid common back injuries and loosen tight muscles and discover how to evaluate your fitness level in order to choose a style of yoga that's best for you, how to incorporate a meditative mindset throughout your daily life, and more.

In addition to the additional articles about yoga that you can find online, you can also view ten short videos that introduce you to great ideas for improving your yoga practice, regardless of your age or physical abilities. Check out these tried-and-true poses and routines at www.dummies.com/ go/yogaaiofd.

Where to Go from Here

This All-in-One is designed so that you get to decide how best to access the information, whether you prefer to read chapters one after the other and follow the yoga routines in order or you're more of a free spirit who jumps from one topic to another as the mood strikes you.

However, if you're a newcomer to yoga, spend some time with Book I, which lays the foundation for yoga practice, and Book II, which explains basic postures and key techniques you need to know for nearly all styles of yoga.

Beyond that, feel free to go wherever you like. Are you interested in basic yoga postures and techniques? Head to Book II. Want to check out some new yoga styles? Book VI offers yoga routines with a modern twist. And if you're not sure where you want to go, use the table of contents or the index to find the information you're looking for.

Book I

Getting Started with Yoga Principles

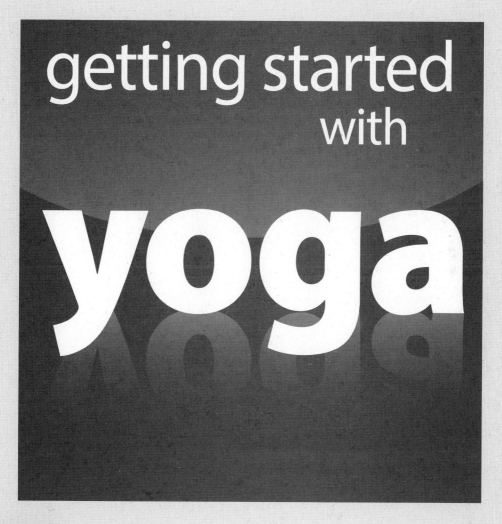

getting started with

yoga

Contents at a Glance

Chapter 1

Yoga 101: Building a Foundation

A lthough *yoga* is now a household word, many people don't know exactly what it is. Far more than just physical exercise, yoga can transform you, even if transformation isn't your intention when you first step onto the mat. This chapter explains what yoga really is, describes how it relates to your health and happiness, and introduces you to the many different branches and approaches to yoga. Yoga really does offer something for everyone.

Whatever your age, weight, flexibility, or beliefs may be, you can practice and benefit from some version of yoga. Yoga may have originated in India, but it's for all of humanity.

Understanding the True Character of Yoga

Whenever you hear that yoga is *just* this or *just* that, your nonsense alert should kick into action. Yoga is too comprehensive to reduce to any one aspect; it's like a skyscraper with many floors and numerous rooms at each level. Yoga isn't *just* gymnastics or stretching, fitness training, a way to control your weight, stress reduction, meditation, or a spiritual path. It's *all* these tools and a great deal more.

Taking a holistic view

The yoga we enjoy today comes from a 5,000-year-old Indian tradition. Some of the exercises look like gymnastics and so, not surprisingly, have made their way into Western gymnastics. These exercises, or postures, help you become (and stay) fit and trim, control your weight, and reduce your stress level. Yoga also offers a whole range of meditation practices, including breathing techniques that exercise your lungs and calm your nervous system, or that charge your brain and the rest of your body with delicious energy.

You can also use yoga as an efficient system of healthcare that has proven its usefulness in both restoring and maintaining health. Yoga continues to gain acceptance within the medical establishment; more physicians are recommending yoga to their patients not only for stress reduction but also as a safe and sane method of exercise and physical therapy (notably, for the back, neck, knees, and hips).

Still, yoga is far more than a system of preventative or restorative healthcare. Yoga looks at health from a broad, holistic perspective that integrative medicine is only now rediscovering. This perspective appreciates the enormous influence of the mind — your psychological attitudes and beliefs — on physical health.

Finding unity

Yoga means "union" or "integration" and also "discipline." The system of yoga, then, is a *unitive, or integrating, discipline*. Yoga seeks unity at various levels. First, it seeks to unite body and mind, which people all too often separate. Some people are chronically "out of the body." They can't feel their feet or the ground beneath them, as if they hover like ghosts just above their bodies. They're unable to cope with the ordinary pressures of daily life, so they collapse under stress. They don't understand their own emotions. Unable to cope with the ordinary pressures of life, they're easily hurt emotionally.

Yoga also seeks to unite the rational mind and the emotions. People frequently bottle up their emotions and don't express their real feelings. Instead, they choose to rationalize away these feelings. Chronic avoidance can become a serious health hazard; if people aren't aware that they're suppressing feelings such as anger, the anger consumes them from the inside out.

Here's how yoga can help you with your personal growth:

- ✔ It can put you in touch with your real feelings and balance your emotional life.

- ✔ It can help you understand and accept yourself so that you feel comfortable with who you are. You don't have to "fake it" or reduce your life to constant role playing.

- ✔ It helps you become more able to empathize and communicate with others.

Yoga is a powerful means of psychological integration. It makes you aware that you're part of a larger whole, not merely an island unto yourself. People can't thrive in isolation. Even the most independent individual is greatly indebted to others. When your mind and body are happily reunited, this union with others comes about naturally. The moral principles of yoga are all-embracing, encouraging you to seek kinship with everyone and everything.

Balancing your life

The Hindu tradition explains yoga as the discipline of balance, another way of expressing the ideal of unity through yoga. Everything in you must harmonize to function optimally. A disharmonious mind is disturbing in itself, but sooner or later, it also causes physical problems. An imbalanced body can easily warp your emotions and thought processes. If you have strained relationships with others, you cause distress not only for them but also for yourself. And when your relationship with your physical environment is disharmonious, well, you trigger serious repercussions for everyone.

Finding yourself: Are you a yogi (or a yogini)?

Someone who's practicing the discipline of balancing mind and body through yoga is traditionally called a *yogi* (if male) or a *yogini* (if female). This book uses both terms. Becoming a *yogi* or *yogini* means you do more than practice yoga postures. Yoginis embrace yoga as a self-transforming spiritual discipline. A yogi who has really mastered yoga is called an *adept*. If such an adept also teaches (and not all of them do), this person is traditionally called a *guru*. The Sanskrit word *guru* literally means "weighty one." According to traditional esoteric sources, the syllable *gu* signifies spiritual darkness, and *ru* signifies the act of removing. Thus, a guru is a teacher who leads the student from darkness to light.

Very few Westerners have achieved complete mastery of yoga, mainly because yoga is still a relatively young movement in the West. So please be careful about anyone who claims to be enlightened or to have been given the title of guru! However, at the level at which yoga is generally taught outside its Indian homeland, many competent yoga teachers or instructors can lend a helping hand to beginners.

A beautiful and simple yoga exercise called the tree (see Book II, Chapter 3) improves your sense of balance and promotes your inner stillness. Even when conditions force a tree to grow askew, it always balances itself out by growing a branch in the opposite direction. In this posture, you stand still like a tree, perfectly balanced.

Yoga helps you apply this principle to your life. Whenever life's demands and challenges force you to bend to one side, your inner strength and peace of mind serve as counterweights. Rising above all adversity, you can never be uprooted. For more strategies on finding balance, relieving stress, and attaining mindfulness, head to Book VII.

Considering Your Options: The Eight Main Branches of Yoga

Picture yoga as a giant tree with eight branches; each branch has its own unique character, but each is also part of the same tree. With so many different paths, you're sure to find one that's right for your personality, lifestyle, and goals. This section outlines the eight main branches of yoga and then delves a little deeper into Hatha Yoga, which is the kind of yoga focused on in this book.

An overview of the types of yoga

Here are the eight principal branches of yoga:

- **Bhakti (bhuk-tee) Yoga, the yoga of devotion:** Bhakti Yoga practitioners believe that a supreme being (the Divine) transcends their lives, and they feel moved to connect or even completely merge with that supreme being through acts of devotion. Bhakti Yoga includes such practices as making flower offerings, singing hymns of praise, and thinking about the Divine.

- **Hatha (haht-ha) Yoga, the yoga of physical discipline:** All branches of yoga seek to achieve the same final goal, enlightenment, but Hatha Yoga approaches this goal through the body rather than through the mind or the emotions. Hatha Yoga practitioners believe that, unless they properly purify and prepare their bodies, the higher stages of meditation and beyond are virtually impossible to achieve; such an attempt is like trying to climb Mt. Everest without the necessary gear or training. This book focuses on this particular branch of yoga.

- **Jnana (gyah-nah) Yoga, the yoga of wisdom:** Jnana Yoga teaches the ideal of *nondualism* — that reality is singular and your perception of countless distinct phenomena is a basic misconception. (What about the chair or sofa you're sitting on? Isn't that real? Jnana Yoga masters answer these questions by saying that all these things are real at your present level of consciousness, but they aren't ultimately real as separate or distinct things. Upon enlightenment, everything merges into one, and you become one with the immortal spirit.)

- **Karma (kahr-mah) Yoga, the yoga of self-transcending action:** Karma Yoga's most important principle is to act unselfishly, without attachment, and with integrity. Karma Yoga practitioners believe that all actions, whether bodily, vocal, or mental, have far-reaching consequences for which practitioners must assume full responsibility.

- **Mantra (mahn-trah) Yoga, the yoga of potent sound:** Mantra Yoga makes use of sound to harmonize the body and focus the mind. It works with *mantras,* which can be a syllable, word, or phrase.

Traditionally, practitioners receive a mantra from their teacher in the context of a formal initiation. They're asked to repeat it as often as possible and to keep it secret. Many Western teachers feel that initiation isn't necessary and that any sound works. You can even pick a word from the dictionary, such as *love, peace,* or *happiness.* From a traditional perspective, such words aren't really mantras, but they can be helpful nonetheless.

- **Raja (rah-jah) Yoga, the royal yoga:** Raja Yoga means literally "royal yoga" and is also known as classical yoga. When you mingle with yoga students long enough, you can expect to hear them refer to the eightfold path laid down in the Yoga-Sutra of Patanjali, the standard work of Raja Yoga, through which the practitioners seek to attain enlightenment. (To discover what these eight limbs are, head to the nearby sidebar "The eight limbs of yoga.")

Book I

Getting Started with Yoga Principles

The sacred syllable *om*

The best-known traditional mantra, used by Hindus and Buddhists alike, is the sacred syllable *om* (pronounced ommm, with a long *o* sound). It's the symbol of the absolute reality — the Self or spirit. It consists of the letters *a, u,* and *m,* joined by the nasal humming of the letter *m.* The *a* corresponds to the waking state, *u* to the dream state, and *m* to the state of deep sleep; the nasal humming sound represents the ultimate reality.

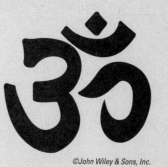

©John Wiley & Sons, Inc.

Another name for this yogic tradition is Ashtanga Yoga (pronounced ahsh-tahng-gah), the "eight-limbed yoga" — from *ashta* (eight) and *anga* (limb). But don't confuse this tradition with the yoga style known as Ashtanga Yoga, which is by far the most athletic of the three versions of Hatha Yoga, combining postures with breathing.

✔ **Tantra (tahn-trah) Yoga (including Laya Yoga and Kundalini Yoga), the yoga of continuity:** Tantra Yoga is the most complex and most widely misunderstood branch of yoga. In the West and India, Tantra Yoga is often confused with "spiritualized" sex; although some (so-called left-hand) schools of Tantra Yoga use sexual rituals, they aren't a regular practice in the majority of (so-called right-hand) schools. Tantra Yoga is actually a strict spiritual discipline involving fairly complex rituals and detailed visualizations of deities. These deities are either visions of the divine or the equivalent of Christianity's angels and are invoked to aid the yogic process of contemplation.

✔ **Guru (goo-roo) Yoga, the yoga of dedication to a yoga master:** In Guru Yoga, your teacher is the main focus of spiritual practice. Such a teacher is expected to be enlightened, or at least close to being enlightened. In Guru Yoga, you honor and meditate on your guru until you merge with him or her. Because the guru is thought to already be one with the ultimate reality, this merger duplicates his spiritual realization in you.

The eight limbs of yoga

In traditional Raja Yoga, students move toward enlightenment, or liberation, through an eight-limb approach:

✔ **Yama (yah-mah):** Moral discipline, consisting of the practices of nonharming, truthfulness, nonstealing, chastity, and greedlessness.

✔ **Niyama (nee-yah-mah):** Self-restraint, consisting of the five practices of purity, contentment, austerity, self-study, and devotion to a higher principle.

✔ **Asana (ah-sah-nah):** Posture, which serves two basic purposes: meditation and health.

✔ **Pranayama (prah-nah-yah-mah):** Breath control, which raises and balances your mental energy, thus boosting your health and mental concentration.

✔ **Pratyahara (prah-tyah-hah-rah):** Sensory inhibition, which internalizes your consciousness to prepare your mind for the various stages of meditation.

✔ **Dharana (dhah-rah-nah):** Concentration, or extended mental focusing, which is fundamental to yogic meditation.

✔ **Dhyana (dhee-yah-nah):** Meditation, the principal practice of higher yoga.

✔ **Samadhi (sah-mah-dhee):** Ecstasy, or the experience in which you become inwardly one with the object of your contemplation. This state is surpassed by actual enlightenment, or spiritual liberation.

Good karma, bad karma, no karma

The Sanskrit term *karma* literally means "action." It stands for activity in general, but also for the "invisible action" of destiny. According to yoga, every action of body, speech, and mind produces visible and also hidden consequences. Sometimes the hidden consequences — destiny — are far more significant than the obvious repercussions. Don't think of karma as blind destiny. You're always free to make choices. The purpose of Karma Yoga is to regulate how you act in the world so that you cease to be bound by karma. The practitioners of all types of yoga seek to not only prevent bad karma but also go beyond good karma, to no karma at all.

But please don't merge with your guru too readily! Guru Yoga is relatively rare in the West, so approach it with great caution to avoid possible exploitation.

Taking a closer look at Hatha Yoga

In its voyage to modernity, yoga has undergone many transformations. One of them was Hatha Yoga, which emerged around 1100 A.D. (This book focuses on this branch of yoga.) The most significant adaptations, however, occurred during the past several decades, particularly to serve the needs or wants of Western students. Of the many styles of Hatha Yoga available today, the following are the best known:

- ✔ **Iyengar Yoga** is the most widely recognized approach to Hatha Yoga. Characteristics of this style include precision performance and the aid of numerous props.

- ✔ **Viniyoga** (pronounced vee-nee yoh-gah) focuses on the breath and emphasizes practicing yoga according to your individual needs and capabilities.

- ✔ **Ashtanga Yoga** is by far the most athletic of the three versions of Hatha Yoga. This version combines postures with breathing.

   Power Yoga is a generic term for any style that closely follows Ashtanga Yoga but doesn't have a set series of postures. It emphasizes flexibility and strength and was mainly responsible for introducing yoga postures into gyms. To find out more about Power Yoga, head to Book IV; Book V offers Yoga with Weights.

- ✔ **Kripalu Yoga** is a three-stage yoga approach. The first stage emphasizes postural alignment and coordination of breath and movement; you hold the postures for a short time only. The second stage adds meditation and prolongs the postures. In the final stage, practicing the postures becomes a spontaneous meditation in motion.

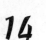

- ✔ **Integral Yoga** aims to integrate the various aspects of the body-mind by using a combination of postures, breathing techniques, deep relaxation, and meditation.

- ✔ **Sivananda Yoga** includes a series of 12 postures, the sun salutation sequence, breathing exercises, relaxation, and mantra chanting.

- ✔ **Ananda Yoga** is a gentle style that prepares students for meditation. Its distinguishing features are the silent affirmations associated with holding the postures. This yoga style includes exercises that involve consciously directing the body's energy (life force) to different organs and limbs.

- ✔ **Kundalini Yoga** isn't only an independent approach of yoga; it's also the name of a style of Hatha Yoga. Its purpose is to awaken the serpent power *(kundalini)* by means of postures, breath control, chanting, and meditation.

- ✔ **Prime of Life Yoga** follows the principle of modifying postures to match the needs and abilities of the student. It offers a safe, user-friendly approach targeted to men and women ages 45 to 75. Hallmarks of this approach are its focus on the breath, function over form, a mix of dynamic and static movement, and Forgiving Limbs. Throughout this book, you can discover aspects of Prime of Life Yoga: Head to Book I, Chapter 3 for information about Forgiving Limbs and explore the basics of the breath in Book II, Chapter 1. For a video of a beginning Prime of Life routine, go to www.dummies.com/go/yogaaiofd.

- ✔ **Somatic Yoga** is an integrated approach to the harmonious development of body and mind, based on both traditional yogic principles and modern psychophysiological research. This gentle approach emphasizes visualization, very slow movement into and out of postures, conscious breathing, mindfulness, and frequent relaxation between postures.

- ✔ **Moksha Yoga** champions a green philosophy. It uses traditional postures in a heated room and includes relaxation periods.

- ✔ **Bikram Yoga** has a set routine of 26 postures. This very vigorous style requires a certain fitness level for participation, especially because it calls for a high room temperature.

Hot Yoga isn't really a style itself; it just means that the practice occurs in a high-temperature room (usually 104 degrees to 109 degrees Fahrenheit). Best known is Bikram Yoga, although other styles also heat the room. For more on Hot Yoga, head to Book VI, Chapter 3.

Finding Your Niche: Four Basic Approaches to Yoga

Since yoga came to the West from its Indian homeland in the late 19th century, it has undergone various adaptations. Broadly, you can look at yoga in four overlapping approaches:

✔ As a method for physical fitness and health maintenance

✔ As a body-oriented therapy

✔ As a comprehensive lifestyle

✔ As a spiritual discipline

The first two approaches are often categorized as Postural Yoga; it contrasts with Traditional Yoga, which generally encompasses the last two approaches. As its name suggests, *Postural Yoga* focuses (sometimes exclusively) on yoga postures. *Traditional Yoga* seeks to adhere to the traditional teachings taught anciently in India. The upcoming sections take a look at the four basic approaches.

Most traditional or tradition-oriented approaches to yoga share two fundamental practices, the cultivation of awareness and relaxation: *Awareness* is the ability to pay close attention to something, to be consciously present, and to be mindful. *Relaxation* is the conscious release of unnecessary tension in the body. Both awareness and relaxation go hand in hand in yoga. Without bringing awareness and relaxation to yoga, the movements are merely exercises — not *yoga*.

Conscious breathing often joins awareness and relaxation as a third foundational practice. Normally, breathing happens automatically. In yoga, you bring awareness to this act, which then makes it a powerful tool for training your body and your mind. You can read much more about these aspects of yoga in Book II, Chapter 1.

Yoga as fitness training

The first approach, yoga as fitness training, is the most popular way Westerners practice yoga. It's also the most radical revamping of Traditional Yoga. More precisely, it's a modification of traditional Hatha Yoga. Yoga as fitness training is concerned primarily with the physical body's flexibility, resilience, and strength.

Fitness is how most newcomers to yoga encounter this great tradition. Fitness training is certainly a useful gateway into yoga, but later, some people discover that Hatha Yoga is a profound *spiritual* tradition. From the earliest times, yoga masters have emphasized the need for a healthy body, but they've also always pointed beyond the body to the mind and other vital aspects of the being.

If what motivates you is the prospect of having tighter buns or improving your golf game, you can certainly find that through yoga. As you progress with a dedicated practice, your body will become stronger and more agile, and your buns will tighten, too. As a "meditation in motion," though, yoga also can impact your performance on the green. The focus and coordination you develop on your yoga mat will spill over to your swing — and to the rest of your life.

Yoga as therapy

The second approach, yoga as therapy, applies yogic techniques to restore health or full physical and mental function. Though the idea behind yoga as a therapy is quite old, it's growing into a whole new professional discipline. Different from even highly experienced yoga teachers, yoga therapists have specialized training to apply the tools of yoga to promote and support healing.

Yoga as a lifestyle

Yoga as a lifestyle enters the proper domain of Traditional Yoga. Although practicing yoga only once or twice a week for an hour or so and focusing on its fitness training aspect is beneficial, you unlock the real potency of yoga when you adopt it as a lifestyle — *living* yoga and practicing it every day through physical exercises and meditation. Above all, when you adopt yoga as a lifestyle, you apply the wisdom of yoga to your everyday life and live with awareness. Yoga has much sage advice about everyday living, including diet and sleep habits, how you relate to others, and where you focus your attention and energy. It offers a total system of conscious and skillful living.

In modern times, a yoga lifestyle includes caring for the ailing environment, an idea especially captured in Green Yoga. Green Yoga incorporates environmental mindfulness and activism in its spiritual orientation. It centers on a deep reverence for all life and a lifestyle of voluntary simplicity; it believes the time has come to make yoga count in more than personal terms. Carpooling or biking to your next class and using an environmentally friendly yoga mat are just a couple of ways to get started.

Yoga as a spiritual discipline

Lifestyle Yoga (see the preceding section) is concerned with healthy, wholesome, functional, and benevolent living. Yoga as a spiritual discipline, the fourth approach, is concerned with all that *plus* the traditional ideal of *enlightenment* — that is, discovering your spiritual nature. This approach is often equated with Traditional Yoga.

Different people understand the word *spiritual* differently. In this context, *spiritual* relates to *spirit,* your ultimate nature. In yoga, it's called the *atman* (pronounced aht-mahn) or *purusha* (poo-roo-shah). According to *nondualistic* (based in one reality) yoga philosophy, the *spirit* is one and the same in all beings and things. It's formless, immortal, superconscious, and unimaginably blissful. It's transcendental because it exists beyond the limited body and mind. You discover the spirit fully in the moment of your enlightenment.

Locating Your Starting Place in the World of Yoga

When you know the lay of the land (see the preceding sections), consider what motivates you to practice yoga, as well as your lifestyle, physical style, and any limitations. Then find the style of yoga and practice environment that are good fits for you. Ask yourself these questions:

- ✔ Are you primarily looking for a method of stress management?
- ✔ Do you need to get your body moving after spending long hours in front of your computer?
- ✔ Do you seek quiet time and decompression after running after the kids all day?
- ✔ Are you drawn to a mental image of yourself with six-pack abs and tight buns?
- ✔ Do you aspire to reach transcendence?
- ✔ Are you a spiritual person in search of an outlet?
- ✔ Are you a secular person who yearns for moments of focus and balance?
- ✔ Do you have health concerns, such as lower back problems, that may limit your movement?
- ✔ Are you an athletic person looking for variety?
- ✔ Have you been a couch potato until now?

If your goals are entirely spiritual, choose a branch of yoga that can best help you achieve those goals. You may resonate with Bhakti Yoga, Jnana Yoga, Raja Yoga, Karma Yoga, or Tantra Yoga. If your main interest is in improving your health or overall physical well-being, or if you primarily want to become fit and flexible, select a style of Hatha Yoga that fits you best. To help you wind down, go with one of the more restorative styles. To get the juices flowing and blood pumping, try one of the flow styles. And Viniyoga and Prime of Life styles of yoga are especially well suited for people with physical concerns such as achy backs and shoulders.

All forms of yoga, when done with intention, can help you relax and give you a feeling of oneness. That oneness is yoga.

Chapter 2

Yoga and the Mind-Body Connection

*Y*ou may not know it, but when you exercise, you have the potential to exercise with your mind as well as your body. And in yoga, the mind plays a bigger part than it does in other exercise disciplines, because one of the goals of yoga is to be self-aware and to develop your relationship with your consciousness in everything you do.

This chapter explores training your mind and some of the mental aspects of yoga. You look into quieting and calming your mind, listening to your body as you exercise, and breaking the mental barriers that keep you from wanting to exercise. You also discover a mental visualization technique for focusing your mind and a special contract-and-release exercise for wringing all the tension from your body.

Taming the Monkey Mind

One of the objects of traditional yoga is to discover how to calm your mind to achieve clarity of thought. An overactive mind is sometimes called a "monkey mind." In traditional yoga, a *monkey mind* is one that swings wildly from branch to branch — that is, from thought to thought — without really considering where it's going. A monkey mind is always busy, so much so that it leaves you feeling exhausted and robs you of your precious energy resources and your ability to concentrate.

Taming a monkey mind isn't easy. It takes time, practice, and, perhaps most importantly, a commitment to discovering how to relax your mind and always remain in the moment. What does "in the moment" mean? It means to be consciously aware of your surroundings and how you feel *now* — not letting your mind drift into memories or fantasies. When you tame the monkey mind, you achieve self-awareness and the ability to think with clarity. You literally pull yourself together, body and mind. For more tips on taming a monkey mind, check out "Bringing Your Mind into the Present Moment" later in this chapter.

Focusing on the Transitions

Yoga masters pay a lot of attention to transitions. The entire yoga philosophy is not about abrupt stops and starts but rather smooth transitions of breath into breath and moment into moment. This philosophy applies to all activities in life — the transition between sleep and wakefulness, the transition between work and play, and even the transition from year to year and decade to decade, for example. In yoga class, it means paying as much attention to getting into and out of a pose as being in the pose itself.

The object is to make all transitions, from the smallest to the largest, smooth and graceful so you maintain your self-awareness and your yoga consciousness as a matter of course, no matter what you do or where you go. When you take on a yoga lifestyle, you strive to make all your activities — all the moments of your life — one vast, inspired moment imbued with yoga consciousness. This effort gives you a greater sense of personal empowerment and freedom of choice as you skillfully live your life. With each breath and each moment leading one to the other, you're fully alive as you embrace your life to its fullest without missing out on a single moment of the journey.

Easier said than done, of course, but practicing yoga can help. To start down the road of greater consciousness, focus on the transition between yoga exercises and how you link one breath to the next. (See Book II, Chapter 1 for breathing details.) Try to create effortless, flowing, graceful transitions between exercises, with as little excess movement as possible. When your mind wanders, as it will, gently pull it back and focus on what you're doing in the present. When you forget to breathe properly, you put more mental effort into breathing next time. You observe your own training, and, in the process, you become your own peak-performance coach. No one knows better than you do whether you're getting the most out of yoga exercises.

By focusing on the transitions between exercises, you can carry vitality, strength, and endurance from one exercise to the next. With enough attention to transitions, you can turn your yoga workout into a living dance, with all the postures connected through balance, presence, attention, and breath. And guess what? You'll even have some fun in the process.

Exercising from the Inside Out

Yoga is different from nearly all forms of exercise in that you do the exercises "from the inside out." In basketball and weightlifting, for example, the object is to do something outside of your body — make a basket or press a certain amount of weight. But in yoga, the object of the exercises is found mostly within, not outside of, the body. Yoga, in all its forms, is a profound technique for getting in touch with your body. As you perform an exercise, you feel and listen to the inner workings of your body. Your body tells you whether you're doing the exercise correctly, and part of your job is to discover how to listen. If you're in tune with yourself — if you feel balanced, if you feel the right combination of muscles at work, if you're pushing yourself precisely to the threshold of your ability — you'll know it.

Exercising from the inside out takes some getting used to for people who aren't accustomed to exercising this way. It requires a fair amount of patience; it requires you to focus within; and, to a certain degree, it requires you to rely on your intuition and to notice the subtle sensations in your body. Although instructors can help you with your posture and movements, knowing whether you're exercising correctly is ultimately up to you, and you'll know because you can feel it. No outside objective — jumping to a certain height, lifting a certain amount of weight — can tell you whether you're on target with an exercise. Only you, your intuition, your innate wisdom, and your intelligence can tell you when you're exercising right. Figuring it out may take some time, and it takes practice, but when you do, it feels great.

Letting Go of "I Can't Do It"

More so than muscle fatigue, what keeps most people from yoga is that broken record that each person has in his or her collection, the one that says over and over and over again, "I can't do it." Exercising is hard in and of itself; attempting a new exercise program may be even harder.

The only way to push aside "I can't do it" is to use your head. When the old record starts playing, take notice and then focus on your breathing. Listen to the air slowly entering and slowly leaving your lungs. This technique helps quiet your mind and keeps the record from playing. It helps you immerse yourself in the exercises. (For more information on breathing during yoga exercises, see Book II, Chapter 1.)

Resistance to exercising can come from many different places. Everyone can find excuses not to exercise. Everyone can think of things he or she would rather do. The easiest way to break through old barriers that your mind has built up against exercise is to take the first step or the first yoga breath. After you get going, you discover that exercising isn't as hard as you thought it was. Let each exercise session act as a new beginning and a fresh start. Take it one breath at a time. Make that your objective. Personal power — your greatest potential — rests within. When you bring what's within out into the world, miracles happen.

Bringing Your Mind into the Present Moment

Bringing your mind into the present moment is easier said than done. All people have distractions that keep them from focusing on the moment. To help you get there, check out the mental visualization technique and the exercise for relieving tension in this section. Turn to these pages when you want to coax yourself into living in the present. The information you find here can help you live life to the fullest by being in the moment.

Visualizing a calmer mind

One way to tame a wild and overly active mind — a monkey mind (see "Taming the Monkey Mind" earlier in this chapter) — is visualization. With *visualization,* you close your eyes and go on a mental journey as a means of calming your mind and achieving a quiet, meditative state of self-awareness. In effect, you become the producer of your own visual effects — a sort of director of your own mental movies. The idea is to reach a state of deep relaxation and focus.

The object of the following visualization is to discover a refuge of calm and quiet within yourself. You need at least 10 minutes for this visualization. Lights, camera, action:

1. **Lie down or sit comfortably in a quiet place.**

   Do your best to find a place where you aren't bothered by cellphones and other distractions.

2. **Notice the tip of your nose and the coolness or warmth of each breath as the stream of air flows in and out of your nostrils.**

3. **Keeping your attention on the tip of your nose, feel the sensations of your lungs as they fill with air and then empty themselves of air.**

   Focus on your lungs for at least six breaths.

4. **Imagine that the innermost center of your body, from your hips up to your shoulders, is a deep pond.**

5. **View this deep pond in your mind and direct your attention to the surface of the pond.**

6. **Notice the currents or waves on the surface of the pond and look toward the sky, above the pond in your mind, and observe any clouds.**

   The clouds represent your emotions, and the surface of the pond represents your thoughts. In the next several steps in the visualization, you sink deeper into the image of the pond and distance yourself from your flow of emotions and the activity of your thoughts.

7. **Visualize dropping a pebble into the pond.**

   In your mind, follow that pebble with all your awareness as it sinks deeper into the pond. Breathe in and out calmly and quietly, remaining aware of the tip of your nose if doing so helps you breathe more calmly and deeply.

8. **As the pebble continues to sink (which represents deeper levels of your awareness), feel a sense of your own depth, the calmness within you, and the stilling and quieting of your mind as the pebble falls into deeper waters of inner knowing.**

9. **Imagine the pebble coming to rest on the bottom of the pond.**

   You're at a point of restfulness in the depths; dwell here for as long as you want.

10. **In the role of an observer, step back from this visualization and notice that you've taken your mind and thoughts into deeper waters.**

    High above, the clouds (your emotions) are still alive and well, and the surface of the pond (your thoughts) is still ripe with currents and activity. Down in the depths, however, you are still and quiet. You've discovered the deeper well of a steady mind and calm deep within you. This state is known as *equanimity,* when the mind is calm and aware.

    Dwell comfortably and securely in this place of calm for as long as you care to remain. Remember: This place of calmness is always there waiting in case you need to visit it.

Releasing tension with a contract-and-release exercise

The object of this contract-and-release exercise is to release tension in your body and bring your mind into the present moment. You isolate different areas of your body one at a time, starting with your toes and working your way up to your head. In each body area, you contract your muscles hard and then gently relax them. The idea is to tense each muscle group hard, without straining, for about five to ten seconds, and then suddenly let go of the tension or contraction. When you release your muscles, you do so fully and abruptly, relaxing and letting your body fall completely limp. In this way, you achieve a state of deeper relaxation, and you systematically relieve tension from different areas of your body.

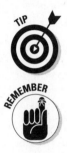

Visualize each muscle group you're working on in your mind's eye before you contract and relax the muscle group. By directing your thoughts into a part of your body, you can discover the nerve pathways necessary for relaxation. You discover how to relax by directing your mental energy toward your body.

Repeat the contract-and-release sequence three times with each part of your body you're working on. Hold the first contraction for five counts, the second for about seven, and the third for about ten. As you do so, inhale through your nose during contractions and exhale through pursed lips after you relax your muscles. Inhale deeply, yet not so deeply that you feel discomfort in your chest or lungs.

This exercise takes a bit of time — perhaps 10 to 20 minutes — but it's well worth the effort. Follow these steps to do the contract-and-release exercise:

1. **Lie down on your back in a quiet, comfortable place, and take a few deep, slow, Abdominal Breaths (Book II, Chapter 1 explains what these breaths are).**

   As you exhale, notice the weight of your body and how that weight is distributed on the carpet or on your yoga mat.

   In the next seven steps, starting with your toes and working upward, contract and relax muscle groups for five seconds.

2. **Direct your attention to your right and left legs and, in a wavelike action that moves from your feet upward, tighten your feet by curling your toes downward, and then relax.**

   If your muscles cramp, relax and gently shake off the cramp or wait until it stops, and then start again. Sometimes the muscles act up because you haven't used them in such a deep way for a while.

3. **Move the contractions up higher, tightening your calf muscles while flexing your toes toward you or turning your toes under (do whichever feels best).**

4. **Move the contraction higher again, engaging the muscles of your thighs all the way up to your hips.**

   You may tighten your buttocks along with your thighs, because the thigh muscles attach to that area. Feel your thigh muscles smoothing out and relaxing completely as you exhale.

5. **Tighten and relax your buttocks, hips, and abdominal areas.**

6. **Contract and release your back and chest.**

   As you relax, imagine a wave of release moving smoothly downward from your chest. Feel the excess tension in your chest flowing away with each exhalation.

7. **Clench your fists and feel the contraction moving up your arms; relax your arms and hands.**

   If you have to lift your arms from the floor, you can do so. Notice the muscles around your shoulder blades pushing in.

8. **Tense and relax the muscles in your neck, forehead, face, and scalp, as well as the muscles around your ears.**

   Be careful not to grind your teeth. Feel the frown lines on your face melting away.

9. **Repeat Steps 2 through 8, holding each muscle contraction for seven counts before releasing.**

10. **Repeat Steps 2 through 8 again, holding each muscle contraction for ten counts before releasing.**

11. **Take a deep, full breath and mentally scan your body for any tension that still remains; notice where you're still holding tight, and contract and relax the muscles there.**

    Feel your body resting deeply.

12. **Inhale and, as you gently hold your breath, contract your muscles everywhere — bottom to top, front to back, inside to outside, outside to inside, forward and back, up and down.**

    Feel a wave of contraction moving from your held breath into every area of your body.

13. **Exhaling quickly through your mouth, release all the muscles you've been contracting.**

    You'll hear a swooshing or deep-releasing *ahh* sound that rises from your belly as you exhale.

14. **Repeat Steps 12 and 13 three times.**

    Finish by resting gently. Let your breathing become natural again. Enjoy the sensations of your body resting on the floor.

Playing a bit of soothing music in the background helps some people with this exercise. And this exercise is a great way to finish off a yoga routine!

Taking a mind-body minute

Have a minute? Take a mind-body adventure. Keep it simple. Allow it to take you where it does each time. The following steps give you one way to enjoy a short mind-body ride.

1. **Sit comfortably on a firm chair with a straight back.**

   Sit up tall, but relaxed so that your spine is straight and comfortable. Put the soles of your feet flat on the floor.

2. **Place your hands on your knees, palms turned upward if you're in need of gathering more energy in, or palms turned down if you need to calm down and ground yourself more.**

   If you take a moment in an office or someplace with people around you and you don't want to stand out, just leave your arms relaxed on your legs.

3. **Close your eyes if you're comfortable with doing so.**

   Otherwise, leave them open, especially if you're around other people. If your eyes are open, turn your mental focus inside away from the bustle around you.

4. **Inhale fully and exhale fully; then let your breath return to a regular pattern, but still deep and regular.**

5. **Feel any heat or energy you can coming up through the soles of your feet; follow the energy with your mind as it travels up your legs, and your spine, stopping to circle around your heart.**

6. **Send the energy circling up into your head, then back down the front of your body, letting it pour out toward your hands, before returning back to your torso.**

   You can pull more energy in through your feet and let it cavort around your body again, or even several times.

7. **To finish, acknowledge that presence of energy and calm, inhale fully again and exhale fully, and come back to the present.**

That's the mind-body minute! Use your mind-body adventure to explore what burbles up on its own, reenergize yourself, meditate to clear your head, or calm yourself.

Chapter 3

Preparing for a Fruitful Yoga Practice

*I*n yoga, what you do and how you do it are equally important, and both mind and body contribute to your actions. Yoga respects the fact that you're a thinking, feeling body as well as a physical one. Full mental participation in even the simplest of physical exercise enables you to tap into your deeper potential as a human being.

This chapter is about cultivating the right attitude toward your yoga practice, which is the best preparation for success in yoga. Try to find your own pace without pushing yourself and risking injury, and leave your competitive spirit to other endeavors. Here, the emphasis is function over form; therefore, a modified version of the "ideal form" of a posture may be the right form for you. You can also find information on a few practical topics, like what to look for in a yoga instructor, whether to join a group or practice on your own, how to make time for yoga, and more.

Cultivating the Right Attitude

Yoga encourages you to examine all your basic attitudes toward life to discover which ones are dysfunctional so that you can replace them with more appropriate ones. One attitude worth cultivating is balance in everything, which is a top yogic virtue (refer to Book I, Chapter 1).

A balanced attitude in this context means that you're willing to build up your yoga practice step by step instead of expecting instant perfection. It also means not basing your practice on incorrect assumptions, including the notion that yoga is about tying yourself in knots. On the contrary, yoga loosens all your bodily, emotional, and intellectual knots. This sections gives you some guidelines for getting in the right yoga mindset.

Leave pretzels for snack time

Many people are turned off by magazine covers showing photographs of experts in advanced postures with their limbs tied in knots. What these publications may fail to disclose is that most of these yogis and yoginis have practiced yoga several hours a day for many years to achieve their level of skill. You don't have to be a pretzel to experience the undeniable benefits of yoga. The benefit you derive from yoga comes from practicing at a level appropriate for you, not from striking an advanced or "ideal" form.

Practice at your own pace

Some people are natural pretzels. If you (like most) aren't inherently noodlelike, regular practice can increase your flexibility and muscular strength. Take a graduated approach. In Book II, you can find all the preparatory and intermediary steps that lead up to the final forms for the various postures. The late yoga master T. S. Krishnamacharya of Chennai (Madras), India, the source of most of the best-known orientations of modern Hatha Yoga, emphasized tailoring yoga instruction to the needs of each individual and advised yoga teachers to take into account a student's age, physical ability, emotional state, and occupation. Follow this sound advice: Proceed gently but steadfastly.

Note: In this book, the exercise descriptions include all the stages of developing comfort with a particular posture. Why? Because asking a middle-aged newcomer to yoga to imitate the final form of many of the postures without providing suitable transitions and adaptations is a prescription for disaster. For instance, in many books on Hatha Yoga, you see the headstand featured quite prominently. This posture has become something of a symbol for yoga in the West. Headstands are powerful postures, to be sure, but they also count among the more advanced poses. Because this book emphasizes exercises that are both feasible and safe, it doesn't include the headstand. Instead, you find several adaptations that are easier to perform and have no risk attached.

Send the scorekeeper home

American children often grow up in a highly competitive environment. From childhood on, they're pressured to do more, push harder, and win. Young athletes grow up with the spirit of competition. Although competition has its place in society, this type of competitive behavior has no place in the practice of yoga.

The idea of *no pain, no gain* — a completely mistaken notion — often reinforces competitiveness. Although pain and discomfort are part of life, you don't have to invite them. The goal of yoga is to still the mind and experience freedom and liberation from suffering. Yoga is about peace, compassion, and harmony — the exact opposite of the competitive mindset. Yoga doesn't require you to fight against anyone, least of all yourself, or to achieve some goal by force. On the contrary, you're invited to be kind to yourself and others and, above all, to collaborate with your body rather than coerce it or do battle with your mind. Therefore, never flog your body; only coax it gently. Follow the motto "No gain from pain."

Picture yourself in the posture

Use visualization when executing postures. For example, before you do the cobra (Book II, Chapter 7), shoulder stand (Book II, Chapter 6), or triangle (Book II, Chapter 3) — or any pose, for that matter — take 10 seconds or so to visualize yourself moving into the final posture. Make your visualization as vivid as possible. Enlist the powers of your mind!

Enjoying a Peaceful and Safe Yoga Practice

As you travel through yogic postures, you begin to build awareness of the communications taking place between your body and mind. Do you feel peacefully removed from the raging storm of life around you, comfortable and confident with your strength, range of motion, flexibility, and steadiness? Or are you painfully noting the slow passage of time, sensing a physical awkwardness or strain in your movements? To help make your yoga experience an expression of peace, calm, and security, listen to your own feelings and sensations, and acknowledge their importance. That positive message is what yoga practice is all about.

Busting the perfect posture myth

The perfect posture is a perfect myth. How can the same posture be perfect for both a 15-year-old athlete and a 60-year-old retiree? As the great yoga master Patanjali explained nearly 2,000 years ago, posture has only two requirements: A posture should be steady and easeful:

- ✔ **Steady posture:** A *steady* posture is a posture that you hold stable for a certain period of time. The key isn't freezing all movement, though. Your posture becomes steady when your mind is steady. As long as your thoughts run wild, including your negative emotions, your body also remains unsteady. As you become more skilled in self-observation, you begin to notice the ever-revolving carousel of your mind and become sensitive to the tension in your body. That tension is what yoga means by *unsteadiness*.

- ✔ **Easeful posture:** A posture is *easeful* when it's enjoyable and enlivening rather than boring and burdensome. An easeful posture increases the principle of clarity — *sattva* — in you. But easefulness isn't slouching. *Sattva* and joy are intimately connected. The more *sattva* is present in your body-mind, the more relaxed and happy you are.

Listening to your body

No one knows your body like you do. The more you practice yoga, the better you become at determining your limitations, as well as your strengths, within each posture. Each posture presents its own unique challenges. You want to feel encouraged to explore and expand your physical and emotional boundaries without risking strain or injury to yourself.

Some teachers speak of practicing at the *edge,* the point at which the intensity of a posture challenges you but doesn't cause you pain or unusual discomfort. The idea is to slowly and carefully push that edge farther back and open up new territory. Cultivate self-observation and pay attention to the feedback from your body to be able to practice at the edge.

Each yoga session is an exercise in self-observation without judgment. Listen to what your body is telling you. Train yourself to become aware of the signals that continually travel from your muscles, tendons, ligaments, bones, and skin to your brain. Be in dialogue with your body instead of indulging in a mental monologue that excludes bodily awareness. Pay particular attention to signals coming from your neck, lower back, jaw muscles, abdomen, and any known problem or tension areas of your body. Here are some suggestions:

✔ If your breathing becomes labored, it usually indicates that, figuratively, you're going over the edge and you may want to back off.

✔ Beginners commonly experience trembling when holding certain yoga postures. Normally, the involuntary motion is noticeable in the legs or arms and is nothing to worry about, as long as you aren't straining. The tremors are simply a sign that your muscles are working in response to a new demand. Instead of focusing on the feeling that you've become a wobbly bowl of jelly, lengthen your breath a little, if you can, and allow your attention to go deeper within. If the trembling starts to go off the Richter scale, either ease up a little or end the posture altogether.

Moving slowly but surely

Most people are usually on automatic with movements that tend to be unconscious, too fast, and not particularly graceful. But all postural movements in yoga are intended to be executed slowly. Consider the advantages of slow motion:

✔ Enhanced awareness, which enables you to listen to what your body is telling you and to practice at the edge.

✔ Safer practice. Slowing down lowers the risk of straining or spraining muscles, tearing ligaments, and overtaxing your heart.

✔ Arrival at a deep stage of relaxation more quickly.

✔ Improved breathing and breathing stamina.

✔ Shared workload among more muscle groups.

For the best results, practice your postures at a slow, steady pace while calmly focusing on your breath and the postural movement (flip to Book II, Chapter 1 for more info on breathing and movement). Resist the temptation to speed up; instead, savor each posture. Relax and be present here and now. If your breathing becomes labored or you begin to feel fatigued, rest until you're ready to go on.

If you find yourself rushing through your program, pause and ask yourself, "Why the hurry?" Here are some strategies that can help you slow down:

✔ **If you're truly short on time,** shorten your program and focus on fewer postures. But if you just can't shake the feeling of being pressured by time, consider postponing your yoga session altogether and practice conscious breathing (discussed in Book II, Chapter 1) while you go about your other business.

✔ **If you're rushing through your program because you're feeling bored or generally distracted,** pause and remind yourself why you're practicing yoga in the first place. Renew your motivation by telling yourself that you have plenty of time to complete your session.

Boredom is a sign that you're detached from your own bodily experience and aren't living in the present moment. Participate fully in the process. As Book II, Chapter 1 explains, full yogic breathing in one of the resting postures has a wonderful calming effect. If you need more than a mental reminder, use one of the relaxation techniques in Book VII, Chapter 2 to slow yourself down.

Practicing function over form with Forgiving Limbs

In yoga, as in life, function is more important than form. The function, not the form, of the posture gives you its benefits. Beginners in particular need to adapt postures to enjoy their function and benefits right from the start.

One useful adaptive device is *Forgiving Limbs*. With Forgiving Limbs, you give yourself permission to slightly bend your legs and arms instead of keeping them fully extended. Bent arms and legs enable you to move your spine more easily, which is the focus of many postures and the key to a healthy spine.

For example, the primary mechanical function of a standing forward bend is to stretch your lower back. If you have a good back, take a moment to see what how Forgiving Limbs works; this adapted posture is safe for beginners:

1. **Stand up straight and, *without forcing anything,* bend forward and try to place your head on your knees, with the palms of your hands on the floor (see Figure 3-1a), or hold the backs of your ankles.**

   Few people can actually do this, especially beginners.

2. **Now stand up again, separate your feet to hip width, and bend forward, allowing your legs to bend until you can place your hands on the floor and almost touch your head to your knees (see Figure 3-1b).**

   When bending forward, be sure not to bounce up and down, as most people are inclined to do. You're not a bungee cord!

As you become more flexible — and you will! — gradually straighten your legs until you can come closer to the ideal posture.

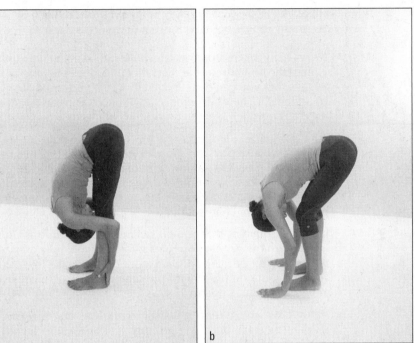

Figure 3-1:
Standing
forward bend
without and
with Forgiving
Limbs.

a

b

Photographs by Adam Latham

Putting safety first

The most important factor for determining the safety of a yoga class is your
personal attitude. If you participate with the understanding that you aren't
competing against the other students or trying to impress the teacher, and
that you also must not inflict pain upon yourself, you can enjoy a safe yoga
practice.

If you haven't exercised for a while, you can expect to encounter your body's
resistance at the beginning. You may even feel a little working soreness
the next day, which just reflects your body's efforts and its adjustment to
the new adventure. But try to avoid discomfort that causes you distress or
increases the likelihood of injury.

The key to avoiding injury is to proceed gently; better to err on the side of
gentleness than to face torn ligaments. Always ease into the postures and
work creatively with your body's physical resistance. Nonharming is an
important moral virtue in yoga, and observing this foremost yoga principle
applies not just to how you treat others but also to how you treat yourself!

Make sure you're physically ready before you begin this new venture with yoga — or any fitness activity, for that matter. Here are some pointers:

✔ **If you have an existing health challenge,** consult your doctor before embarking on your new activity. Keep in mind that one of the bounties of yoga is that you can benefit from it even if your medical history includes hypertension, heart problems, arthritis, or chronic back pain. You just need to approach it with respect for your body's needs and limits as well as its possibilities.

✔ **If you have any physical limitations (recent surgeries; knee, neck, or back problems; and so on),** be sure to inform the center and the teacher beforehand. In a classroom setting, instructors have to split their attention among many students; your upfront communication can help prevent personal injury.

If a teacher insists that you do an exercise or a routine that feels very uncomfortable or that you think may hurt you, take a break on your mat or, if that isn't possible, just walk out of the class. Try to stay cool, and register your complaint with the school afterward. Fortunately, this situation rarely happens.

✔ **If you have any serious physical limitations or concerns,** consider working closely with a competent yoga therapist to create just the right routines and to monitor your progress.

Ready, Set, Yoga: Dealing with the Practicalities

This section gives you everything you need to prepare for your yoga practice, whether you opt to take part in a class or practice solo. Here you discover information about the gear you want to have, how to find enough time to practice, how to cultivate an attitude that helps you get the most out of your practice, and more.

Finding suitable yoga instruction

Although you can explore some basic practices by reading about them (this book makes sure of that!), a full-fledged, safe yoga routine really requires proper instruction from a qualified teacher. This section helps you determine what kind of class to seek out.

Most people go for group instruction, but if you can afford private lessons, even a few sessions can be extremely beneficial. Importantly, if you have a serious health challenge, you need to work privately with a yoga therapist. After a few classes and with the benefit of an instructor's step-by-step guidance, you can certainly continue practicing and exploring yoga on your own (see the section "Going for it on your own" later in this chapter). Indeed, practicing on your own between classes is a great way to solidify yoga as an integral part of your life. However, if your solo practice is in lieu of class attendance, consider checking in with a teacher every so often, just to make sure you haven't acquired any bad habits in your practice style along the way.

Checking out centers, classes, and teachers

These days, it seems you can find a yoga class on every corner in large cities, so urbanites have lots of choices. But even country folks should be able to find an option that works.

Check out your local YMCA/YWCA, adult education center, or local health club to see what any of these has to offer. (If you go the health club route, however, make sure the teacher is really qualified. How much training has he had? Has she been certified by a recognized or registered yoga teacher training school or instructor?) You can also explore online yoga sites that offer taped or streamed yoga classes. Many sites offer classes in a range of styles for a variety of abilities and preferences.

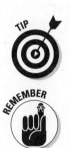

Why not put the word out that you're looking? You may get lots of referrals and suggestions. You can also search online for studios and classes in your area.

Visit a few places and teachers before you commit to a course or a series of classes. When you visit a yoga center or classroom, pay attention to how the staff treats you and how you respond to the people attending class. Stroll around the facility and feel its overall energy. First impressions are often (although not always) accurate. Some teachers even let you quietly look in on a class, although others find this practice too distracting for their students.

When checking out a yoga center, don't hesitate to ask questions of the instructor or other staff members about any concerns you have. In particular, find out what style of Hatha Yoga the center offers. Some styles — notably Ashtanga, or Power, Yoga — demand athletic fitness (head to Book IV for more on Power Yoga). Others embody a more relaxed and adaptable approach. If you're not familiar with the style of a particular school, don't hesitate to ask for an explanation (check out the explanation of styles in Book I, Chapter 1). Yoga practitioners are usually pretty friendly folk, eager to answer your questions and put your mind at ease.

Backyard studios and home classes

Throughout the world, many yoga teachers hold sessions in their homes or in backyard studios. Don't let this practice turn you off; you may find a great opportunity. Some of the most dedicated yoga teachers work this way because they want to avoid commercialism and the details of administering a full-scale center. Backyard studios often offer a great sense of community, and you can also expect lots of valuable personal attention from the teacher because the groups tend to be smaller than in larger centers.

Getting an impression of the teacher

A good yoga teacher is an example of what yoga is all about: a balanced person who's skillful in the postures, courteous of and thoughtful toward others, and adaptive and attentive to everyone's individual needs in class. Check out the teacher's credentials to be sure she has been properly trained or is certified in one of the established traditions.

Steer clear of teachers who have taken only a few workshops on yoga or received their diplomas after a three-day course. They may be excellent aerobics instructors who know nothing about yoga. Also avoid the drill sergeant type or anyone who makes you feel intimidated about your level of skill in performing the postures. By the way, under no circumstances must you allow your instructor to push or coerce you into a posture that doesn't feel right or that causes you pain.

Making sure the course fits your experience level

If you're a beginner, look for a beginner's course. You're likely to feel more comfortable in a group that's starting at the same skill level instead of being surrounded by advanced practitioners who can perform difficult postures easily and elegantly. Beginner's classes are sometimes advertised as *Easy Does It Yoga* or *Gentle Yoga*.

As a beginner, stay away from overly large classes (more than 20 students) or mixed-level classes that lump together yoga freshmen with postgraduates. Though some highly skilled and experienced teachers can manage such classes well, chances are that the teacher can't give you the attention you need to ensure your safety. If you find yourself as a newbie in a large class, let the teacher know you're a beginner, and bring up any physical limitations you may have. Then stake out a spot where the instructor can observe you throughout the class, or at least from time to time.

Taking cost into account

In general, group yoga classes are pretty affordable. The cheapest classes are usually available at adult education centers and at community and senior centers. YWCA classes also tend to be reasonably priced. If you have a health club membership, check to see whether your gym includes free yoga classes as part of the package. Most regular yoga centers in metropolitan areas charge an average of $15 to $20 per class; some offer package deals that can lower the cost per class. A one-time drop-in fee (for anyone who hasn't committed to taking more than one class) is usually a few dollars higher. Some schools offer the first class free, and others may charge as much as $25. On the other end, many yoga studios now offer community classes at a reduced fee or on a donation basis. Obviously, private lessons are quite a bit more expensive than group classes and range from $50 to $250.

When you're considering a commitment to a yoga center, check into the larger packages — they're often a good investment.

Deciding what to wear and packing your yoga class kit

Yoga practitioners wear a wide variety of exercise clothing. When selecting your own yoga wardrobe, your most important consideration needs to be whether the clothing allows you to move and breathe freely. Another practical matter is dressing for the temperature of the room. Have an extra layer that you can wear in the beginning until you warm up and that you can put back on toward the end as you cool down.

Although many yoga centers furnish mats as well as blocks, straps, blankets, and bolsters, consider bringing your own if you're serious about your yoga practice (and if you're concerned about hygiene). Note, however, that not every teacher uses props to the same extent, and the need for these various yoga helpers varies with the style of the class (as discussed in Book I, Chapter 1) and the teacher's preferences.

Before attending a class, find out what kind of floor it practices on. If the floor is carpeted, a towel or a sticky mat works. A hardwood floor may require more padding, especially if your knees are sensitive. In that case, bring along a thick yoga mat or a rug remnant that's a little longer than your height and a little wider than your shoulders. A folded blanket is also helpful if you need a pad under your head when you're lying down. If you tend to get cold, bring along a blanket to cover yourself during final relaxation. You want to make this item your own because you use it not just for support but also to cover your body.

Making time for yoga practice

For centuries, the traditional time for yoga practice has been sunrise and sunset, which are thought to be especially auspicious. Today's busy lifestyles, however, can undermine your best intentions, so be pragmatic and arrange your yoga practice at your convenience. Just keep in mind that, statistically, you have a 30 percent greater chance of accomplishing a fitness goal if you practice in the morning. More important than holding tight to a preset time is just making sure that you work yoga into your schedule *somewhere* — and stick with it.

Practicing at roughly the same time during the day can help you create a positive habit, which may make maintaining your routine easier. Experiment to see what works in your life, and stick to it. Mix and match from these suggestions:

✔ A short daily practice of 10 to 15 minutes

✔ A yoga class two or three times per week

✔ Short breathing and meditation breaks throughout the day

The amount of time you dedicate to yoga is a personal choice — no need to feel guilty about your decision. Guilt is counterproductive and has no place in yoga practice.

Going for it on your own

If you live in an isolated area and don't have easy access to a yoga instructor or class, don't be disheartened. You still have several choices that can help you begin your yogic journey. Here's some advice:

✔ **Video, DVD, and so on:** If you opt for this particular approach, consider this recommendation: After you learn a routine, begin listening only to the instructor's voice rather than focusing on the screen. Yoga emphasizes more inner work than outer activity, and watching the screen interferes with this process. Listening to a disembodied voice works better. (According to yoga, the eye is an active and even aggressive sense, whereas the ear is a more passive receptor.) CDs can also work well for this reason, as long as they're accompanied by informative illustrations.

✔ **Books and magazines:** You may find that you prefer a good yoga book to magazine or newspaper articles, simply because creating a book usually requires more in-depth, detailed consideration of subject matter and presentation. Plus, books have fewer advertisements taking up valuable space than periodicals do. But don't discount the value of a newsletter from a backyard yoga studio. The publication can be a real find if it comes from a legitimate source.

The difficulty with self-tutoring at the beginning is that you may have trouble judging good form from bad — and by *good,* read "safe." A good form is also one that helps you build your foundation for more advanced practice, not one that aims to fit the common stereotype of what yoga is "supposed to" look like. You need time to understand how your body responds to the challenge of a posture and determine the proper adjustments for your body's own optimal form.

Some people use a mirror to check the postures, but that tells only one side of the story. More importantly, it externalizes the whole process too much. Become comfortable with checking from the inside, through inwardly *feeling* your body. Until you're proficient at doing so, seek out a competent instructor if at all possible. Another person sees you objectively — from all sides — and can thus give you valuable feedback about your body's specific resistances and requirements.

Book I

Getting Started with Yoga Principles

Book II

Basic Yoga Techniques and Postures

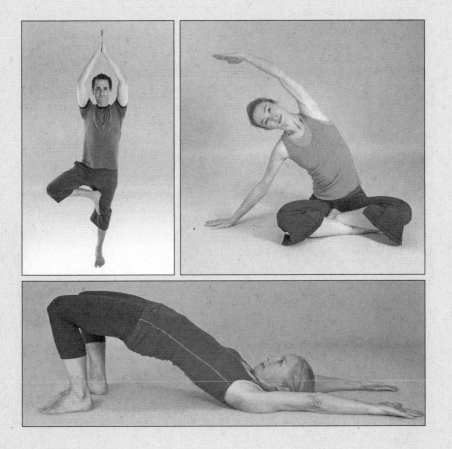

Contents at a Glance

Chapter 1

The Fundamentals of Yogic Breathing

*I*n the ancient Sanskrit language, the word for "breath" is the same as the word for "life" — *prana* (pronounced prah-nah) — which translates into what is known as vital force, your life force. This gives you a good clue about how important yoga thinks breathing is for your well-being. Yoga practiced without conscious breathing (which awakens *prana)* is like putting an empty pot on the stove and hoping for a delicious meal.

In this chapter, you discover how to use conscious breathing in conjunction with the yoga postures. This chapter also introduces several breathing exercises that you do seated either on a chair or in one of the yoga sitting postures (if you're up to that).

Breathing Your Way to Good Health

Most people's breathing habits are quite poor and to their great disadvantage. Shallow breathing, which is common, doesn't efficiently oxygenate the ten pints of blood circulating in your arteries and veins. Consequently, toxins accumulate in the cells. Before you know it, you feel mentally sluggish and emotionally down, and eventually organs begin to malfunction. Poor breathing is also known to cause and increase stress, which itself shortens your breath and increases your level of anxiety.

You can help alleviate stress through the simple practice of yogic breathing. Among other benefits, breathing loads your blood with oxygen, which, by nourishing and repairing your body's cells, maintains your health at the most fundamental level. Is it any wonder that the breath is the best tool you have to profoundly affect your body and mind?

The masters of yoga discovered the usefulness of the breath thousands of years ago and have perfected a system for the conscious control of breathing. In yoga, consciously regulated breathing has three major applications:

- ✔ In conjunction with the various postures, to achieve the deepest possible effect and to prepare the mind for meditation
- ✔ As breath control (called *pranayama,* pronounced prah-nah-yah-mah), to invigorate your vitality and reduce your anxiety
- ✔ As a healing method in which you consciously direct the breath to a particular part or organ of the body, to remove energetic blockages and facilitate healing

During your normal breathing, you may notice a slight natural pause between inhalation and exhalation. This pause becomes important in yogic breathing; even though it lasts only one or two seconds, the pause is a natural moment of stillness and meditation. If you pay attention to this pause, it can help you become more aware of the unity among body, breath, and mind — all of which are key elements in your yoga practice. With the help of a teacher, you also can discover how to lengthen the pause during various yoga postures to heighten its positive effects.

Practicing safe yogic breathing

As you look forward to the calming and restorative power of yogic breathing, take time to reflect on a few safety tips that can help you enjoy your experience:

- ✔ If you have problems with your lungs (such as a cold or asthma), or if you have heart disease, consult your physician before embarking on breath control, even if you're under the supervision of a yoga therapist.
- ✔ Don't practice breathing exercises when the air is too cold or too hot. Also avoid practicing in polluted air, including the smoke from incense.
- ✔ Don't strain your breathing; remain relaxed while doing the breathing exercises.
- ✔ Don't overdo the number of repetitions. Stay within the guidelines for each exercise.
- ✔ Don't wear constricting clothing.

Reaping the physical benefits of yogic breathing

Besides benefiting your mental outlook, yoga breathing techniques offer many benefits to your health. Here are a handful of them:

- ✔ **Metabolism:** Breathing well supports the function of the digestive, respiratory, circulatory, and hormonal systems and may be helpful in promoting metabolic balance.

- ✔ **Detoxification:** When you exhale, you release carbon dioxide (a waste product of your body's natural metabolism) that has been passed from your bloodstream into your lungs. By expelling air from the deepest recesses of your lungs, you expel more carbon dioxide and you enable your lungs to take in more oxygen.

- ✔ **Oxygenation:** The supply of oxygen to your brain and the muscles of your body increases. Oxygen enables your body to metabolize vitamins, minerals, and other nutrients.

- ✔ **Organ massage:** Each time you inhale, your diaphragm descends and your abdomen expands. This action massages your intestines, heart, and other organs near your diaphragm. Proper breathing helps to promote improved circulation in these organs. What's more, it helps to strengthen and tone your abdominal muscles.

- ✔ **Posture:** The breathing techniques encourage good posture. Poor posture can be a cause of incorrect breathing.

According to the yoga tradition, each person is allotted a certain number of breaths, and after you exceed this number, your time on earth is finished. People who breathe hurriedly and shallowly use up their allotment of breaths quickly, but if you breathe slowly and consciously, your breath allotment lasts for many years. Let this thoughtful idea remind you how valuable and life-expanding each breath may be. Developing a breath that's balanced, steady, and rhythmic — one that's never forced but deep and full — helps you live a long and healthy life.

Understanding the emotional benefits of yogic breathing

Psychologically, people tend to use the diaphragm as a lid to bottle up their undigested or unwanted emotions of anger and fear. Chronic contraction of the diaphragm makes it inflexible and blocks the free flow of energy between the abdomen (the nether region of the bowels) and the chest (the feelings associated with the heart). Yogic breathing helps restore flexibility and function to the diaphragm and removes obstructions to the flow of physical and emotional energy. You can then experience liberation of your emotions, which can lead you to integrate them with the rest of your life.

Deep breathing not only affects the organs in your chest and abdomen but also reaches down into your gut emotions. Don't be surprised if sighs and perhaps even a few tears accompany the tension release your breath work achieves. These are welcome signs that you're peeling off the muscular armor you have placed around your abdomen and heart. Instead of feeling concerned or embarrassed, rejoice in your newly gained inner freedom! Yoga practitioners know that real men (and women) do cry.

Starting Out with Focus Breathing

Before you delve into the specific kinds of yogic breathing — or if you've had a little difficulty synchronizing yourself with the rhythm of the complete yoga breathing techniques — you may first want to try a simpler method called *focus breathing*. Focus breathing is a great stepping stone to all the other techniques. The following list walks you through the phases of focus breathing:

- ✔ **Phase 1:** During your yoga practice, simply follow the directions about when to inhale and exhale for each posture, breathe only through the nose, and make the breath a little longer than normal. That's all you have to do! Don't worry about where the breath is starting or ending — just breathe slowly and evenly. (The chapters of Book II present the basic postures.)

- ✔ **Phase 2:** When you're used to the Phase 1 practice, just add a short pause of one or two seconds after inhalation and another one after exhalation.

- ✔ **Phase 3:** When you're comfortable with the practices of Phases 1 and 2, add drawing in the belly during exhalation without force or exaggeration.

A Variety of Yoga Breathing Techniques

The breathing techniques presented here are designed to relax and energize you. You can practice these breathing techniques by themselves or as you do your yoga routines and workouts. Get to know each technique so that you can call on it when you need it. After experimenting for a while, you discover the breath that feels best to you while you're working out. Although several workouts in this book offer a suggestion for a certain breath, feel free to substitute a breath you prefer. You can also do these breathing techniques while you're sitting, lying down, or standing.

No matter which breathing technique you undertake, follow these basic breathing guidelines:

Book II

Basic Yoga Techniques and Postures

- ✓ **Breathe through your nose unless told to breathe through your mouth.** Nostril breathing slows the process down. It also helps to filter and warm the air as it enters your body. A few classical yogic techniques for breath control, however, require you to breathe through the mouth. When a mouth-breathing technique is presented, the instructions alert you to that fact.

- ✓ **Listen to yourself breathe.** By listening to your breathing, you begin to control your breathing, and, in turn, you notice that you can gently shift your mood or disposition in subtle ways. Working gently with the sound and the sensations of your breath, you can subtly control how your body feels.

- ✓ **Breathe rhythmically.** If your breath stops or sounds rough, short, or shallow, it's a sign that you may be pushing too hard as you exercise.

- ✓ **Concentrate on making a smooth transition between each inhalation and exhalation — focus on the point of stillness where one becomes the other.** Don't hold your breath at the top of an inhalation; ride it a bit over the top and then smoothly turn it into an exhalation. At the bottom of an exhalation, ride it out just a bit as well, and then smoothly transition into a natural inhalation.

- ✓ **Never force your breath beyond the natural capacity of your lungs.** Full, rhythmic, gentle breathing without strain is the goal of yoga breathing.

- ✓ **Never force your lungs to inhale or expel air.** Feel your lungs filling evenly and calmly in all directions — up, down, into each side, forward, and back.

- ✓ **Don't practice yoga breathing in uncomfortable places where the air is too cold or too hot.** Like Goldilocks's porridge, the air should be "just right." Find a place that feels comfortable to you.

- ✓ **Straighten your posture.** If you slouch, let your belly hang out, round your shoulders, or stand without distributing and balancing the weight of your body properly, you can't breathe well. If your posture is poor, you're crowding or collapsing your lungs and diminishing their capacity to take in oxygen.

The Complete Breath

Most people are either shallow chest breathers or shallow belly breathers. Yogic breathing incorporates a complete breath that expands both the chest and the abdomen on inhalation either from the chest down or from the abdomen up. The Complete Breath engages your entire respiratory system. Besides raising and gently opening your collarbone and rib cage area, you engage your abdomen evenly and activate your diaphragm naturally, thus creating a full and deep breath. If you do no other yoga exercise, the complete yoga breath — integrally combined with relaxation — can still be of invaluable benefit to you.

Ideally, you should inhale and exhale six times per minute when using the Complete Breath. Breathing through your nostrils, you inhale four to six counts at minimum, and you exhale six to ten counts at minimum. Of course, this is the ideal, but if you're new to yoga, inhale as many counts as you can without straining, and try to reach the four- to six-count minimum.

Yogic breathing involves breathing much more deeply than usual, which, in turn, brings more oxygen into your system. Don't be surprised if you feel a little lightheaded or even dizzy in the beginning. If this situation happens during your yoga practice, just rest for a few minutes or lie down until you feel like proceeding. Remind yourself that you don't need to rush.

Belly-to-chest breathing

In belly-to-chest breathing, you really exercise your chest and diaphragm muscles as well as your lungs, and you treat your body with oodles of oxygen and life force *(prana)*. When you're done, your cells are humming with energy, and your brain is grateful to you for the extra boost. You can use this form of breathing before you begin your relaxation practice, before and where indicated during your practice of the yoga postures, and whenever you feel so inclined throughout the day. You don't necessarily have to lie down as described in this exercise; you can be seated or even walking. After practicing this technique for a while, you may find that it becomes second nature to you.

1. **Lie flat on your back, with your knees bent and your feet on the floor at hip width, and relax.**

   Place a small pillow or folded blanket under your head if you have tension in your neck or if your chin tilts upward. Place a large pillow under your knees if your back is uncomfortable.

2. **Inhale while expanding your abdomen, your ribs, and then your chest; pause for a couple of seconds.**

3. **Exhale while releasing your chest and shoulder muscles, gently and continuously contracting or drawing in your abdomen; pause again for a couple of seconds.**

4. **Repeat Steps 2 and 3 from 6 to 12 times.**

You can greatly enhance the value of this exercise and others by fully participating with your mind. Feel the air fill your lungs. Feel your muscles work. Feel your body as a whole. Visualize precious life energy entering your lungs and every cell of your body, rejuvenating and energizing you. To help you experience this exercise more profoundly, keep your eyes closed. Place your hands on your abdomen and feel it expand upon inhalation.

Chest-to-belly breathing

Folks in the West sit in chairs and bend forward too much. The daily sitting routine begins in the early morning when they go to the bathroom and then lean over the sink to brush their teeth and then continues throughout the day, usually ending as they sit in front of the television at home until their eyes get blurry. The chest-to-belly breathing emphasizes arching the spine and the upper back to compensate for all this bending forward throughout the day, and it also works well for moving into and out of yoga postures. Chest-to-belly breathing is also an excellent energizer in the morning; you can do it even before you hop out of bed. Don't do this exercise late at night, though, because it's likely to keep you awake.

You can practice the following exercise lying down, seated, or even while walking.

1. **Lie flat on your back, with your knees bent and your feet on the floor at hip width, and relax.**

   Place a small pillow or folded blanket under your head if you have tension in your neck or if your chin tilts upward. Place a large pillow under your knees if your back is uncomfortable.

2. **Inhale while expanding the chest from the top down and continuing this movement downward into the belly; pause for a couple of seconds.**

3. **Exhale while gently contracting and drawing the belly inward, starting just below the navel; pause for a couple of seconds.**

4. **Repeat Steps 2 and 3 from 6 to 12 times.**

Book II

Basic Yoga Techniques and Postures

The Abdominal Breath

Do the Abdominal Breath when you're feeling tension, stress, or fatigue. This breath relaxes you. A few minutes of deep abdominal breathing can help bring greater connectedness between your mind and your body. The goal is to shift from upper chest, short, shallow breathing to deeper abdominal breathing. Concentrate on your breath and try to breathe in and out gently through your nose. With each breath, allow any tension in your body to slip away. After you start breathing slowly with your abdominals, sit quietly and enjoy the sensation of physical relaxation.

Follow these steps to practice the Abdominal Breath:

1. **Lie on your back or sit comfortably in a chair.**

2. **Place one hand on your abdomen just above your pubic bone and below your navel; place your other hand on your solar plexus right beneath your breastbone.**

3. **Listening to your breath, inhale slowly and deeply through your nostrils — so deeply that your belly expands and you feel a wave of breath moving into the bottom, or lowest recesses, of your lungs.**

   Get down to the bottom of your lungs with this inhalation, going as low and as deep inside your lungs as you can. You can feel the rounding of your abdomen in your hands such that your hands rise a bit and your abdominal cavity pushes upward. Meanwhile, your chest opens and expands gently as if your abdomen is a balloon filling with air evenly and equally in all directions.

4. **At the top of your inhalation, find the point of transition where the inhale becomes an exhale.**

   At the top of every breath is a point of passage, the place where the inhale ends and the exhale begins. Find that place within your lungs and pause a moment to notice how your breath gently begins to shift in a new direction.

5. **To a count of six to eight (or more) seconds, exhale fully through your nostrils.**

   Feel your whole body releasing tension and letting go. Allow your body, including your arms and legs, to relax and go limp.

Do ten slow, full Abdominal Breaths.

The Abdominal Breath is *very* relaxing. It really works when done well, and for that reason, you may not want to practice it while you're driving.

The Ocean Breath

The Ocean Breath — sometimes called "rib breathing" or the "upward-moving breath" — oxygenates your blood, stimulates your circulation, and gives you a burst of energy.

You emit a sound during the Ocean Breath — the sound (you guessed it) of an ocean breeze. You stay in your chest and fill your lungs from the diaphragm upward. To stay inflated, your lungs rely on a vacuumlike action inside your chest, and then you push out a full, deep, and complete exhalation through your nostrils. This breath is different from the Complete Breath because you mostly engage your chest and rib cage, and you gently contract your abdomen.

Book II

Basic Yoga Techniques and Postures

Follow these steps to practice the Ocean Breath:

1. **Stand or sit comfortably with your spine straight.**

2. **Place your arms on your chest with the fingers of your right hand tucked into your left armpit and the fingers of your left hand tucked into your right armpit.**

3. **Close your eyes or gaze straight ahead with your windpipe open, your jaw and mouth relaxed, and your chin pointing gently downward.**

4. **Inhale to a count of six to ten, engaging the sipping muscles in the back of your throat as if you're sipping through a straw, and feel your ribs opening and your breath filling to the top of your lungs.**

   Inhale to whichever count you can manage best.

   Pay attention to the tip of your nose as you inhale. It enhances the sensation of filling your chest all the way up.

5. **Gently, but with some commitment and determination, exhale steadily through your nostrils until the exhale is complete.**

   Feel your breath passing from the back of your throat, across the roof of your mouth, and out your nostrils. You hear a hissing sound, something similar to the sound of a hose when you turn it on and the water begins rushing out.

   Never push too hard; this breath is dynamic, but never forced. Feel yourself releasing the air. When you push the air out, your abdominal muscles come into play a bit more. The exhale is something like a volcanic eruption that begins at the diaphragm and rises with increasing strength.

Take 10 Ocean Breaths; pause to rest; do 10 more; pause to rest again; and if you like the results, do 10 more for a total of 30 breaths. Then you can let your abdomen relax and your breath normalize once again.

Perfecting the Ocean Breath takes time, especially when you try smoothing out the transition between inhaling and exhaling, but stick with it. As yoga teacher Sherri Baptiste says, "Breath into breath, moment into moment."

The Balancing Breath

The object of the Balancing Breath is to develop a conscious control of your breathing. Try this simple breathing technique when you feel tired or overwhelmed or when you just want to clear your head for a moment.

Follow these steps to practice a Balancing Breath:

1. **Sit, lie down, or stand with your shoulders, mouth, and jaw relaxed.**

   Your choice: Gaze softly straight ahead or close your eyes. Make sure your back is erect but not rigid.

2. **To a count of four, slowly inhale through your nose.**

   Feel your breath expanding into your abdomen, mid-body (the diaphragm area), and upper chest. Without forcing, engage and gently fill your lungs to their full capacity.

3. **To a count of four, exhale slowly through your nose, drawing your abdomen gently in and up to help send the breath smoothly out.**

   Although your breath empties from your lungs, focus on releasing it first with your abdomen, and then with your diaphragm, and then with your upper chest. Emit all the air from your lungs.

Practice the Balancing Breath six to ten times — inhaling to a count of four and exhaling to a count of four — pause to rest for a moment, and then do another six to ten Balancing Breaths.

The Cleansing Breath

The purpose of the Cleansing Breath is to clean and clear out your lungs. This breath is unique, because instead of exhaling through your nose, you exhale through your mouth as you purse your lips. Pursing your lips creates pressure on your airways and helps keep them open so stale air can exit your lungs. It feels almost as though you're releasing pent-up emotions when you do the Cleansing Breath. In effect, you emit a "sigh of relief."

If you can, practice the Cleansing Breath outside in the fresh morning air. Follow these steps to practice a Cleansing Breath:

1. **Inhale a Complete Breath comfortably through your nostrils to the count of four to six.**

   You can find the Complete Breath in the section "The Complete Breath" earlier in this chapter.

2. **Gently purse your lips as you strongly exhale to a count of four.**

   Exhale vigorously so you make a loud whooshing sound. Feel your breath rising from the bottom to the top of your lungs in a dynamic and complete release. Refreshing, isn't it? You feel as though you're cleansing your entire system.

   Gently contracting your abdominal muscles as you exhale helps push the air out.

Complete this breath four to six times.

The Vitality Breath

The Vitality Breath sends energy to all parts of your body and makes you feel more alive.

Follow these steps to practice the Vitality Breath:

1. **Stand upright with your feet spread wider than your hips and your toes pointing forward.**

   Make sure your body weight is well-balanced between both legs.

2. **While inhaling a Complete Breath through your nostrils to the count of four, extend your arms straight out in front of you, palms facing upward.**

   This is the starting position.

   For an explanation of the Complete Breath, refer to the section "The Complete Breath" earlier in this chapter. Although you hold your arms in front of you, you should hold them in a relaxed manner.

3. **Exhale slowly through your mouth or through pursed lips as you draw your hands toward your body along the sides of your rib cage and gradually contract the muscles of your arms and hands.**

   By the time your arms and hands reach the sides of your body, contract your muscles so that your fists are clenched. Put some force into it.

Book II

Basic Yoga Techniques and Postures

At this point, your fists should be tightly clenched, and you should feel a driving force or sense of inner release as you exhale.

4. **Relax your arms and hands as you deeply inhale, slowly unclench your fists, and return to the starting position (see Step 2).**

Imagine that you're taking in this breath through your hands and heart.

Repeat Steps 2 through 4 six to eight times to complete six to eight Vitality Breaths.

Seeing How Breath and Postural Movement Work Together

In yoga, breathing is just as important as the postures, described in Book II. How you breathe when you're moving into, holding, or moving out of any given posture can greatly increase the efficiency and benefits of your practice. Consider some basic guidelines:

✔ **Let the breath initiate the movement.** The breath is the initiator or activator of the posture or exercise (that is, it leads the movement) by a couple of moments. It activates the action or flow of postures. When you inhale, the body opens or expands, and when you exhale, the body folds or contracts.

✔ **In the beginning, let the breath dictate the length of the postural movement.** For example, if you're raising your arms as you inhale and you run out of breath before you reach your goal, just pause your breathing for a moment and bring your arms back down as you exhale. With practice, your breath will gradually get longer.

✔ **Let the breath itself be your teacher.** When your breath sounds labored, you need to back off or come out of a posture.

✔ **Breathe in four directions.** Normally, when people move, they tend to hold or strain their breath. In yoga, you simply follow the natural flow of the breath. As a rule, adopt this pattern:

• Inhale when moving into back bends (see Figure 1-1a).

• Exhale when moving into forward bends (see Figure 1-1b).

• Exhale when moving into side bends (see Figure 1-1c).

• Exhale when moving into twists (as shown in Figure 1-1d).

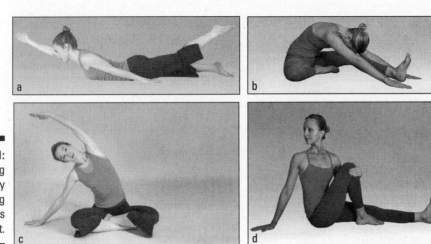

Figure 1-1:
Breathing
properly
during
postures is
important.

Photographs by Adam Latham

Chapter 2

Please Be Seated

In This Chapter

▶ Using good technique to gain physical and spiritual benefits

▶ Executing fundamental sitting postures

*Y*our everyday sitting preferences have a decided effect on your capacity to feel steady and comfortable in the yoga postures, whether standing or sitting. If you're new to yoga and its sitting postures, you'll soon discover that a lifetime of chair sitting exacts a stiff price. Your work with the postures in this book can help you gradually improve your floor sitting, but until you're ready to make the transition to the floor, use a chair when you sit for formal practice. After all, two of the largest yoga organizations in the world, Self-Realization Fellowship (SRF) and Transcendental Meditation (TM), encourage their Western practitioners to use a chair for meditation and breathing exercises.

This chapter describes a variety of sitting postures that you can use for relaxation, meditation, breath control, and various cleansing practices — or as a starting point for other postures.

Yoga uses many other sitting postures as well; you can gradually add to your basic repertoire as your joints become more flexible and your back muscles gain strength.

Understanding the Philosophy of Sitting

Beyond increasing strength and flexibility, yoga postures, or *asanas* (pronounced ah-sah-nahs) in Sanskrit, help you get in tune with yourself, your body, and your environment. Traditionally, the main purpose of *asana* is to prepare the body to sit quietly, easily, and steadily for breathing exercises and meditation. So when you're in the right position, you can begin to see yourself as one with your environment.

Yogic postures are more than mere bodily poses; they're also expressions of state of mind. An *asana* is poise, composure, carriage — all words suggesting an element of balance and refinement. The postures demonstrate the profound

Asana by any other name

The term *asana* simply means "sitting." It can denote both the surface you sit on and the bodily posture. An alternative term is *tirtha,* or "pilgrimage center," which suggests that practitioners should approach yoga postures not casually but respectfully, with great mental focus. Some postures are called *mudras* (pronounced moo-drahs), or "seals," because they're especially effective in keeping the life energy *(prana)* sealed within the body. Adopting these postures leads to greater vitality and better mental focus. Life energy is everywhere, both inside and outside the body, but you must properly harness it within the body to promote health and happiness.

connection between body and mind. Flopping down on a chair isn't yoga, but when you sit with intention, awareness, and balance, it is.

The way you sit is an important foundation technique for these practices; when you perform them properly, the sitting postures act as natural "tranquilizers" for the body — and when the physical vehicle is still, the mind soon follows.

If your knees are more than a few inches higher than your hips when you sit cross-legged on the floor, it's an indication that your hip joints are tight. If you try to sit for a long time in this position for meditation or breathing exercises, you may well end up with an aching back. Don't feel bad; you're not alone. Accept your current limitations in this area and use a prop, like a firm cushion or thickly folded blanket, to raise your buttocks off the floor high enough to drop your knees at least level with your hips.

Adding Variety to Your Sitting Postures

Some contemporary Hatha Yoga manuals feature more than 50 sitting postures, which demonstrate not only the inventiveness of yoga practitioners but also the body's amazing versatility. But half a dozen yogic sitting postures are plenty for your repertoire. This section describes some good sitting postures and shows you how to execute them.

For postures that involve sitting on the floor, raising your buttocks off the floor on a firm cushion or thickly folded blanket is helpful because it allows you to sit in a comfortable and stable position without slumping. Also, be sure to alternate the cross of your legs from day to day when practicing any of the sitting postures; you don't want to become lopsided.

Differentiating between gripping and contracting muscles

Like turning off your gray matter, relaxing your muscles can be oh-so-easy and oh-so-difficult, partly because of its contradictory nature. You have to contract muscles to accomplish a movement. How do you lift a leg in a yoga balance if you don't contract a muscle to get it there?

Okay, okay, you don't just flop like a fish. Still, you can use your muscles in one of two ways:

✔ **Gripping:** Muscle use often accompanied by clenched teeth, a clamped jaw, or clenched, white-knuckled fingers. Not to mention all the surrounding muscles also getting tight even when they don't need to. This builds tension and usually stops conscious breathwork.

✔ **Contracting:** Using a specific muscle without involving your entire body and all the muscles not involved in that movement — including your clenched jaw. This usually allows relaxation and continued full and deep breathing.

Have you ever floated on your back in water? If you fight the water, flailing and splashing, you can't begin to float. But if you just relax and breathe, you can float effortlessly — even though, of course, you do use some muscular contraction. That's what you need to do in most of yoga exercises — float effortlessly, using only the muscles needed in a mindful and focused way and leaving the others to come along for the ride.

Book II

Basic Yoga Techniques and Postures

Chair-sitting posture

Cultural habits inspire most Westerners to sit in a chair when they meditate, so floor sitting is usually something folks have to work up to with practice. Over time, your *asana* practice can help you build comfort with sitting on the floor for exercises. As Figure 2-1 shows, your ear, shoulder, and hip are in alignment, as viewed from the side. The following steps walk you through the chair-sitting posture:

1. **In a sturdy, armless chair, sit near the front edge of the seat without leaning against the chair back.**

   Make sure your feet are flat on the floor. If they don't quite reach, support them with a block, folded blanket, or book.

2. **Rest your hands on your knees with your palms down, and then close your eyes.**

3. **Rock your spine a few times, alternately slumping forward and arching back to explore its full range of motion.**

   Settle into a comfortable upright position midway between the two extremes.

4. **Lift your chest, without exaggerating the gentle inward curve in your lower back, and balance your head over your torso.**

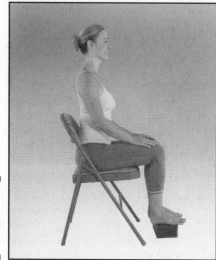

Figure 2-1
The chair-
sitting
posture.

Photograph by Adam Latham

The easy posture: Sukhasana

According to yoga master Patanjali, a posture must be "steady" *(sthira)* and "easeful" *(sukha)* (refer to Book I, Chapter 3). The basic yoga sitting position is called, appropriately, the easy/easeful posture *(sukhasana)*; Westerners sometimes call it the tailor's seat. If you're a beginner, start your floor sitting practice with the easy posture, which Figure 2-2 illustrates.

The easy posture is a steady and comfortable sitting position for meditation and breathing exercises. The posture also helps you become more aware of and actually increase the flexibility in your hips and spine. It's good preparation for more advanced postures.

Here's how it works:

1. **Sit on the floor with your legs straight out in front of you; place your hands on the floor beside your hips, with your palms down and fingers pointing forward.**

   Shake your legs up and down a few times to get the kinks out.

2. **Cross your legs at the ankles with the left leg on top and the right leg below.**

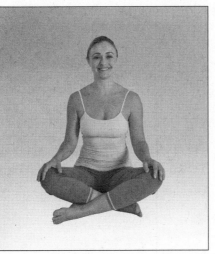

Book II

Basic Yoga
Techniques
and
Postures

Figure 2-2
Be sure
you're
steady and
comfortable
in the easy
posture.

Photograph by Adam Latham

3. **Press your palms on the floor, and slide each foot toward the opposite knee until your right foot is underneath your left knee and your left foot is underneath your right knee.**

4. **Lengthen the spine by stretching your back in an upward motion, and balance your head over your torso.**

The thunderbolt posture: Vajrasana

The thunderbolt posture is one of the safest sitting postures for students with back problems. *Vajrasana* increases the flexibility of your ankles, knees, and thighs; improves circulation to the abdomen; and aids in digestion.

As traditionally taught, you drop your chin to your chest, extend your arms, and lock your elbows. Try this modification instead, which is more relaxing for beginners: Rest your hands on your knees with your palms down and elbows bent, and keep your head upright.

Use the following steps to practice this posture:

1. **Kneel on the floor and sit back on your heels; position each heel under the buttocks on the same side, and rest your hands on the tops of your knees, with your elbows bent and your palms down.**

2. **Lengthen your spine by stretching your back in an upward motion, balance your head over your torso, and look straight ahead, as in Figure 2-3.**

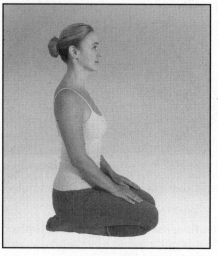

Figure 2-3
A safe sitting posture for lower back problems.

Photograph by Adam Latham

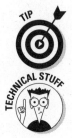

If you have trouble sitting back on your heels because of tightness in your thigh muscles or pain in your knees, put a cushion or folded blanket between your thighs and calves. Increase the thickness of your lift until you can sit comfortably. If you feel discomfort in the fronts of your ankles, put a rolled towel or blanket underneath them.

The Sanskrit word *vajra* (pronounced vahj-rah) means "thunderbolt" or "adamantine." So this posture is also known as the adamantine posture.

The auspicious posture: Svastikasana

Before its perversion in Nazi Germany, the *svastika* served as a solar symbol for good fortune. It has the same meaning in yoga. The term is made up of the prefix *su* ("good") and *asti* ("is") — hence, "It's good."

The *svastikasana* improves the flexibility of the hips, knees, and ankles and also strengthens the back. The following instructions help you get the hang of this posture.

1. **Sit on the floor with your legs straight out in front of you; place your hands on the floor beside your hips, with your palms down and fingers pointing forward.**

   Shake your legs up and down a few times to get the kinks out.

2. **Bend your left knee, and place the sole of your left foot against the inside of your right thigh, with your left heel close to your groin.**

   If this step is difficult, don't use this pose.

3. **Bend your right knee toward you, and take hold of your right foot with both hands.**

4. **Grip the front of your ankle with your right hand and the ball of your big toe with your left hand; slide the little-toe side of your foot between your left thigh and calf until only your big toe is visible, and wiggle the big-toe side of your left foot up between the right thigh and calf if you can.**

5. **Rest your hands on your knees, with your arms relaxed and palms down.**

6. **Lengthen your spine by stretching your back in an upward motion, balance your head over your torso, and look straight ahead, as in Figure 2-4.**

Note: In the classic posture, the chin rests on the chest with the arms straight down and palms open in *jnana mudra* at the knees. The bottom (left) foot is pulled up and wedged between the right calf and the thigh.

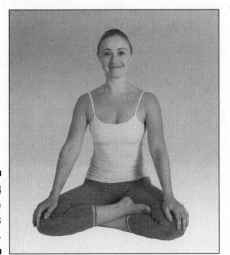

Figure 2-4
The auspicious posture.

Photograph by Adam Latham

Jnana mudra (pronounced gyah-nah moo-drah), or "wisdom seal," is one of several hand positions used in yoga. To do this *mudra,* bring the tip of your index finger to the tip of your thumb to form a circle; extend the three remaining fingers, keeping them close together. This hand gesture makes a good circuit, sealing off the life energy *(prana)* in your body.

The perfect posture: Siddhasana

The Sanskrit word *siddha* (pronounced sidd-hah) means both "perfect" and "adept." In yoga, an *adept* isn't just a skillful practitioner but rather an accomplished master who has attained inner freedom.

Many yoga masters in bygone eras preferred this posture and used it often in place of the lotus posture. This book doesn't cover the half lotus or the full lotus position because they're suitable only for more experienced students.

The *siddhasana* improves the flexibility of your hips, knees, and ankles, and strengthens the back. It differs from *svastikasana* in that you tuck your feet into your thighs between the thighs and calves on both sides. The posture is considered the perfect meditation posture for anyone practicing celibacy. *Siddhasana* is also beneficial for men with various prostate problems.

Here's how you do it:

1. **Sitting on the floor with your legs straight out in front of you, place your hands at your sides (close to your hips), with your palms down and fingers forward.**

   Shake your legs out in front of you a few times.

2. **Bend your left knee, and bring your left heel into your groin near the *perineum* (the area between the anus and the genitals).**

   Stabilize your left ankle with your left hand.

3. **Bend your right knee and slide your right heel toward the front of your left ankle.**

4. **Lift your right foot, position your right ankle just above your left ankle, and bring your right heel into the genital area.**

5. **Tuck the little-toe side of your right foot between your left thigh and your calf.**

6. Place your hands, palms down, on the same-side knee, with your arms relaxed.

7. Straighten and extend your back and neck, bringing your head up nice and tall; look straight ahead, as in Figure 2-5.

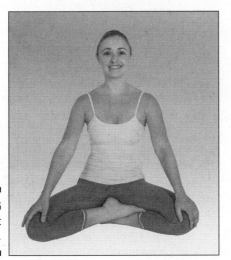

Figure 2-5
The perfect posture.

Photograph by Adam Latham

Book II

Basic Yoga Techniques and Postures

You can use a cushion to raise your hips so they're level with your knees.

Note: In the classic posture, which isn't recommended for beginners, the chin rests on the chest, the arms are straight down, the elbows are locked, and the palms are open in *jnana mudra* (discussed in the preceding section) at the knees. The big-toe side of the left foot is pulled up and wedged between the right calf and the thigh.

Persuading posture trainer

To help you incorporate the basics of a good seated posture, try the persuading posture trainer (see Figure 2-6). The name is fitting because this exercise helps you overcome bad posture habits, and it relieves stress and tension in your shoulders and arms. Try it after a hard day's work. It's a good way to relax and get your body and head straight.

Figure 2-6
The
persuading
posture
trainer
lets you
experience
the feeling
of sitting
correctly.

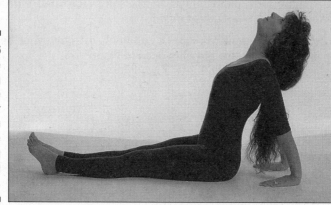

Photograph by Raul Marroquin

Use these steps to practice the persuading posture trainer:

1. **Sit on the floor in the easy posture; relax and take a few slow, deep breaths.**

   Sit with both legs extended straight in front of you, your spine straight, and your shoulders back. Keep your feet pointing upward and slightly flexed as you fold your hands in your lap.

2. **Extend your arms behind your torso, fingers facing forward, bend your elbows, and place your palms on the floor.**

3. **Slide your hands backward about 2 feet behind you so that your arms are fully extended but your elbows aren't locked; expand your chest and allow your torso to lean backward.**

4. **Keep your vision forward and hold this position for 2 to 5 deep breaths; relax, placing your hands back into your lap, and repeat Steps 2 through 4.**

Chapter 3

Standing Tall

*T*he simple act of standing upright brings your spine, muscles, tendons, and ligaments into play. Ordinarily, these parts do their assigned tasks quite automatically. But to stand efficiently and elegantly, you also need to bring awareness to the act, and that's where yoga enters the picture. In this chapter, you can find ten of the most common and favored yoga standing postures to practice. They can help you discover the art of standing consciously, efficiently, and beautifully.

Standing Strong

The yogic standing postures make up the foundation of *asana* practice. You may hear that you can derive everything you need to master your physical practice from the standing postures. The standing postures help you strengthen your legs and ankles, open your hips and groin, and improve your sense of balance. In turn, you develop the ability to "stand your ground" and "stand at ease," which are important aspects of the yogic lifestyle. The standing postures are versatile. You can use them in the following ways:

✔ As a general warm-up for your practice.

✔ In preparation for a specific group of postures (think of the standing forward bends, for example, as a kind of on-ramp to the seated forward bends, which you can find in Book II, Chapter 7).

✔ To counterbalance another posture, such as a back bend or side bend. For more information, see Book II, Chapter 7.

✔ For rest.

✔ As the main body of your practice.

You can creatively adapt many postures from other groups to a standing position, which you can then use as a learning (or teaching) tool or for therapeutic purposes. Consider, for example, the well-known cobra posture, a back bend that many beginning students find hard on the lower back (see Book II, Chapter 7). By performing this same posture in a standing position near a wall, you can use the changed relationship to gravity, the freedom of not having your hips blocked by the floor, and the pressure of the hands on the wall to free your lower back. Then you can apply this newly won understanding about your back in your practice of the more demanding traditional form of the cobra posture — or any other posture that you choose to modify at the wall. (For more on Yoga against the Wall, head to Book VI, Chapter 2.)

Exercising Your Standing Options

This section introduces you to ten standing postures and describes the step-by-step process for each exercise. You can also find discussions on the benefits and the classic (traditionally taught) version of the posture. If you're a beginner, avoid the classic version because, in most cases, the postures are more difficult and sometimes risky. Here are a few tips before you get started with the standing postures:

- Many of these postures start in the mountain posture, so be sure to check out the "Mountain posture: Tadasana" section.

- When you try the postures on your own, follow the instructions for each exercise carefully, including the breathing. Always move into and out of the posture slowly and pause after the inhalation and exhalation (flip to Book II, Chapter 1 for more on breathing). Complete each posture by relaxing and returning to the starting place.

- When you bend forward from all the standing postures, start with your legs straight (without locking your knees), and then soften, or slightly bend, your knees when you feel the muscles pulling in the back of your legs.

- When you come up out of a standing forward bend, do so in one of these three ways:

  - The easiest and safest way is to roll your body up like a rag doll, stacking your vertebrae one on top of the other, with your head coming up last.

  - The next level of difficulty is to bring your arms up from the sides like wings as you inhale and raise your back.

  - The third and most challenging way is to start with the inhalation and extend your arms forward and up alongside your ears. Then continue raising the upper, middle, and lower back until you're straight up and your arms are overhead, if possible.

Mountain posture: Tadasana

The mountain posture is the foundation for all the standing postures. *Tadasana* aligns the body, improves posture and balance, and facilitates breathing.

1. **Stand tall but relaxed, with your feet at hip width (down from the sits bones, not the outer curves), and hang your arms at your sides, with your palms turned toward your legs.**

   The *sits bones,* also known as the *ischial tuberosity,* are the bony parts you feel underneath the flesh of your buttocks you when you sit up straight on a firm surface.

2. **Visualize a vertical line connecting the opening in your ear, your shoulder joint, and the sides of your hip, knee, and ankle.**

   Look straight ahead, with your eyes open or closed, as in Figure 3-1.

3. **Remain in this posture for 6 to 8 breaths.**

Note: In the classic version of this posture, the feet are together and the chin rests on the chest.

Book II

Basic Yoga
Techniques
and
Postures

Figure 3-1:
Start your
standing
postures
with the
mountain
posture.

Photograph by Adam Latham

Standing forward bend: Uttanasana

The Sanskrit word *uttana* (pronounced oo-tah-nah) means "extended," and this posture certainly fits that bill. The standing forward bend (see Figure 3-2) stretches the entire back of the body and decompresses the neck (makes space between the vertebrae), thus freeing the cervical spine and allowing the neck muscles to relax. It also improves overall circulation and has a calming effect on the body and mind. The following steps walk you through the process.

Be careful of all forward bends if you have a disc problem. If you're unsure, check with your doctor or health professional.

1. **Start in mountain posture and, as you inhale, raise your arms forward and then up overhead (see Figure 3-2a).**

2. **As you exhale, bend forward from your hips.**

   When you feel a pull in the back of your legs, soften your knees (as in the Forgiving Limbs discussion in Book I, Chapter 3) and hang your arms.

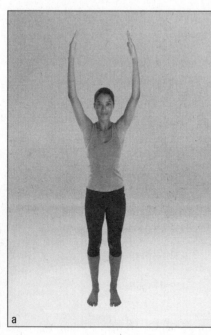
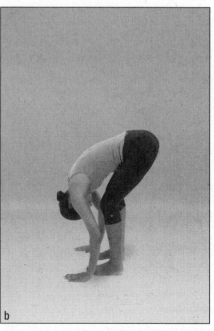

Figure 3-2:
The standing forward bend.

a

b

Photographs by Adam Latham

3. **If your head isn't close to your knees, bend your knees more.**

   If you have the flexibility, straighten your knees but keep them soft. Relax your head and neck downward, as Figure 3-2b illustrates.

4. **As you inhale, roll up slowly, stacking the bones of your spine one at a time from bottom to top, and then raise your arms overhead.**

   Rolling is the safest way to come up. If you don't have back problems, after a few weeks, you may want to try the two more advanced techniques discussed earlier in the section.

5. **Repeat Steps 1 through 4 three times, and then stay in the folded position (Step 3) for 6 to 8 breaths.**

Note: In the classic posture, the feet are together and the legs are straight. The forehead presses against the shins, and the palms are on the floor.

Half standing forward bend: Ardha uttanasana

The Sanskrit word *ardha* (pronounced ahrd-ha) means "half." The half standing forward bend strengthens your legs, back, shoulders, and arms, and improves stamina.

1. **Start in the mountain posture and, as you inhale, raise your arms forward and then up overhead, as in the standing forward bend (see the preceding section).**

2. **As you exhale, bend forward from your hips; soften your knees and hang your arms.**

3. **Bend your knees and, as you inhale, raise your torso and arms up from the front so that they're parallel to the floor, as in Figure 3-3.**

   If you have any back problems, keep your arms back by your sides; then, over a period of time, gradually stretch them out to the sides like a *T* and eventually in front of you so they're parallel to the floor.

4. **Bring your head to a neutral position so that your ears are between your arms; look down and a little forward.**

   To make the posture easier, move your arms back toward your hips instead of having them extend forward or out to the sides — the farther back, the easier.

5. **Repeat Steps 1 through 4 three times, and then stay in Step 4 for 6 to 8 breaths.**

Note: In the classic version of this posture, the feet are together and the legs and arms are straight.

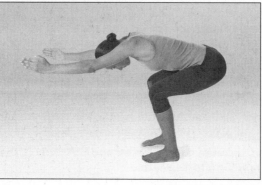

Figure 3-3: The half standing forward bend is great for stamina.

Asymmetrical forward bend: Parshva uttanasana

The asymmetrical forward bend stretches each side of the back and hamstrings separately. The Sanskrit word *parshva* (pronounced pahr-shvah) means "side" or "flank," and this posture indeed opens the hips, tones the abdomen, decompresses the neck, improves balance, and increases circulation to the upper torso and head.

1. **Stand in the mountain posture and, as you exhale, step forward about 3 to 3½ feet (or the length of one leg) with your right foot.**

   Your left foot turns out naturally, but if you need more stability, turn it out even more — but not past 45 degrees.

2. **Place your hands on the top of your hips, and square the front of your pelvis; release your hands and hang your arms.**

3. **As you inhale, raise your arms forward and then overhead, as in Figure 3-4a.**

4. **As you exhale, bend forward from the hips, soften your right knee and both arms, and hang down, as Figure 3-4b illustrates.**

   If your head isn't close to your right knee, bend your knee more. If you have the flexibility, straighten your right knee — but keep it soft.

5. **As you inhale, roll up slowly, stacking the bones of your spine one at a time from the bottom up, and then raise your arms overhead; relax your head and neck downward.**

   Rolling up is the safest way to come up, but if you don't have back problems, you may want to try the more advanced techniques covered earlier in the section after a few weeks.

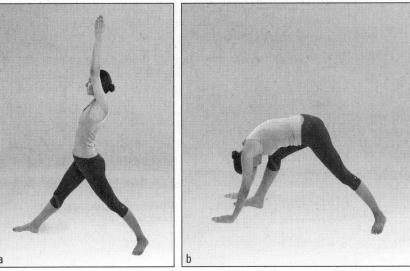

Figure 3-4:
This exercise stretches each side of the back and hamstrings separately.

a

b

Photographs by Adam Latham

6. **Repeat Steps 3 and 4 three times, and then stay in Step 4 for 6 to 8 breaths.**

7. **Repeat the same sequence on the left side.**

Note: In the classic version of this posture, both legs are straight and the forehead presses against the forward leg.

To make the posture more challenging, square your hips forward and rotate your back foot inward.

Triangle posture: Utthita trikonasana

The Sanskrit word *utthita* (pronounced oot-hee-tah) means "raised," and *trikona* (pronounced tree-ko-nah) means "triangle." The triangle posture stretches the sides of the spine, the backs of the legs, and the hips. It also stretches the muscles between the ribs (the *intercostals*), which opens the chest and improves breathing capacity.

1. **Stand in the mountain posture, exhale, and step out to the right about 3 to 3½ feet (or the length of one leg) with your right foot.**

2. **Turn your right foot out 90 degrees. On your left foot, have your toes turned slightly in rather than straight ahead.**

An imaginary line drawn from the right heel (toward the left foot) should bisect the arch of the left foot.

3. **Face forward and, as you inhale, raise your arms out to the sides parallel to the line of the shoulders (and the floor) so that they form a *T* with your torso (see Figure 3-5a).**

4. **As you exhale, reach your right hand down to your right shin as close to the ankle as is comfortable for you, and then reach and lift your left arm; as much as you can, bring the sides of your torso parallel to the floor.**

   Bend your right knee slightly, as in Figure 3-5b, if the back of your leg feels tight.

5. **Soften your left arm and look up at your left hand.**

   If your neck hurts, look down or halfway down at the floor.

6. **Repeat Steps 3 through 5 three times, and then stay in Step 5 for 6 to 8 breaths.**

7. **Repeat the same sequence on the left side.**

Note: In the classic version of this posture, the arms and legs are straight and the trunk is parallel to the floor. The right hand is on the floor outside the right foot.

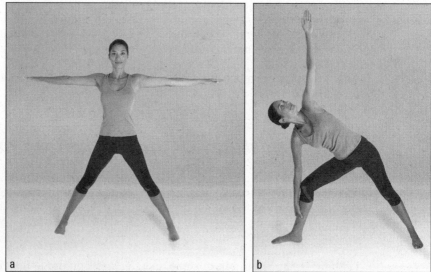

Figure 3-5:
The side-bending triangle opens the chest so you can breathe deeply.

a

b

Photographs by Adam Latham

Reverse triangle posture: Parivritta trikonasana variation

The Sanskrit word *parivritta* (pronounced pah-ree-vree-tah) means "revolved," which makes perfect sense with this posture. The action of twisting and untwisting increases circulation of fresh blood to the discs between the spinal vertebrae (intervertebral discs) and keeps them supple as you grow older. The reverse triangle also stretches the backs of your legs, opens your hips, and strengthens your neck, shoulders, and arms.

1. **Standing in the mountain posture, exhale and step the right foot out to the right about 3 to 3½ feet (or the length of one leg).**

2. **As you inhale, raise your arms out to the sides parallel to the line of your shoulders (and the floor) so that they form a *T* with your torso, as Figure 3-6a illustrates.**

3. **As you exhale, bend forward from your hips and then place your right hand on the floor near the inside of your left foot.**

4. **Raise your left arm toward the ceiling and look up at your left hand; soften your knees and your arms, and then bend your left knee, or move your right hand away from your left foot (and more directly under your torso), as in Figure 3-6b, if necessary.**

If you feel neck strain, turn your head toward the floor.

Book II

Basic Yoga Techniques and Postures

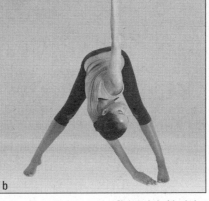

Figure 3-6: The reverse triangle posture.

a

b

Photographs by Adam Latham

5. **Repeat Steps 2 through 4 three times, and then stay in Step 4 for 6 to 8 breaths.**

6. **Repeat the same sequence on the left side.**

Note: In the classic version of this posture, the feet are parallel and the legs and arms are straight. The torso is parallel to the floor, and the bottom hand rests lightly outside the opposite side foot.

Warrior 1: Vira bhadrasana 1

The Sanskrit word *vira* (pronounced vee-rah) is often translated as "hero," and *bhadra* (pronounced bhud-rah) means "auspicious." This posture, also known as just *warrior,* strengthens your legs, back, shoulders, and arms; opens your hips, groin, and chest; increases strength and stamina; and improves balance. As its name suggests, this posture instills a feeling of fearlessness and inner strength. For pointers on moving into this posture, go to http://www.dummies.com/go/yogaaiofd.

1. **Stand in the mountain posture and, as you exhale, step forward approximately 3 to 3½ feet (or the length of one leg) with your right foot (see Figure 3-7a).**

   Your left foot turns out naturally, but if you need more stability, turn it out more (so that your toes point to the left).

2. **Place your hands on the top of your hips, and square the front of your pelvis; release your hands and hang your arms.**

3. **As you inhale, raise your arms forward and overhead, and bend your right knee to a right angle (so that your knee is directly over your ankle and your thigh is parallel to the floor), as in Figure 3-7b.**

   If your lower back is uncomfortable, lean your torso slightly over your forward leg until you feel a release of tension in your back.

4. **As you exhale, return to the starting place in Figure 3-7a; soften your arms and face your palms toward each other, and look straight ahead.**

5. **Repeat Steps 3 and 4 three times, and then stay in Step 3 for 6 to 8 breaths.**

6. **Repeat Steps 1 through 5 on the left side.**

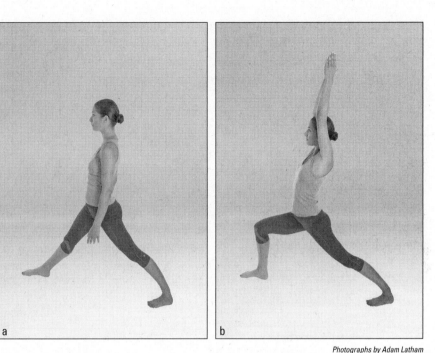

Book II

Basic Yoga
Techniques
and
Postures

Figure 3-7:
The
warrior is a
position of
power and
strength.

Photographs by Adam Latham

Warrior II: Vira bhadrasana II

Like the warrior I posture covered in the preceding section, warrior II strengthens your legs, back, shoulders, and arms. It focuses more on your hips and groin, and it increases strength and stamina; it also improves balance. Use the following steps as your guide.

1. **Stand in the mountain posture; exhale and step out to the right about 3 to 3½ feet (or the length of one leg) with your right foot.**

2. **Turn your right foot out 90 degrees, and have the toes of your left foot turned slightly in rather than forward.**

   An imaginary line drawn from your right heel toward your left foot should bisect the arch of your left foot.

3. **Face forward and, as you inhale, raise your arms out to the sides, parallel to the line of your shoulders (and the floor), so that they form a *T* with your torso (see Figure 3-8a).**

4. **As you exhale, turn your right foot out 90 degrees and bend your right knee over your right ankle so that your shin is perpendicular to the floor, as in Figure 3-8b; if possible, bring your right thigh parallel to the floor.**

5. **Repeat Steps 3 and 4 three times, keeping your arms in a *T*; then turn your head to the right, looking out over your right arm, and stay for 6 to 8 breaths.**

6. **Repeat Steps 1 through 5 on the left side.**

Be careful not to force your hips open; doing so may cause problems with your knees.

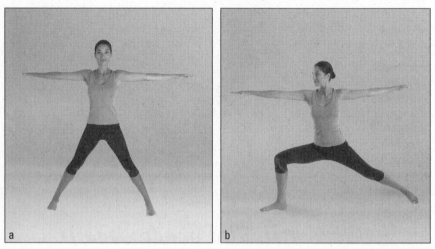

Figure 3-8: Warrior II.

Photographs by Adam Latham

Standing spread-legged forward bend: Prasarita pada uttanasana

The Sanskrit word *prasarita* (pronounced prah-sah-ree-tah) means "outstretched," and *pada* (pronounced pah-dah) means "foot." This posture, also called the wide-legged standing forward bend, stretches your hamstrings and your *adductors* (on the insides of the thighs) and opens your hips. The hanging forward bend increases circulation to your upper torso and lengthens your spine. Figure 3-9 illustrates this posture.

1. **Stand in the mountain posture, exhale, and step your right foot out to the right about 3 to 3½ feet (or the length of one leg).**

2. **As you inhale, raise your arms out to the sides, parallel to the line of your shoulders (and the floor), so that they form a *T* with your torso.**

3. **As you exhale, bend forward from the hips and soften your knees.**

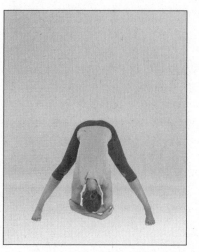

Figure 3-9: This posture is a great way to release pressure in your lower back.

Photograph by Adam Latham

4. **Hold your bent elbows with the opposite-side hands, and hang your torso and arms.**

5. **Stay in Step 4 for 6 to 8 breaths.**

Note: In the classic version of this posture, the legs are straight, the head is on the floor (and the chin presses the chest), and the arms reach back between the legs, with the palms on the floor.

Half chair posture: Ardha utkatasana

The Sanskrit word *ardha* (pronounced ahrd-ha) means "half," and *utkata,* (pronounced oot-kah-tah) translates as "powerful." The half chair posture strengthens the back, legs, shoulders, and arms and builds overall stamina. If you find this posture difficult or you have problem knees, you may want to skip this position for now and return to it after your leg muscles become a little stronger. Don't overdo this exercise (either by holding the position too long or by repeating it more than recommended), or you'll have sore muscles the next day. But there's no harm in experiencing some muscle soreness, either, especially if you haven't exercised in a long time. Check out Figure 3-10 for guidance.

1. **Start in the mountain posture and, as you inhale, raise your arms forward and up overhead, with your palms facing each other.**

2. **As you exhale, bend your knees and squat halfway to the floor.**

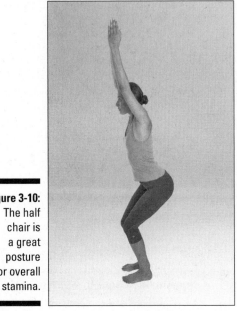

Figure 3-10:
The half chair is a great posture for overall stamina.

Photograph by Adam Latham

3. **Soften your arms, but keep them overhead; look straight ahead.**

4. **Repeat Steps 1 through 3 three times, and then stay in Step 3 for 6 to 8 breaths.**

Note: In the classic version of this posture, the feet are together and the arms are straight, with the fingers interlocked and the palms turned upward. The chin rests on the chest.

Downward-facing dog: Adhomukha shvanasana

The Sanskrit word *adhomukha* (pronounced ahd-ho-mook-hah) means "downward facing," and *shvan* (pronounced shvahn) means "dog." Inspired by a dog's leisurely stretching, the downward-facing dog practice stretches the entire back of your body and strengthens your wrists, arms, and shoulders. This posture is a good alternative for beginning students who aren't yet ready for inversions like the handstand and headstand. Because the head is lower than the heart, this *asana* circulates fresh blood to the brain and acts as a quick pick-me-up when you're fatigued.

1. **Start on your hands and knees; straighten your arms, but don't lock your elbows (see Figure 3-11a).**

   Be sure that the heels of your hands are directly under your shoulders, with your palms on the floor, your fingers spread, and your knees directly under your hips. Emphasize pressing down with the thumbs and index fingers, or the inner web of your hand.

2. **As you exhale, lift and straighten (but don't lock) your knees; as your hips lift, bring your head to a neutral position so that your ears are between your arms.**

3. **Press your heels toward the floor and your head toward your feet, as in Figure 3-11b.**

   If your hamstrings feel tight, try putting a little bend in your knees to help you straighten your spine.

   Don't complete Step 3 if doing so strains your neck.

Book II

Basic Yoga
Techniques
and
Postures

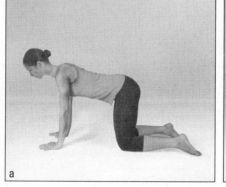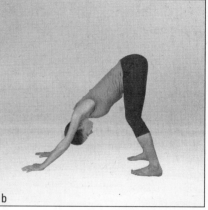

Figure 3-11:
Challenge
yourself in
downward-
facing dog,
but don't
strain.

a

b

Photographs by Adam Latham

4. **Repeat Steps 1 through 3 three times, and then stay in Step 3 for 6 to 8 breaths.**

Note: In the classic posture, the feet are together and flat on the floor, the legs and arms are straight, and the top of the head is on the floor, with the chin pressed to the chest.

Be careful not to hold this posture too long if you have problems with your neck, shoulders, wrists, or elbows.

Chapter 4

Steady as a Tree: Mastering Balance

. . . .

In This Chapter
▶ Understanding the psychology of balance
▶ Practicing balancing exercises

. . . .

Balance (called *samata* [sah-mah-tah] or *samatva* [sah-mah-tvah] in Sanskrit) is fundamental to yoga. A balanced approach to life includes being even-tempered and seeing the great unity behind all diversity. Balance translates to being nonjudgmental and treating others with equal fairness, kindness, and compassion.

One way to begin to gain this balance is to practice balancing postures. Remember, according to yoga, body and mind form a working unit. Imbalances in the body are reflected in the mind, and vice versa. This chapter emphasizes the importance of balance in yoga and offers six postures that provide you with a *samata* sampling.

Getting to the Roots of the Posture

When you look at a tree, you see only what's above ground — the vertical trunk, with its crown of branches and foliage, and maybe a few chirping birds. Trees appear to just perch atop the soil, and you wonder how in the world such a top-heavy thing can stay upright. Well, everyone knows that the secret of the tree's equilibrium is its underground network of roots that anchor the visible part of the plant solidly into the earth. In the balancing postures, you, too, can discover how to grow your "roots" into the earth and stand as steady as a tree.

The balancing postures can be the most fun and the most dramatic of all the postures. Although they're relatively simple, they can produce profound effects. As you may expect, they work to improve your overall sense of physical balance, coordination, and grounding. With awareness in these three areas, you can move more easily and effectively, whether you're going about your daily business or are engaged in activities that call for great coordination, such as sports or dance. The yogic balancing postures also have therapeutic applications, such as with back problems or in retraining whole muscle groups.

When you improve your physical balance naturally, you can expect to enjoy improved mental balance. The balancing postures are exceptional seeds for concentration, and when you master them, you earn confidence and a sense of accomplishment.

Balancing Postures for Graceful Strength

Contemporary life is highly demanding and stressful; if you're not properly grounded, you face a constant risk of being pushed out of balance. *Grounding* means being centered and firm without being inflexible, knowing who you are and what you want, and feeling that you're empowered to achieve your life goals. A good way to begin your grounding work is to improve your physical sense of balance. Improving your balance helps you synchronize the movement of your arms and legs, giving you poise. When you can stand and move in a more balanced manner, your mind is automatically affected. You *feel* more balanced.

A sense of balance is connected with the inner ears. Your ears tell you where you are in space. The ears are also connected with *social space;* if you aren't well balanced, you may feel — or actually *be* — a bit awkward in your social relationships. Balancing and grounding work can remedy this discomfort. Only when you can stand still — in balance — can you also move harmoniously in the world.

The postures in this section appear in order of ease, starting with simple exercises and moving to more advanced ones. If you try the postures individually rather than as part of a sequence, try to hold each posture for 6 to 8 breaths. Breathe freely through the nose, and pause briefly after inhalation and exhalation.

Warrior at the wall: Vira bhadrasana III variation

The Sanskrit word *vira* (pronounced vee-rah) means "hero." *Bhadra* (pronounced bhud-rah) means "auspicious." This posture improves your overall balance and stability. It strengthens the legs, arms, and shoulders, and stretches the thighs — both front and back — and the hips. As with the other one-legged balancing poses, this posture enhances focus and concentration. Check out the following steps:

1. **Stand in the mountain posture (see Book II, Chapter 3), facing a blank wall about 3 feet away.**

2. **As you exhale, bend forward from the hips and extend your arms forward until your hands are touching the wall; adjust so that your legs are perpendicular and your torso and arms are parallel with the floor.**

   Depending on your balance, you may prefer to have your palms flat against the wall or touch only with your fingertips.

3. **As you inhale, raise your left leg back and up until it's parallel to the floor (see Figure 4-1).**

4. **Stay in Step 3 for 6 to 8 breaths; repeat with the right leg.**

Book II

Basic Yoga Techniques and Postures

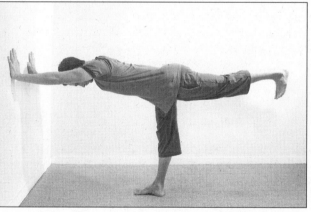

Figure 4-1: A safe balancing posture for beginners.

Photograph by Adam Latham

Balancing cat

The balancing cat posture strengthens the muscles along the spine (the *paraspinals*), as well as the arms and the shoulders, and it opens the hips. The posture enhances focus and concentration and also builds confidence.

1. **Beginning on your hands and knees, position your hands directly under your shoulders, with your palms down, your fingers spread on the floor, and your knees directly under your hips; straighten your arms, but don't lock your elbows.**

2. **As you exhale, slide your left hand forward and your right leg back, keeping your hand and your toes on the floor.**

3. **As you inhale, raise your left arm and right leg to a comfortable height, as Figure 4-2 illustrates.**

4. **Stay in Step 3 for 6 to 8 breaths, and then repeat Steps 1 through 3 with opposite pairs (right arm and left leg).**

This posture is a variation of *cakravakasana* (pronounced chuk-rah-vahk-ah-sah-nah). The *cakravaka* is a particular kind of goose, which, in India's traditional poetry, is often used to convey "love bird." Apparently, when these birds have paired up and then are separated, their heartache causes them to call to each other.

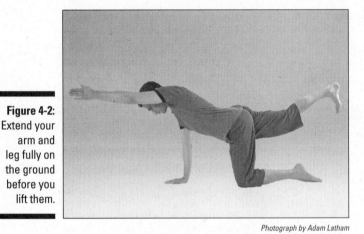

Figure 4-2:
Extend your arm and leg fully on the ground before you lift them.

Photograph by Adam Latham

The tree posture: Vrikshasana

The Sanskrit word *vriksha* (pronounced vrik-shah) means "tree." The tree posture improves overall balance, stability, and poise. It strengthens your legs, arms, and shoulders, and opens your hips and groin. Like the other one-legged balancing poses, it also enhances focus and concentration and produces a calming effect on your body and mind. Here's how it works:

1. **Stand in the mountain posture (see Book II, Chapter 3 for this posture).**

2. **As you exhale, bend your right knee and place the sole of your right foot, toes pointing down, on the inside of your left leg between your knee and your groin.**

3. As you inhale, bring your arms over your head and join your palms together.

4. Soften your arms, and focus on a spot 6 to 8 feet in front of you on the floor (see Figure 4-3).

5. Stay in Step 4 for 6 to 8 breaths, and then repeat with the opposite leg.

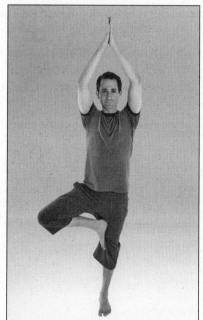

Figure 4-3:
Focus on a spot 6 to 8 feet in front of you; concentrate and breathe slowly.

Photograph by Adam Latham

Note: In the classic (traditionally taught) version of this posture, the arms are straight and the chin rests on the chest.

If you have limited flexibility in your hips and have difficulty getting your foot all the way up to your thigh in Step 2, you can place the foot of your bent leg between your knee and ankle. Just take care not to place your foot directly against your knee joint.

The karate kid

The karate kid posture improves overall balance and stability. It strengthens the legs, arms, and shoulders, and opens the hips. As with the other one-legged balancing postures, the karate kid enhances focus and concentration.

1. **Stand in the mountain posture, described in Book II, Chapter 3.**

2. **As you inhale, raise your arms out to the sides, parallel to the line of your shoulders (and the floor), so that they form a _T_ with your torso.**

3. **To steady yourself, focus on a spot on the floor 10 to 12 feet in front of you.**

4. **As you exhale, bend your left knee, raising it toward your chest; keep your right leg straight (see Figure 4-4).**

5. **Stay in Step 4 for 6 to 8 breaths; repeat with the right knee.**

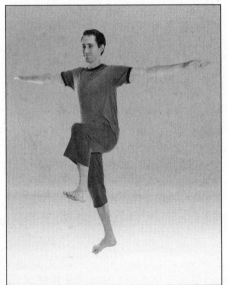

Figure 4-4:
The karate
kid.

Photograph by Adam Latham

The Sanskrit name for this pose is _utthita hasta padangusthasana_ variation.

Standing heel-to-buttock

The standing heel-to-buttock posture improves your overall balance and stability. This posture strengthens your legs, arms, and shoulders and stretches your thighs. As with the other one-legged balancing poses, this posture enhances focus and concentration as well. Here's how it works:

1. **Stand in the mountain posture (see Book II, Chapter 3).**

2. **As you inhale, raise your left arm forward and overhead.**

3. **To steady yourself, focus on a spot on the floor 10 to 12 feet in front of you.**

4. **As you exhale, bend your right knee and bring your right heel toward your right buttock, keeping your left leg straight; grasp your right ankle with your right hand, as Figure 4-5 illustrates.**

5. **Stay in Step 4 for 6 to 8 breaths; repeat Steps 1 through 5 with your left foot.**

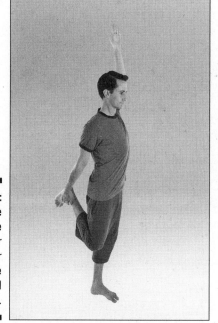

Figure 4-5: This pose can improve your balance for the more advanced postures.

Photograph by Adam Latham

Scorpion

The scorpion posture improves overall balance and stability. This posture, which is a variation of *cakravakasana,* strengthens your shoulders; improves the flexibility of your hips, legs, and shoulders; and enhances focus and concentration.

1. **While on your hands and knees, position your hands directly under your shoulders, with your palms down, fingers spread on the floor, and knees directly under your hips; straighten your arms, but don't lock your elbows.**

2. **Place your right forearm on the floor, with your right hand just behind your left wrist; reach behind you with your left hand, twisting the torso slightly to the left, and grab your right ankle.**

3. **As you inhale, lift your right knee off the floor, raise your chest until it's parallel to the floor, and look up; find a comfortable height for your chest and raised leg, and steady yourself by pressing your right forearm and thumb on the floor (see Figure 4-6).**

4. **Stay in Step 3 for 6 to 8 breaths, and then repeat Steps 1 through 4 on the opposite side (with your left forearm and left leg).**

Figure 4-6:
Steady yourself by pressing your right forearm and thumb into the floor.

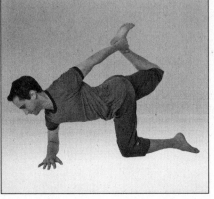

Photograph by Adam Latham

Chapter 5

Absolutely Abs

Many Eastern systems of spiritual exercise and healing consider the lower abdomen to be the vital center of your whole being — body, mind, and spirit. Westerners, on the other hand, think much differently about their bellies, tending to see them as mere food bags or as waste-processing stations.

Many people have a love-hate relationship with their bellies. Although people may be obsessed with having the "perfect" midriff, they tend to neglect or even abuse this area of their bodies. On the inside, they stuff the belly with way too much junk food. On the outside, they let it grow slack. But as the yoga masters warn, when this area is polluted by impurities, it becomes a seat of sickness.

Apart from diseases, weak bellies (and belly muscles) contribute significantly to lower back problems. Studies indicate that 80 percent of the American population has had, is having, or will have back problems. Back-related problems are the second-leading cause of missed workdays, trailing only respiratory problems or the common cold.

This chapter walks you through some yoga exercises that focus on the abdomen so that you can keep this vital area of your body strong and healthy.

Taking Care of the Abdomen: Your Business Center

The abdomen is an amazing enterprise, with its complex food-processing plant (the stomach), several subsidiary operations (liver, spleen, kidneys, and so on), and a 25-foot-long sewer system (the intestines). Poor diets and eating habits lead to annoying and sometimes deadly serious digestive and elimination problems, including constipation, diarrhea, irritable bowel syndrome, and colon cancer. Regular yoga practice can help you take care of your abdominal organs so they can function well and take care of you without the aid of antacids, digestive enzyme supplements, or laxatives.

The following section describes exercises that work with three sets of abdominal muscles:

- The *rectus abdominis,* which is strung vertically along the front of the belly from the bottom of the sternum to the pubis
- The internal and external *obliques,* which, as their name suggests, take an "oblique" course along the side of the belly from the lower ribs to the top rim of the pelvis
- The *transversalis abdominis,* which lies behind the internal obliques

You may hear these three abdominals called the "stomach muscles," which is really a misnomer. The actual stomach muscles line the baglike stomach and are active only during digestion. Of course, the yogic exercises also positively affect the abdominal organs (stomach, spleen, liver, and intestines). If you take care of your abdominal muscles and the organs they protect — through exercise and proper diet — you've accomplished much of the work to stay healthy.

Navel secrets, declassified

After a doctor or midwife severs a newborn's umbilical cord, thus creating his navel, no one pays much attention to this birth socket. Yet the navel is a very important feature of your anatomy. According to yoga, a special psycho-energetic center is located at the navel. This center is known as the *manipura-cakra* (pronounced mah-nee-poo-rah-chuk-rah), which means literally "center of the jeweled city."

The center corresponds to (but isn't identical with) the *solar plexus,* which is a large network of nerves that has been called the body's second brain. The *manipura-cakra* controls the abdominal organs and regulates the flow of energy through the entire body. The navel center is associated with emotions and the will. You can have "too much navel" (be pushy) or "not enough navel" (be a pushover).

Exercising Those Abs

These yogic postures for the abdominal muscles incorporate a team approach that values slow, conscious movement; proper breathing mechanics; and the use of sound. The emphasis here is on the *quality* of the movement rather than sheer quantity. A few movements done with diligent attention are much safer and more effective than dozens and even hundreds of mindless repetitions. Conscious breathing, especially the gentle tightening of the front belly on each exhalation, can encourage and then sustain the strength and tone of the abdominals. The use of sound further enhances this kind of breathing.

Carrying a powerful center

Contrary to what many people believe, your legs don't power you through movements, nor do your arms power you. Your brain isn't even what powers you. Your physical (and mental) power center is in your core. Right smack in the center of your body, basically around your belly button and abdominals; that's your *core* and that's where your *power center* is.

If you try to walk, balance, stand up from sitting, reach to a cabinet, or do any kind of common sports or daily-life movement without your core engaged, you aren't able to move smoothly or strongly. No matter what you do, imagine its movement stems from your center, your power center, and not from the limb doing the action.

Try this little game to understand the importance of using your core:

1. **Stand up, and pick up one foot so that you're doing a stork imitation, letting your**
abdominals hang out and your whole body sag.

   Toppling over, are you?

2. **Pull in your abdominals and turn on all circuits in your power center by focusing all your energy right to your core.**

   Balancing is easier, yes?

Physically, dancers and other movement artists use their core's power to allow them to perform sensational feats. Mindfully, your core is the fountain of all your body's energy and, according to the theories of some mind-body practices, the core must be worked and massaged so that you can break free of pain, fill yourself with positive energy, successfully complete a move, or find the true meaning of bliss.

Exploring push-downs

Push-downs strengthen the abdomen, especially the lower abdomen. In addition to a floor exercise, you can do push-downs in a seated position by pushing your lower back against the back of your chair. You can perform this exercise sitting in a car, on a plane, or at the office.

1. **Lie on your back with your knees bent and your feet on the floor, at hip width.**

   Rest your arms near your sides, palms down.

2. **As you exhale, push your lower back down to the floor for 3 to 5 seconds (see Figure 5-1).**

3. **As you inhale, release your back.**

4. **Repeat Steps 2 and 3 six to eight times.**

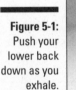

Figure 5-1:
Push your lower back down as you exhale.

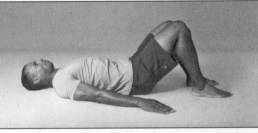

Photograph by Adam Latham

Trying yogi sit-ups

Yogi sit-ups strengthen the abdomen, especially the upper abdomen, the *adductors* (insides of your legs), the neck, and the shoulders.

1. **Lie on your back with your knees bent and your feet on the floor, at hip width.**

2. **Turn in your toes "pigeon-toed" and bring your inner knees together.**

3. **Spread your palms on the back of your head, with your fingers interlocked, and keep your elbows wide.**

4. **As you exhale, press your knees firmly, tilt the front of your pelvis toward your navel, and, with your hips on the ground, slowly sit up halfway.**

   Keep your elbows out to the sides, in line with the tops of your shoulders. Look toward the ceiling. Don't pull your head up with your arms; instead, support your head with your hands and come up by contracting the abdominal muscles, as in Figure 5-2.

5. **As you inhale, slowly roll back down.**

6. **Repeat Steps 4 and 5 six to eight times.**

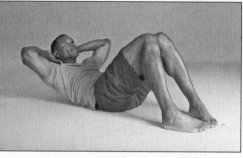

Figure 5-2:
Let your eyes
follow the
ceiling as you
sit up.

Photograph by Adam Latham

The sound of yoga

A very busy, well-known movie producer from Malibu suffered from a chronic neck and stress condition, and he also had what his girlfriend referred to as a "little jelly belly." Regular sit-ups to tighten his abs just aggravated his neck problem. But with a 12-minute, twice-a-day yoga routine that included the yogi sit-back and the use of sound (both discussed in this chapter), his neck problem went away, and his belly firmed up nicely. He liked using sound so much that many members of his movie crew joined him in the afternoon for "a little sound."

Strengthening with yogi sit-backs

Yogi sit-backs strengthen both the lower and upper abdomen. This posture is a variation of *navasana*. The Sanskrit word *nava,* pronounced nah-vah, means "boat."

1. **Sit on the floor with your knees bent and your feet on the floor, at hip width.**

2. **Extend your arms and place your hands on the floor, palms down.**

3. **Bring your chin down, and round your back in a *C* curve, as in Figure 5-3a.**

4. **As you inhale, roll slowly onto the back of your pelvis, dragging your hands along on the floor (see Figure 5-3b).**

   Keep the rest of your back off the floor to maintain the contraction of the abdominals, but don't strain to hold this position; if you have any negative symptoms, don't use this posture.

5. **As you exhale, roll up again, sliding your hands forward.**

6. **Repeat Steps 4 and 5 six to eight times.**

Figure 5-3:
Bring your chin down, and keep your back rounded in a *C* curve.

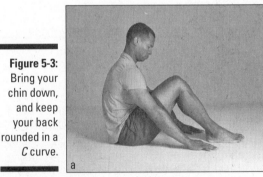
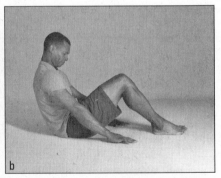

a b

Photographs by Adam Latham

Sit-backs are easier on the neck than most sit-ups. However, if you have lower back problems, be cautious with sit-backs. If you notice any pain in your back, just stop and work with the other exercises in this chapter instead.

Creating variety with extended leg slide-ups

A variation of *navasana,* the extended leg slide-ups strengthen both the upper and lower abdomen, as well as the neck.

TIP

If this pose bothers your neck, support your head by putting both hands behind it. If the problem persists, stop.

1. **Lie on your back with your knees bent and your feet flat on the floor, at hip width.**

2. **Bend your left elbow, and place your left hand on the back of your head just behind your left ear.**

3. **Raise the left leg as close to vertical (90 degrees) as possible, but keep your knee slightly bent.**

4. **Draw the top of your foot toward your shin, to flex your ankle, and place your right palm on your right thigh near your pelvis, as Figure 5-4a illustrates.**

5. **As you exhale, sit up slowly halfway and slide your right hand toward your knee.**

   Keep your left elbow back in line with your shoulder, and look at the ceiling. Don't throw your head forward (see Figure 5-4b for the proper positioning).

6. **Repeat Steps 1 through 5 six to eight times, and then repeat Steps 1 through 6 on the other side.**

Book II

Basic Yoga Techniques and Postures

Figure 5-4:
Work the abs and the hamstrings.

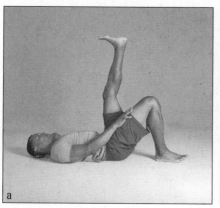

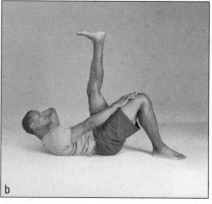

a

b

Photographs by Adam Latham

Arching with the suck 'em up posture

The suck 'em up posture strengthens and tones the abdominal muscles and the internal organs. The posture is especially beneficial for relieving constipation.

1. **Start on your hands and knees, with your hands just below your shoulders and your knees at hip width.**

2. **Inhale deeply through your nose.**

3. **Exhale through your mouth, and hump your back like a camel as you bring your chin down.**

   When you've fully exhaled, don't immediately inhale; hold your breath where it is and then suck your belly up toward your spine (see Figure 5-5).

   Wait 2 to 3 seconds with the belly up and breath restrained, as long as you don't end up gasping for air.

Figure 5-5:
Make sure you exhale fully before you suck your belly up.

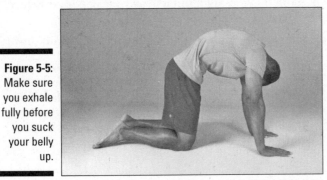

Photograph by Adam Latham

4. **As you inhale, return to the starting position and then pause for a breath or two.**

5. **Repeat Steps 2 through 4 four to six times, pausing for a breath or two between each repetition.**

Do this exercise only on an empty stomach, and avoid it if you're having stomach pain or cramps of any kind because it may intensify the symptoms. Also avoid this exercise during menstruation.

Exhaling "soundly"

The use of sound exercise strengthens and tones the abdomen and its internal organs, in addition to strengthening the muscles of the diaphragm.

1. **Sit in a chair or on the floor with your spine comfortably upright.**

   If you find yourself slumping, sit on a folded blanket.

2. **Place the palm of your right hand on your navel so that you can feel your belly contracting as you exhale.**

3. **Take a deep inhalation through your nose; as you exhale, make the sound *ah, ma,* or *sa*.**

   Continue sounding this consonant for as long as you can do so comfortably.

4. **Repeat Steps 2 and 3 six to eight times.**

   Pause for a resting breath or two between each sound.

If you're on a detox program of any kind and the use of sound gives you a headache, work with the other exercises in this chapter instead.

Chapter 6

Looking at the World Upside-Down: Safe Inversion Postures

In This Chapter

▶ Making heads or tails of the yogic principle of reversal

▶ Working with leg inversions

▶ Gravitating toward shoulder stands

Thousands of years ago, the yoga masters made an amazing discovery: By tricking the force of gravity with the help of inversion exercises, you can reverse the effects of aging, improve your health, and add years to your life.

To picture how inversions work, take a look at a jug of unfiltered apple juice sitting on the grocery store shelf. Gravity has pulled the solids in the juice to the bottom of the jug, diluting the liquid near the top. If you turn the bottle upside-down, gravity pulls the bottom sediment toward the top of the inverted jug, remixing the juice with the pulp of the apples. In a similar way, when you turn yourself upside-down, the sediments — mostly blood and *lymph* (a clear, yellowish fluid similar to blood plasma) — that have collected in your lower limbs during a long day of uprightness sink toward your head and revitalize your entire body and mind, helping you face your fears and reversing the tide of stagnation and mental negativity.

The idea that you must practice the headstand to be a "real yogi" just isn't true. In fact, you can practice a variety of inversions other than the headstand. This chapter describes inverted exercises that impart the benefits without the risk. Use yogic breathing (see Book II, Chapter 1) to boost their beneficial effect, and grab a prop as necessary to facilitate the postures and ensure easy breathing.

Avoid the headstand unless an experienced teacher supervises your efforts. The neck is designed to support the 8 pounds of the head, not the 100 or more pounds of the body. Approach the headstand cautiously and only after proper preparation.

Getting a Leg Up on Leg Inversions

Effective inversions can actually be quite simple. This section describes four postures that don't require you to literally turn yourself upside-down to enjoy the numerous benefits of an inversion.

Avoid all inverted postures if you have an acute headache or if you experience sudden pain while performing the exercise.

Feel free to luxuriate in the two supported inversions; they're both held longer than other poses.

Legs up on a chair

The legs up on a chair posture improves circulation to your legs, hips, and lower back, and has a calming effect on your nervous system. It also helps alleviate symptoms of PMS in women and prostatitis in men.

To enjoy these benefits, do the following:

1. **Sit on the floor in a simple cross-legged position, facing a sturdy chair, and lean back onto your forearms.**

2. **Slide your buttocks along the floor toward the chair.**

3. **While exhaling, lift your feet off the floor and place your heels and calves on the chair seat.**

   You want your thighs and shins to be at a right angle.

4. **Lie back on the floor with your arms near your sides, palms down or up, as in Figure 6-1.**

5. **Stay in Step 4 for 2 to 10 minutes.**

This posture is a variation of the *classic* (traditionally taught) posture of *urdhva prasarita padasana* (pronounced oord-hvah prah-sah-ree-tah pahd-ah-sah-nah), which means "upward extended foot posture."

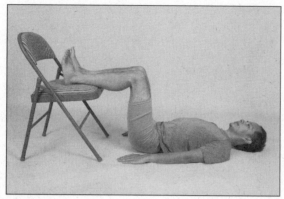

Figure 6-1:
The legs up
on a chair
posture.

Photograph by Adam Latham

Legs up on the wall

Legs up on the wall, which is a variation of *urdhva prasarita padasana,* improves circulation to the legs, hips, and lower back, and has a calming effect on the nervous system. It, too, helps alleviate symptoms of PMS in women and prostatitis in men.

Try it for yourself by following these steps:

1. **Sit sideways with your right side as close to the wall as possible, with both legs extended forward (see Figure 6-2a).**

2. **As you exhale, swing both legs up on the wall and lie flat on your back.**

   Extend your legs up as far as possible. Extend your arms comfortably at your sides, palms down, and relax (see Figure 6-2b).

3. **Stay in Step 2 for 2 to 10 minutes.**

The happy baby

A variation of *urdhva prasarita padasana,* the happy baby posture improves circulation in the legs, arms, hips, and lower back, and has a calming effect on the nervous system. It also improves the range of motion of the ankles, toes, wrists, and fingers.

Here's how it works:

1. **Lying on your back with your knees bent and feet flat on the floor, place your arms at your sides with your palms down.**

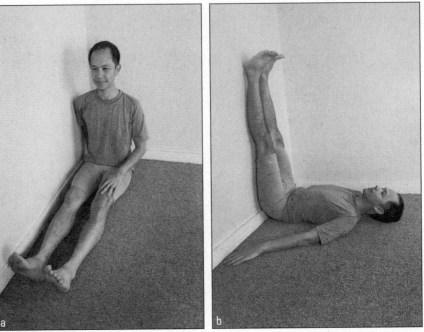

Figure 6-2:
The legs up
on the wall
posture.

Photographs by Adam Latham

2. **As you exhale, extend your legs and arms up vertically.**

   Keep your limbs relaxed (check out the discussion of Forgiving Limbs in Book I, Chapter 3) as you hold them up.

3. **With your feet, toes, hands, and fingers, draw circles in the air both clockwise and counterclockwise, as in Figure 6-3.**

   You can make your hands and feet go in different directions at the same time. Breathe freely. Keep your arms and legs up as long as you feel comfortable, and then return to the starting position.

4. **Repeat Steps 2 and 3 three to five times, but don't hold the limbs up for more than a total of 5 minutes; you don't want to tire yourself out or strain your back.**

Avoid this posture if you have lower back problems.

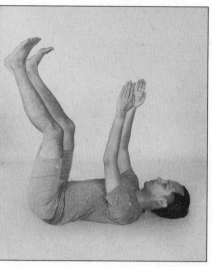

Figure 6-3:
Enjoy the freedom of movement in your ankles and wrists.

Photograph by Adam Latham

Standing spread-legged forward bend at the wall

The standing spread-legged forward bend at the wall, which is a variation of *prasarita pada uttanasana* (described in Book II, Chapter 8), improves circulation in your head and stretches your spine and hamstrings.

Follow these easy steps:

1. **Stand with your back 4 to 12 inches from a sturdy wall, separate your feet to a comfortably wide stance, and then lean your buttocks back against the wall.**

2. **As you exhale, bend forward from the hips and hang your arms and head down.**

   If your hands touch the floor, grasp your elbows with opposite-side hands and let your forearms hang. Keep your knees soft, and relax your neck and head, as in Figure 6-4.

3. **Stay in Step 2 for 2 to 3 minutes; use any of the yoga breathing techniques covered in Book II, Chapter 1.**

If you feel light-headed when doing this pose or any other inversion exercise, reduce the duration for now and then increase the time gradually.

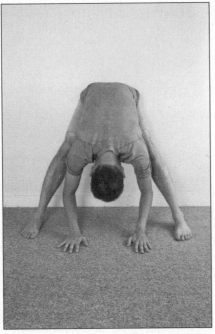

Figure 6-4:
The standing spread-legged forward bend at the wall.

Photograph by Adam Latham

Trying a Trio of Shoulder Stands

These shoulder stands go from easiest to toughest. Each of these three shoulder stands provides common benefits: improved circulation to your legs, hips, back, neck, heart, and head. The postures all stimulate your endocrine glands and improve your lymphatic drainage, enhance elimination, and produce a calming and rejuvenating effect on your nervous system. The wall provides a useful prop for the easier two variations; when you're ready, you can advance with confidence to *viparita karani,* the half shoulder stand.

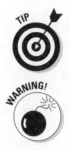

Because of the neck's vulnerability, precede these postures with a dynamic (or moving) bridge posture (see Book III, Chapter 1), to prepare the neck and follow it with a short rest, and then use a dynamic cobra posture (see Book II, Chapter 7) to compensate.

Don't attempt any of these postures if you're pregnant; have high blood pressure or a hiatal hernia; are even moderately overweight; have glaucoma, diabetic retinopathy, or neck problems; or are in the first few days of your period. Also, don't use a mirrored wall — you can injure yourself if you fall.

Half shoulder stand at the wall

This posture is a variation of *viparita karani* (see "Half shoulder stand: *Viparita karani*" later in this chapter) and is perhaps the easiest way to pick up the half shoulder stand in a step-by-step manner. The wall provides support as you build experience with the shoulder stand exercises.

In all the half shoulder stand variations, make sure to keep your head and neck straight. Never turn your head while in any of these postures.

Here's how you do it:

1. **Lie on your back with your knees bent, your feet flat on the floor, your toes just touching the base of a sturdy wall, and your arms extended along the sides of your torso, with your palms down.**

2. **Place your soles up on the wall so that your bent knees form a right angle (with your thighs parallel to each other and your shins perpendicular to the wall), as in Figure 6-5a.**

   You may need to slide your buttocks closer to or farther away from the wall to get the angle just right.

3. **As you inhale, press down with your hands, push your feet to the wall, and lift your hips as high as you comfortably can (see Figure 6-5b).**

4. **Bend your elbows and bring your hands to your lower back.**

   Press your elbows and the backs of your upper arms onto the floor for support. Relax your neck (see Figure 6-5c).

5. **As you exhale, take one foot off the wall and extend that leg until you're looking straight up at the tip of your big toe, as in Figure 6-5d.**

   You can use just one leg at a time and switch, or you can raise both legs together. If you alternate legs, divide the time evenly between each leg.

6. **Stay in Step 4 or 5 for as long as you feel comfortable, or up to 5 minutes; use the yoga breathing techniques in Book II, Chapter 1.**

   When you want to come back down, slowly place one foot and then the other on the wall, and finally lower your pelvis slowly to the floor.

Book II

Basic Yoga Techniques and Postures

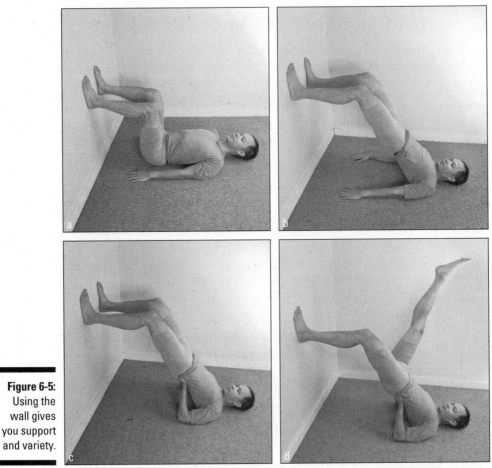

Figure 6-5:
Using the
wall gives
you support
and variety.

Photographs by Adam Latham

Reverse half shoulder stand at the wall

The reverse half shoulder stand at the wall (see Figure 6-6b) is also a variation of *viparita karani,* discussed in the following section. Some people find this exercise easier than the half shoulder stand at the wall. Try them both and see which one is more comfortable for you.

To try this one, follow these steps:

1. **Lie on your back with your head toward the wall at a full arm's distance from the wall; bring your arms back and rest them along the sides of your body, palms down.**

Your legs can be straight, or you can bend your knees with your feet flat on the floor at hip width if it feels better for your back.

Finding the correct distance from the wall depends on the length of your arms. Try these three different measurements: touching the wall with your fingers extended (see Figure 6-6a), touching with the knuckles of your fists, and touching with the backs of your hands.

2. **As you exhale, push your palms down, draw your knees in and up, and raise your hips to a comfortable angle of 45 to 75 degrees.**

   After your legs are up, be sure that they're straight but that your knees aren't locked. Your knees, not your feet, should be over your head in this modified shoulder stand.

Book II

Basic Yoga Techniques and Postures

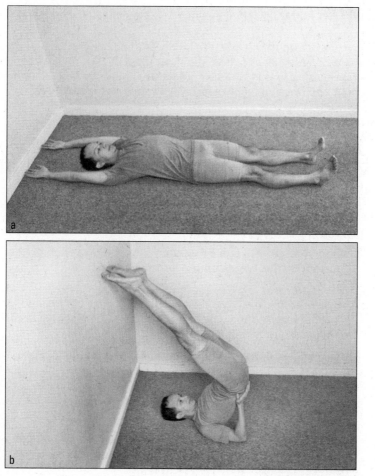

Figure 6-6: Using the wall as a prop for a reverse half shoulder stand.

Photographs by Adam Latham

3. **Bend your elbows and bring your hands to the back of your pelvis; then slide your hands up to your lower back.**

   Press your elbows and the backs of your upper arms onto the floor for support.

4. **Let your toes slowly and gently touch the wall for support; relax your neck (see Figure 6-6b).**

5. **Stay in Step 4 for as long as you feel comfortable, or up to 5 minutes.**

6. **When you want to come down, ease your hips to the floor with the support of your hands, and then bend your knees and lower your feet to the floor.**

Half shoulder stand: Viparita karani

You can work up to this posture by developing comfort with the half shoulder and reverse half shoulder stands at the wall (see the corresponding sections earlier in this chapter). It lets you enjoy the benefits of inversion without compressing your neck as a full shoulder stand does.

When you feel you're ready, follow these steps:

1. **Lie on your back with your knees bent and your feet flat on the floor at hip width; rest your arms along the sides of your body, with your palms down.**

2. **As you exhale, push your palms down, draw your bent knees in and up, and then straighten your legs as you raise your hips to a comfortable angle of 45 to 75 degrees (see Figure 6-7a).**

3. **Bend your elbows and bring your hands to the back of your pelvis; then slide your hands up to your lower back.**

   Make sure your legs are straight but your knees aren't locked, and keep your feet directly above your head. Press your elbows and the backs of your upper arms onto the floor for support. Relax your neck. Figure 6-7b shows this portion of the posture.

4. **Stay in Step 3 for as long as you feel comfortable, or up to 5 minutes.**

5. **When you want to come down, first ease your hips to the floor with the support of your hands, and then bend your knees and lower your feet to the floor.**

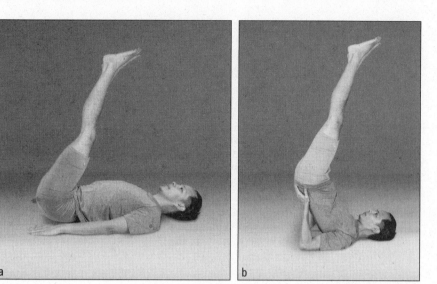

Figure 6-7:
The half
shoulder
stand.

a   b

Photographs by Adam Latham

Book II

Basic Yoga
Techniques
and
Postures

Time out for a language lesson

In Sanskrit — the language of yoga — the accents are not in the traditional English positions of second or third syllables, so watch your automatic responses when you say these aloud. You may hear these said different ways, but try to let the words sort of roll off your tongue in one fell swoop without a huge emphasis on any syllable. And let all the syllables lengthen gracefully rather than grind or swell to stops as is common in English.

Now, where were we? Oh, yeah, postures. . . .

✔ **Asana (ah-sah-nah):** This literally means "posture." A posture can be standing; it can be sitting, but it is a stationary posture. In Yoga, a descriptive Sanskrit word is tacked onto the front of the word *asana* to create a specific posture. For example, one you see early and often in this book is *tadasana*

(tah-dah-sah-nah). In Sanskrit, *tada* means palm tree, which is a tall, stately tree. And that's what tadasana is: a tall stately posture (called *mountain posture* in its English translation).

✔ **Chakra (tshah-kra):** A *chakra* is a center of energy between the top of your head and the base of your spine. Chakra literally means "wheel." Think of these centers of energy as little pinwheels. If the wind stops or you hold an end of one tip, it stops turning or turns very slowly. Same with your energy centers, which are thought to be wheels that whirl actively — unless your energy is blocked.

✔ **Mudra (moo-drah):** A mudra is normally a hand gesture added to a posture. However, it's not just any hand gesture, but rather one

(continued)

(continued)

that is said to seal or lock the life energy inside the body. It is said that when the life energy escapes, it can cause ill health and unhappiness. *Namaste* (see the following item) is a mudra.

✔ **Namaste (nah-mah-stay):** Whether you want to find a spiritual balance through yoga or you just want to work out, you use *namaste.* It is a simple prayerlike position with your hands in front of your breastbone, thumbs touching the breastbone, fingers and palms pressed together, and elbows high. Many asanas or vinyasas (see the last item on this list) start or finish with a position that includes namaste. Perhaps you've been in traditional exercise classes where everybody applauds at the end? Well, in yoga, you find a quick moment of quiet with your hands in namaste and then all students bow slightly toward the teacher and say, "Namaste" as the teachers also

bows slightly in return saying, "Namaste." It translates loosely as "May the divine light be with you" or "I salute the divine light within you." A nice parting word, blessing, and thank you, don't you think?

✔ **Pranayama (prah-nah-yah-mah):** As one word, this means "breath control." Controlling your breath (see Book II, Chapter 1) helps you concentrate and boosts your health. This word stems from *prana,* which means "life force" or "life energy." You help your life force and energy flow smoothly without hurdles and bumps by using good breath control.

✔ **Vinyasa (vee-nyah-sah):** This means "sequence" and is used quite a bit in certain styles of Hatha Yoga where smoothly linking together asanas into a vinyasa is a basic tenet of the practice. No matter what style you practice, try linking together your asanas (postures) for flow.

Chapter 7

Classic Bending Floor Postures

*T*he backbone enables you to bend forward, backward, and sideways, and it also allows you to twist. You perform all these motions every day, but you may do them unconsciously and without adequate muscular support. Yoga uses the natural movements of the spine to train the various muscles supporting it, which contributes to a healthy back and prevents back pain.

This chapter presents a variety of yogic bends. Think of them as simple extensions of the breath. Inhalation takes you naturally into a back bend, and exhalation takes you into a forward bend (for more on breath and movement, flip to Book II, Chapter 1). You can perform bending postures from many different positions — standing, kneeling, sitting, lying, or even turned upside-down (see Book II, Chapter 6). Because the upright bending postures are covered in Book II, Chapter 3, and the most popular bends for warm-up in Book II, Chapter 2, this chapter highlights the classic bending postures that you do on the floor.

From a yogic point of view, the spine is the physical aspect of a subtle energetic pathway that runs from its base to the crown of the head. This pathway is known as the *central channel,* or *sushumna-nadi* ("gracious conduit," pronounced soo-shoom-nah nah-dee). In traditional Hatha Yoga and Tantra Yoga, the awakened "serpent power," or *kundalini-shakti,* rises through this channel. When this power of pure consciousness reaches the crown of the head, you experience a sublime state of ecstasy.

Bending over Backward

Daily life entails a lot of forward bending: putting on a pair of pants, tying shoelaces, picking things up from the floor, working at your computer, gardening, playing sports, and so on. A forward bend closes the front of the torso, shortens the front of the spine, and rounds the back. This closing and rounding is exaggerated by the unhealthy habit of bending forward from the waist rather than from the hip joints. Bending forward in the wrong way day in and day out can lead to spinal problems.

Over the years, this waist-bending habit leads to what is often called a *stoop*, characterized by a sunken chest, a forward-leaning head, aches and pains, and shallow breathing. The antidote for the cumulative effects of forward bending is the regular practice of yoga back bends, which stretch the front of the torso (and spine). Back bends are expansive, extroverted postures that can trigger powerful emotions. (See for yourself: Take a deep inhalation right now and notice how your torso and spine naturally extend during this active, opening phase of the breathing cycle, inviting you to bend backward.)

The major back bends usually come toward the middle of a yoga routine so that you have plenty of time to prepare for these movements and to compensate afterward (see Book II, Chapter 10 for more on preparation and compensation). The next section presents some of the classic floor back bends.

When you lie face down on the floor, raise your chest and head, and use your arms in some fashion, you're doing some form of the cobra posture. When you raise just your legs, or a combination of your legs, chest, and arms, you're performing some form of the locust posture. To make these cobra and locust postures easier, place a small pillow or a folded blanket underneath you between your abdomen and your chest. You can move the blanket a little forward or backward to suit your needs.

Move slowly and cautiously in all the cobra and locust postures. Avoid any of the postures that cause pain in your lower back, upper back, or neck.

Cobra I: Salamba bhujangasana

The cobra posture increases the flexibility and strength of the muscles of the arms, chest, shoulders, and back. Cobra I especially emphasizes the upper back. The cobra opens the chest, increases lung capacity, and stimulates the kidneys and the adrenals. When doing cobra postures, try keeping the buttocks soft; this method can be more therapeutic to the back.

PLAY THIS!

This first cobra posture is also called the sphinx. It's a variation of *bhujangasana,* which is described in the next section. To see how to move into this posture, check out the video at www.dummies.com/go/yogaaiofd.

1. **Lie on your abdomen, with your legs spread at hip width and the tops of your feet on the floor.**

2. **Rest your forehead on the floor, and relax your shoulders; bend your elbows and place your forearms on the floor, with your palms turned down and positioned near the sides of your head (see Figure 7-1a).**

3. **As you inhale, engage your back muscles, press your forearms against the floor, and raise your chest and head.**

   Look straight ahead, as in Figure 7-1b. Keep your forearms and the front of your pelvis on the floor, make sure your bent elbows are directly below or slightly in front of your shoulders, and be mindful of relaxing your shoulders.

Book II

Basic Yoga Techniques and Postures

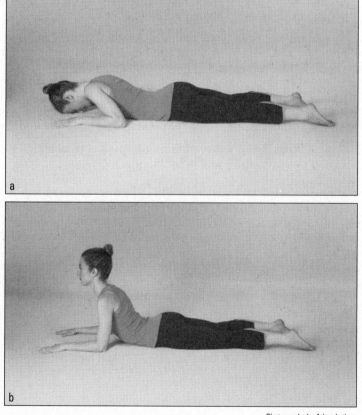

Figure 7-1:
Cobra I emphasizes the upper back and is easier than cobra II.

Photographs by Adam Latham

4. **As you exhale, lower your torso and head slowly back to the floor.**

5. **Repeat Steps 3 and 4 three times, and then stay in Step 3 (the last raised position) for 6 to 8 breaths.**

If you have lower back problems, separate your legs wider than your hips, let your heels turn out, and let your toes turn in.

Cobra II: Bhujangasana

This posture rewards you with most of the same benefits as cobra I, described in the preceding section. In addition, cobra II emphasizes flexibility in your lower back.

1. **Lie on your abdomen, with your legs spread at hip width and the tops of your feet on the floor.**

2. **Bend your elbows and place your palms on the floor, with your thumbs near your armpits; rest your forehead on the floor and relax your shoulders, as in Figure 7-2a.**

3. **As you inhale, press your palms against the floor, engage your back muscles, and raise your chest and head; look straight ahead (see Figure 7-2b).**

   Keep the top front of your pelvis on the floor, and relax your shoulders. Unless you're very flexible, keep your elbows slightly bent.

4. **As you exhale, slowly lower your torso and head back to the floor.**

5. **Repeat Steps 3 and 4 three times, and then stay in Step 3 (the last raised position) for 6 to 8 breaths.**

Note: In the *classic* (traditionally taught) posture, the inner legs are joined and the knees are straight. The head is in alignment with the spine, and the eyes look forward. The palms are on the floor close to the sides of the torso near the navel, the elbows are slightly bent, and the shoulders are relaxed.

If you move your hands farther forward, you make the cobra less difficult; if you move your hands farther back, you increase the difficulty.

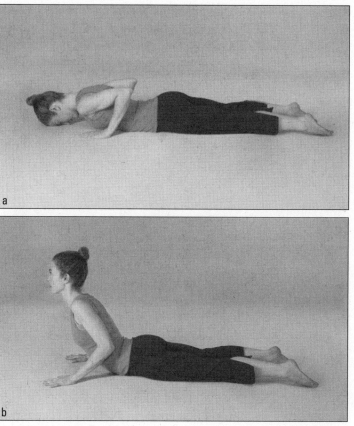

Book II

Basic Yoga Techniques and Postures

Figure 7-2: Cobra II emphasizes flexibility in the lower back.

Photographs by Adam Latham

Cobra III

Cobra III, which is another version of the classic *bhujangasana,* is unique because it doesn't ask you to place your hands on the floor. The emphasis is on strengthening both the lower and upper back.

1. **Lie on your abdomen, with your legs spread at hip width and the tops of your feet on the floor; rest your forehead on the floor.**

2. **Extend your arms back along the sides of your torso, with your palms on the floor, as in Figure 7-3a.**

3. **As you inhale, raise your chest and head, and sweep your arms like wings out to the sides and then all the way forward; your palms can touch or face each other a few inches apart.**

   Keep your legs on the floor, as in Figure 7-3b.

4. As you exhale, sweep your arms back, and lower your torso and your head slowly to the floor.

5. Repeat Steps 3 and 4 three times, and then stay in Step 3 (the last raised position) for 6 to 8 breaths.

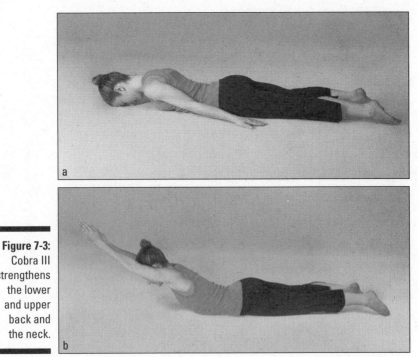

Figure 7-3:
Cobra III strengthens the lower and upper back and the neck.

Photographs by Adam Latham

Locust I: Shalabhasana

The locust posture strengthens the entire torso, including the lower back and the neck, as well as the buttocks and the legs. It also improves digestion and elimination. In locust postures, the buttocks are firm.

1. Lie on your abdomen, with your legs spread at hip width and the tops of your feet on the floor; rest your forehead on the floor.

2. Extend your arms along the sides of your torso, with your palms on the floor.

To make the pose easier, try turning the palms up.

3. **As you inhale, raise your chest, head, and one leg up and away from the floor as high as is comfortable for you (see Figure 7-4a).**

   Consider trying this posture with blankets for more personal comfort. Figure 7-4b shows you the basic blanket positioning, although you can shift it as necessary.

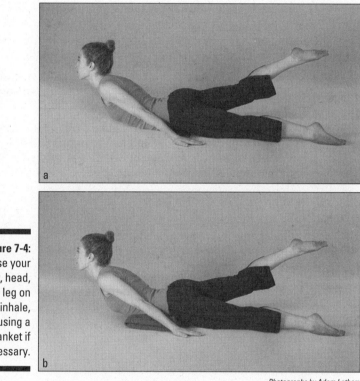

Figure 7-4: Raise your chest, head, and leg on an inhale, using a blanket if necessary.

Photographs by Adam Latham

Book II

Basic Yoga Techniques and Postures

4. **As you exhale, lower your chest, head, and leg together slowly to the floor, and repeat Steps 3 and 4 with the other leg.**

5. **Repeat Steps 3 and 4 three times, and then stay in Step 3 (the last raised position) for 6 to 8 breaths.**

You can increase the level of difficulty by raising both legs at the same time in Step 3. *Note:* In the classic posture, the inner legs are joined and the knees are straight.

Locust II

This posture, which is another variation of *shalabhasana,* also teaches the two sides of the body how to work independently of one another. Many back problems result from imbalances in the muscle system on each side of the spine. Health professionals often call this situation an *asymmetrical problem.* Locust II helps bring your back into symmetry again and also improves your coordination.

1. **Lie on your abdomen, with your legs spread at hip width and the tops of your feet on the floor; rest your forehead on the floor.**

2. **Extend your right arm forward, with your palm resting on the floor; bring your left arm back along the left side of your torso, with the back of your hand on the floor (see Figure 7-5a).**

3. **As you inhale, slowly raise your chest, head, right arm, and left leg up and away from the floor as high as is comfortable for you; try to keep your upper right arm and ear in alignment, and raise your left foot and right hand to the same height above the floor (see Figure 7-5b).**

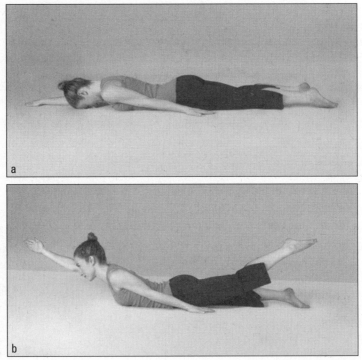

Figure 7-5:
This posture balances the muscles on each side of your back.

Photographs by Adam Latham

4. **As you exhale, slowly lower your right arm, chest, head, and left leg to the floor at the same time.**

5. **Repeat Steps 3 and 4 three times, and then stay in Step 3 for 6 to 8 breaths.**

6. **Repeat Steps 1 through 5 with opposite pairs (left arm and right leg).**

Be careful with locust variations that lift just the legs. Lifting only the legs increases interabdominal and chest pressure, heart rate, and tension in the low back and neck.

Locust III: Superman posture

This posture, a further variation of *shalabhasana,* gets its name from the image of Superman flying through the air at warp speed, with his arms extended out in front leading the way. It's the most strenuous back bend because fully extending your arms and legs as in Figure 7-6 puts quite a load on your entire back. Use this pose only when you're comfortable with locust I and II.

This posture is physically challenging. Don't attempt it if you have back or neck problems.

1. **Lie on your abdomen, with your legs spread at hip width and the tops of your feet on the floor; extend your arms back along the sides of your torso, with your palms on the floor, and rest your forehead on the floor (see Figure 7-6a).**

2. **As you inhale, raise your chest, legs, and head; sweep your arms like wings out to the sides and then all the way forward, as Figure 7-6b illustrates.**

In the beginning, try sweeping your arms only halfway forward in a *T* position; it allows your back muscles to gradually become accustomed to the posture's physical demands.

3. **As you exhale, sweep your arms back and slowly lower your torso, legs, and head to the floor at the same time.**

4. **Repeat Steps 2 and 3 three times, and then stay in Step 2 (the last raised position) for 6 to 8 breaths.**

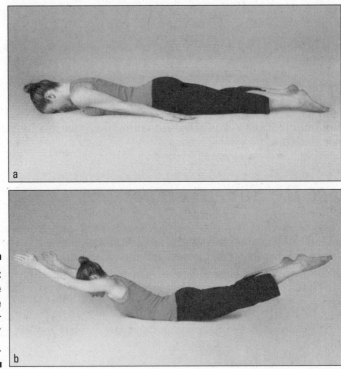

Figure 7-6:
Make sure
you're
ready for
this "super"
posture.

Photographs by Adam Latham

Bending from Side to Side

The spinal column can move in four basic ways: forward *(flexion)*, backward *(extension)*, sideways *(lateral flexion)*, and twist *(rotation)*. The side bend is often the least practiced in yoga. This missed opportunity is unfortunate because side bends help stretch and tone the muscles along the sides of the abdomen, rib cage, and spine to keep your waist trim, your breathing full, and your spine supple. A true side bend fully contracts one side of the body while expanding the other. This section covers some safe, creative ways to use side bends on the floor.

Seated side bend

This seated side bend is a great way to ease into the position if you're not used to bending from side to side. Just follow these steps:

1. **Sit comfortably in a simple cross-legged position; place your right palm on the floor, near your right hip.**

   Check out Book II, Chapter 2 for some appropriate seated positions.

2. **As you inhale, raise your left arm out to the side and above your head beside your left ear.**

3. **As you exhale, slide your right hand across the floor out to the right, letting your torso, head, and left arm follow as you bend to the right (see Figure 7-7).**

   Don't let your buttocks come off the floor as you bend.

Book II

Basic Yoga
Techniques
and
Postures

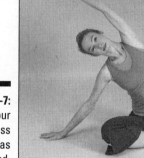

Figure 7-7:
Slide your
hand across
the floor as
you bend.

Photograph by Adam Latham

4. **As you inhale, return to the upright position (as you were at the start of Step 2).**

5. **Repeat Steps 2 through 4 three times, and then stay in the bent position (Step 3) for 6 to 8 breaths.**

6. **Repeat Steps 1 through 5 on the other side.**

All-fours side bend

Many people with back or hip problems have a hard time sitting upright on the floor. The all-fours position gives the spine more freedom and is an easier side bend from the floor.

1. **Start on your hands and knees, with your knees below your hips and your hands below your shoulders, with your palms on the floor.**

   Straighten your elbows, but don't lock them. Look straight ahead.

2. **As you exhale, bend your head and torso sideways to the right, and look toward your tailbone (see Figure 7-8).**

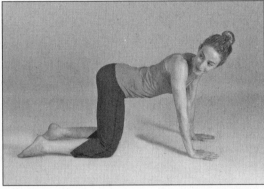

Figure 7-8:
Look back
as you bend.

Photograph by Adam Latham

3. **As you inhale, return to the starting position in Step 1.**

4. **Repeat Steps 2 and 3 three times, and then stay in Step 2 for 6 to 8 breaths.**

5. **Repeat Steps 2 through 4 on the other side.**

Folded side bend

The Sanskrit word *bala* (pronounced bah-lah) means "child." This practice was inspired by a baby's folded position in the womb. The benefits of this side bend, which is a variation of *balasana,* the child's posture (see Book II, Chapter 10 for this posture), are the same as for the seated side bend earlier in this chapter.

1. **Sit on your heels with your toes pointing back, and fold forward by laying your abdomen on your thighs and your forehead on the floor; extend your arms forward with your palms on the floor, as in Figure 7-9a.**

2. As you exhale, stay in the folded position and slide your upper torso, head, arms, and hands to the right as far as possible, as in Figure 7-9b; wait for a few seconds and, again, with another exhalation, slide farther to the right if you can do so without straining.

3. Return to center and repeat the sequence to the left side, staying in Step 2 for 6 to 8 breaths on each side.

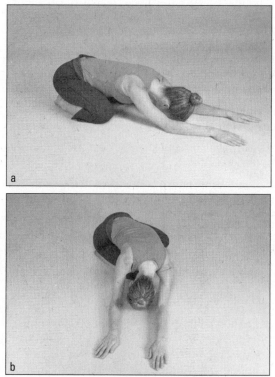

Figure 7-9:
Wait a few moments before you stretch farther on each side.

Photographs by Adam Latham

Bending Forward

Forward bends are usually a good way to begin any movement routine (unless you're dealing with spinal disc injuries or certain other back problems). Back bends are the lively extroverts of the *asana* family, and forward bends are the retiring introverts; you always perform them with an exhalation — the passive, contracting phase of the breathing cycle.

Be very careful of all the seated forward bends if you have disc-related back problems.

If you have a problem sitting upright on the floor in the seated forward bend or in any of the following forward-bending postures, raise your hips with folded blankets or firm pillows.

Seated forward bend: Pashcimottanasana

The seated forward bend intensely stretches the entire back side of the body, including the back of the spine and legs. It also tones the muscles and organs of the abdomen and creates a calming and quieting effect.

1. **Sit on the floor, with your legs at hip width and comfortably stretched out in front of you; bring your back up nice and tall, and place your palms on the floor near your thighs.**

2. **As you inhale, raise your arms forward and overhead until they're beside your ears, as in Figure 7-10a.**

   Keep your arms and legs soft and slightly bent in Forgiving Limbs, described in Book I, Chapter 3.

3. **As you exhale, bend forward from the hips; bring your hands, chest, and head toward your legs; rest your hands on the floor or on your thighs, knees, shins, or feet.**

   If your head isn't close to your knees, bend your knees more until you feel your back stretching (see Figure 7-10b).

4. **Repeat Steps 2 and 3 three times, and then stay folded (Step 3) for 6 to 8 breaths.**

Note: In the classic posture, the inner legs are joined, the knees are straight, and the ankles are extended so that the toes point up. The chin rests on the chest, the hands hold the sides of the feet, the back is extended forward, and the forehead is pressed against the legs.

Head-to-knee posture: Janushirshasana

The head-to-knee posture keeps your spine supple, stimulates the abdominal organs, and stretches your back, especially on the side of the extended leg. It also activates the central channel *(sushumna-nadi)*. As the introduction to this chapter explains, the *central channel* is the pathway for the awakened

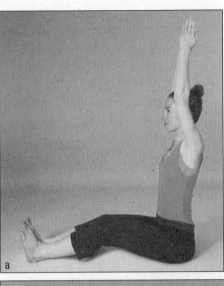

Book II

**Basic Yoga
Techniques
and
Postures**

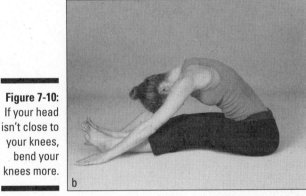

Figure 7-10:
If your head
isn't close to
your knees,
bend your
knees more.

Photographs by Adam Latham

energy of pure consciousness (called *kundalini-shakti*), which leads to
ecstasy and spiritual liberation.

Follow these steps to achieve this posture:

1. **Sit on the floor, with your legs stretched out in front of you, and then
   bend your left knee and bring your left heel toward your right groin.**

2. **Rest your bent left knee on the floor (but don't force it down), and
   place the sole of your left foot on the inside of your right thigh.**

   The toes of the left foot point toward the right knee.

3. **Bring your back up nice and tall; as you inhale, raise your arms forward and overhead until they're beside your ears, as Figure 7-11a shows.**

   Keep your arms and your right leg soft and slightly bent in Forgiving Limbs, described in Book I, Chapter 3.

4. **As you exhale, bend forward from the hips, bringing your hands, chest, and head toward your right leg; rest your hands on the floor or on your thigh, knee, shin, or foot.**

   If your head isn't close to your right knee, bend your knee more until you feel your back stretching on the right side (see Figure 7-11b).

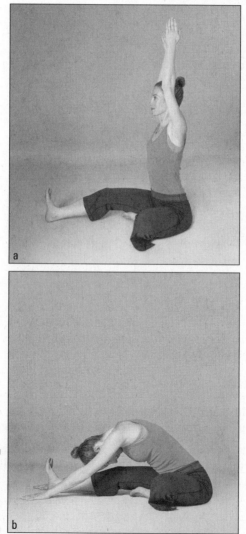

Figure 7-11:
The head-
to-knee
posture.

Photographs by Adam Latham

5. **Repeat Steps 3 and 4 three times, and then stay in Step 4 (the final forward bend) for 6 to 8 breaths.**

6. **Repeat Steps 1 through 4 on the opposite side.**

Keep your back muscles as relaxed as possible.

The great seal: Mahamudra

Ancient Hatha Yoga texts give high praise to the volcano posture. It strengthens the back, stretches the legs, and opens the hips and chest. This posture is unique in that it has qualities of both a forward bend and a back bend. When used with special locks *(bandhas)* that contain and channel energy in the torso, this technique has both cleansing and healing effects.

Book II

Basic Yoga Techniques and Postures

1. **Sitting on the floor, with your legs stretched out in front of you, bend your left knee and bring your left foot toward your right groin.**

2. **Rest your bent left knee on the floor to the left (but don't force it down), and place the sole of your left foot on the inside of your right thigh, with your heel in your groin.**

   The toes of the left foot point toward the right knee.

3. **Bring your back up nice and tall; as you inhale, raise your arms forward and overhead until they're beside your ears.**

   Keep your arms and the right leg soft and slightly bent in Forgiving Limbs, described in Book I, Chapter 3. Refer to Figure 7-11a in the preceding section, if necessary.

4. **As you exhale, bend forward from the hips, lift your chest forward, and extend your back without letting it round; place your hands on your right knee, shin, or toes, and look straight ahead (see Figure 7-12).**

5. **Repeat Steps 3 and 4 three times, and then stay in Step 4 for 6 to 8 breaths.**

6. **Repeat the same sequence on the opposite side.**

Note: In the classic posture, the front leg and the arms are straight, and the hands are holding the toes of the front leg. The back is extended, and the chin is pressed onto the chest. The abdominal muscles are pulled up into the abdominal cavity, and the anal sphincter is tightened.

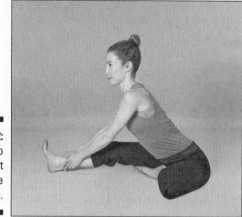

Figure 7-12:
The volcano
is a great
all-inclusive
posture.

Photograph by Adam Latham

Wide-legged forward bend:
Upavishta konasana

The wide-legged forward bend stretches the backs and insides of the legs (hamstrings and adductors) and increases the flexibility of the spine and hip joints. It improves circulation to the entire pelvic region, tones the abdomen, and has a calming effect on the nervous system. Note, though, that muscle density may make this posture difficult for most men.

1. **Sit on the floor, with your legs straight and spread wide apart (but not more than 90 degrees).**

   Because this posture is challenging, give yourself an advantage by pulling the flesh of the buttocks (you may know them as "cheeks") out from under the *sits bones* (the bones directly under that flesh; they're also known as the *ischial tuberosities*) and bending your knees slightly. Alternatively, sit on some folded blankets.

2. **As you inhale, raise your arms forward and overhead until they're beside your ears.**

   Keep your elbows soft and your legs slightly bent in Forgiving Limbs, described in Book I, Chapter 3. Bring your back up nice and tall (see Figure 7-13a).

3. **As you exhale, bend forward from the hips and bring your hands, chest, and head toward the floor.**

   Rest your extended arms and hands palms down on the floor. If you have the flexibility, place your forehead on the floor as well, as in Figure 7-13b.

4. **Repeat Steps 2 and 3 three times, and then stay in Step 3 (the folded position) for 6 to 8 breaths.**

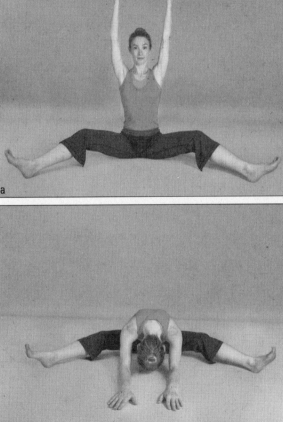

Figure 7-13:
The wide-legged forward bend.

Photographs by Adam Latham

Note: In the classic posture, the legs are straight, with the toes vertical; the chin and chest are on the floor; and the arms are extended forward, with the palms joined.

The wide-legged forward bend is also called the *lifetime posture* because it can take a whole lifetime to master. But don't worry if you don't quite reach mastery. Some yogis believe that if you don't master the pose in this lifetime, you can try again in the next lifetime.

Chapter 8

Several Twists on the Yoga Twist

In This Chapter

▶ Enjoying spinal fitness — with a yogic twist

▶ Introducing six simple twists

*I*magine you're cleaning the kitchen with a wet sponge. After you mop up some spills, the sponge gets dirty. You hold it under the kitchen faucet, turn on the water, and squeeze out the dirty water. As you release the pressure on the sponge, it sucks up some clean water. You're ready to start again.

This description is a lot like how yogic twists work on the spine. The pulpy pads *(discs)* between the individual bones have no direct blood supply of their own after about age 20, so they depend on your everyday movements to help them wring out the accumulated wastes and soak up a fresh supply of blood and other reviving fluids. Over time, if you don't continually squeeze and soak your discs, they tend to harden and dry out, like a sponge left unused for a few days. Consequently, your spine stiffens up and shrinks.

Twists are an important component of any yoga practice. They clean out the discs and help keep them firm and supple; massage the internal organs, such as your intestines and kidneys; stoke the inner fire of digestion; and stretch and strengthen the muscles of your back and abdomen.

This chapter features seated twists, which emphasize the upper spine, and reclining twists, which emphasize the lower spine.

Approach all twists with caution if you're suffering from disc problems anywhere in your spine. Consult your physician, chiropractor, or physical therapist, or work with a reputable yoga therapist after you have a diagnosis.

Trying Simple Upright Twists

When done properly, yogic twisting postures strengthen your body, especially the weak spots (notably the lower back). Although twisting is part of your everyday movements, unless your muscles are well trained, you can easily injure yourself. The exercises in this section can help you get your back in tip-top shape as you look forward to enjoyment and enlightenment along the way.

Easy chair twist

This seated posture is an excellent way for a beginner to safely achieve a good twist before moving on to more complex methods of twisting. And you can use this simple, effective posture to liberate your spine while at the office without drawing too much attention to yourself. Your spine will thank you!

Twist mainly from your shoulders; the head and neck come along for the ride.

1. **Sit sideways on a chair, with the chair back to your left, your feet flat on the floor, and your heels directly below your knees.**

2. **Exhale, turn to the left, and hold the sides of the chair back with your hands.**

3. **As you inhale, extend or lift your spine upward.**

4. **As you exhale, twist your torso and head farther to the left, as in Figure 8-1.**

5. **Repeat Steps 1 through 4, gradually twisting farther with each exhalation, for 3 breaths (don't force it); then hold the twist for 6 to 8 breaths.**

6. **Repeat Steps 1 through 5 on the opposite side.**

If your feet aren't comfortably on the floor for the easy chair twist, elevate them with a folded blanket or a phone book.

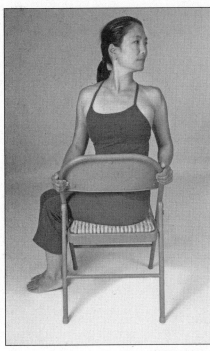

Book II

Basic Yoga Techniques and Postures

Figure 8-1: Easy chair twist.

Photograph by Adam Latham

Easy sitting twist

When you can twist comfortably while seated on a chair (see the preceding section), you can transfer that skill to the floor and try the following exercise. Its effect is similar to that of the easy chair twist, and it fits nicely into a regular yoga practice, a large part of which you can do on the floor.

1. **Sit on the floor with your legs in a simple cross-legged position, and extend your spine upward, nice and tall.**

2. **Place your left hand palm down on top of your right knee.**

3. **Place your right hand palm down on the floor behind your right hip, to prop yourself up.**

4. **As you inhale, extend your spine upward.**

5. **As you exhale, twist your torso and head to the right (see Figure 8-2).**

6. **Repeat Steps 4 and 5 for 3 breaths, gradually twisting farther with each exhalation (don't force it); then hold the twist for 6 to 8 breaths.**

7. **Repeat Steps 1 through 6 on the opposite side.**

TIP

If you have difficulty sitting upright in this seated twist, use blankets or pillows under your bottom to make your hips even with your knees.

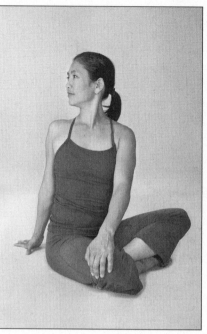

Figure 8-2:
The easy
sitting twist.

Photograph by Adam Latham

The sage twist

The easy chair twist and the easy sitting twist (in the preceding sections) are the simplest yogic twists. By changing the position of your legs, you alter the level of difficulty and also enhance the overall benefit. The sage twist does just that to give you extra rewards for your investment.

1. **Sit on the floor with both legs extended forward; bend your right knee and place your right foot on the floor just inside your left thigh, with your toes facing forward.**

2. **Place your right hand, palm down, on the floor behind you; wrap the palm of your left hand around the side of your right knee.**

3. **As you inhale, extend or lift your spine upward.**

4. **As you exhale, twist your torso and head to the right, as in Figure 8-3.**

5. Repeat Steps 3 and 4, gradually twisting farther with each exhalation, for 3 breaths (don't force it); then hold the twist for 6 to 8 breaths.

6. Repeat Steps 1 through 5 on the opposite side.

If you have difficulty sitting upright in this seated twist, sit on blankets or pillows until your hips are even with your knees.

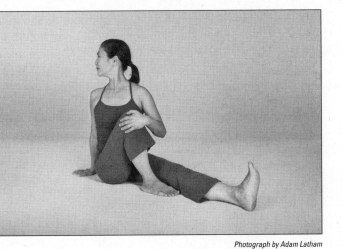

Figure 8-3: Beginners can enjoy benefits from this sage twist variation.

Photograph by Adam Latham

This posture is a variation of the classic posture *maricyasana*. The Sanskrit word *marici* (pronounced mah-ree-chee) means "ray of light" and is the name of an ancient sage.

Twisting while Reclining

The remaining exercises in this chapter call for you to lie down. You can harvest all kinds of benefits from them, including a delicious feeling of release in your spine.

Bent leg supine twist

The bent supine twist is a variation of the classic posture known as *parivartanasana*. The Sanskrit word *parivartana* (pronounced pah-ree-vahr-tah-nah) means "turning."

This posture has a calming effect on the lower back. Here's how you do it:

1. **Lie on your back with your knees bent and feet on the floor at hip width, and extend your arms from your sides like a *T* (in line with the top of your shoulders), with your palms down.**

2. **As you exhale, slowly lower your bent legs to the right side while turning your head to the left (see Figure 8-4).**

   Keep your head on the floor.

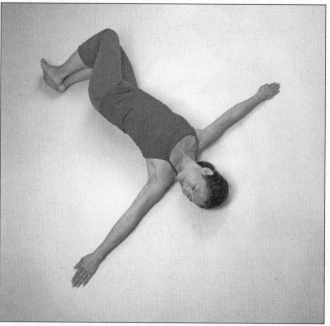

Figure 8-4:
Turn your head in the opposite direction of your legs.

Photograph by Adam Latham

3. **As you inhale, bring your bent knees back to the middle.**

4. **As you exhale, slowly lower your bent knees to the left while turning your head to the right.**

5. **Repeat Steps 1 through 4, alternating three times slowly on each side; then hold one last twist on each side for 6 to 8 breaths.**

The Swiss army knife

This posture, a variation of the classic *jathara parivritti,* tones the abdominal organs and intestines and also stretches the lower back and hips. *Jathara parivritti* (pronounced jat-hah-rah pah-ree-vree-tee) means "belly twisting." Just follow these steps:

1. **Lie flat on the floor with your legs straight down, and extend your arms out from your sides like a *T* (in line with the top of your shoulders), with your palms up.**

2. **Bend your right knee, and draw your thigh into your abdomen.**

3. **As you exhale, slowly lower your bent right leg to the left side and extend it a comfortable distance.**

4. **Extend your left arm on the floor along the left side of your head (palm up), and then turn your head to the right, as in Figure 8-5.**

   Keep your head on the floor, and try to visualize lines of energy going out through your arms and legs.

Book II

Basic Yoga Techniques and Postures

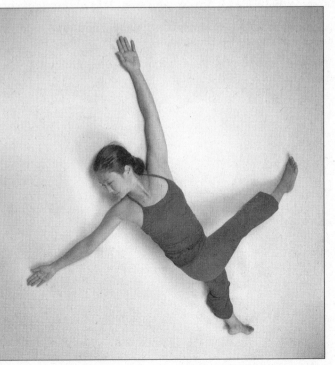

Figure 8-5: Extend your arm and turn your head the opposite way.

Photograph by Adam Latham

5. Relax and stay in Step 4 for 6 to 8 breaths.

6. Repeat Steps 1 through 5 on the opposite side.

Extended legs supine twist: Jathara parivritti

If you enjoy practicing the Swiss army knife (see the preceding section), you're likely to enjoy this slightly more demanding exercise. This variation of *jathara parivritti* gives you the same benefits as the Swiss army knife but creates an even more pronounced stretch of the lower back and hips. Of course, stretching is good for your muscles and your spine, too. The following steps show you how it works:

1. Lie on your back with your knees bent and your feet on the floor at hip width, and extend your arms out from your sides like a *T* (in line with the top of your shoulders), with your palms down.

2. Bend your knees and draw both thighs into your abdomen.

3. As you exhale, slowly lower your bent legs to the right side.

4. Extend both legs a comfortable distance, and then turn your head to the left, as Figure 8-6 illustrates.

   Keep your head on the floor. If this posture is difficult, try bending both legs a little more.

Figure 8-6:
Keep your head on the floor as you turn it and extend your legs.

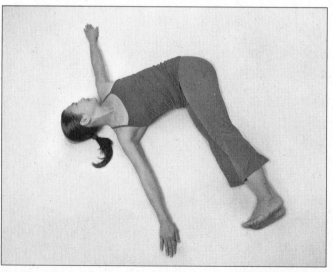

Photograph by Adam Latham

5. **Relax and stay in Step 4 for 6 to 8 breaths.**

6. **Repeat Steps 1 through 5 on the opposite side.**

Note: In the *classic* (traditionally taught) version of this posture, the knees are straight and the joined legs are resting on the floor. The arms are straight and extended to the sides at right angles to the torso. The hand on the same side of the extended legs holds the top foot.

Chapter 9

Dynamic Postures: The Rejuvenation Sequence and Sun Salutation

*T*he sun has long captured humanity's attention for its life-giving power, but you don't have to be a sun worshiper to benefit from yoga's sun salutation (*surya namaskara,* pronounced soor-yah nah-mahs-kah-rah). This exercise — a special sequence of postures — is considered so profound that many people practice it on its own. It works well (with modifications) for people of all ages, from children to seniors. Respected for its excellent effects, the sun salutation reputedly provides an array of physical benefits, such as stretching the spine and strengthening the muscles that support it; improving posture, coordination, and endurance; and improving lung function and oxygen delivery to cells. Yoga masters claim that the sun salutation, which links body, mind, and breath, has deeper psychological and spiritual implications because it stimulates subtle vital energies leading to states of higher awareness.

The sun salutation helps you remember the yogic idea that your body is condensed sunlight. The saluting gesture, called *namaskara mudra* in Sanskrit (pronounced nah-mahs-kah-rah mood-rah), is a salute to the highest aspect within yourself — the spirit.

Warming Up for the Sun: Rejuvenating in 9 Steps

Do you need a more user-friendly version of the sun salutation? Do you have a hard time kneeling (as the 7-step sun salutation requires later in this chapter) or stepping through (as the 12-step sun salutation requires later in this chapter)? Then try the 9-step rejuvenation sequence, direct from California, using the focus breathing technique from Book II, Chapter 1. For help with the rejuvenation sequence, check out the video at www.dummies.com/go/yogaaiofd.

1. **Stand in the mountain posture, with your feet at hip width and arms at your sides (see Figure 9-1a).**

2. **As you inhale, slowly raise your arms out from the sides and overhead (see Figure 9-1b); then pause.**

3. **As you exhale, bend forward from the waist and bring your head toward your knees; bring your hands forward and down toward the floor in the standing forward bend (see Figure 9-1c).**

   Keep your arms and legs soft (see Book I, Chapter 3 for an explanation of Forgiving Limbs); then pause.

4. **Bend your knees quite a bit and, as you inhale, sweep your arms out from the sides and raise halfway up with your arms in a *T* (half forward bend), as in Figure 9-1d; then pause briefly.**

5. **As you exhale, fold all the way down again and hang your arms in the standing forward bend (see Figure 9-1e).**

6. **As you inhale, sweep your arms from the sides like wings, and bring your torso all the way up again, standing with your arms overhead in the standing arm raise (see Figure 9-1f).**

7. **As you exhale, bend your knees and squat halfway to the floor.**

   Soften your arms, but keep them overhead; look straight ahead (see Figure 9-1g).

8. **As you inhale, bring your torso all the way up again, standing with your arms overhead in the standing arm raise (see Figure 9-1h).**

9. **As you exhale, bring your arms back to your sides, as in Step 1 (see Figure 9-1i).**

Repeat the entire sequence six to eight times slowly.

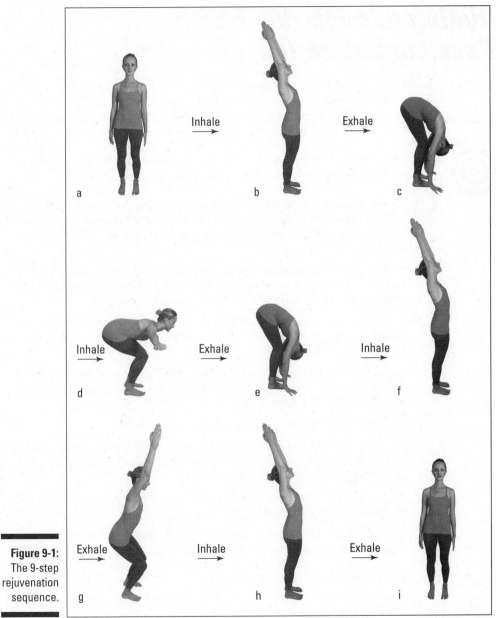

Figure 9-1:
The 9-step rejuvenation sequence.

Photographs by Adam Latham

To make the sequence harder on the last round, stay for 6 to 8 breaths in the half forward bend (Step 4), the standing forward bend (Step 5), and the half squat or half chair (Step 7). To make it much harder, do the entire sequence standing on your toes.

Gliding through the 7-Step Kneeling Salutation

If you aren't quite ready to tackle the 12-step sun salutation, the following 7-step variation can give you many benefits and also help you get in shape for the standing variety. Use focus, chest-to-belly, or belly-to-chest breathing techniques from Book II, Chapter 1, and follow these steps.

Just follow your breath — inhale when you're opening, exhale when you're folding. Move slowly, pausing after each inhalation and exhalation.

1. **Sit on your heels in a bent-knee position, bring your back up nice and tall, and place your palms together in the prayer position, with your thumbs touching the sternum (breastbone) in the middle of your chest (see Figure 9-2a).**

2. **As you inhale, open your palms and slightly raise your arms forward and then overhead; raise your buttocks away from your heels, arch your back, and look up at the ceiling, as in Figure 9-2b.**

3. **As you exhale, bend forward slowly from the hips, placing your palms, forearms, and then forehead on the floor; pause, relaxing your hips, as Figure 9-2c shows.**

4. **Slide your hands forward on the floor until your arms are extended; slide your chest forward, bending your elbows slightly, and arch up into cobra II (see Figure 9-2d).**

   Flip to Book II, Chapter 8 for instructions on cobra II.

5. **As you exhale, turn your toes under, raise your hips, extend your legs, and bring your chest down, keeping both hands on the floor for the downward-facing dog (see Figure 9-2e).**

6. **As you inhale, bend your knees to the floor, with your gaze toward the floor, slightly in front of you, as in Figure 9-2f.**

7. **As you exhale, sit back on your heels and return your hands to the prayer position, as in Step 1 (see Figure 9-2g).**

Repeat the entire sequence 3 to 12 times.

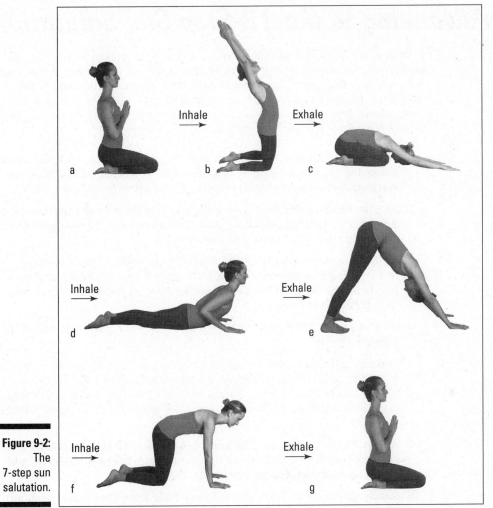

Photographs by Adam Latham

Figure 9-2:
The 7-step sun salutation.

If you're not able to sit on your heels in Steps 1 and 7, simply keep your palms in the prayer position and stand on your knees instead. You can also fold a blanket under your knees for comfort. If you find this 7-step salutation too difficult for you, head to the following section and try Steps 1 through 3 only of the 12-step version until you're ready to do more.

Advancing to the 12-Step Sun Salutation

To enjoy the greatest benefit from this sequence (as well as all your yoga postures), execute each part with full participation of your mind. When you stand, really stand; plant your feet firmly on the ground. When you bend or stretch, bend or stretch with complete attention. Your mind makes your practice not only elegant but also potent. Use any of the yoga breathing techniques from Book II, Chapter 1, and follow these steps:

1. **Start in a standing position, with your feet at hip width, and place your palms together in the prayer position, with your thumbs touching the sternum (breastbone) in the middle of your chest (see Figure 9-3a).**

2. **As you inhale, open your palms slightly and raise your arms forward and overhead; arch your back and look up toward the ceiling without throwing your head back (see Figure 9-3b).**

3. **As you exhale, bend forward from the hips, soften your knees (as in Forgiving Limbs, which Book I, Chapter 3 covers), and place your hands on the floor; bring your head as close as possible to your legs, as Figure 9-3c shows.**

4. **As you inhale, bend your left knee and step your right foot back into a lunge.**

   Make sure that your left knee is directly over your ankle and your thigh is parallel to the floor so that your knee forms a right angle. Your gaze should be downward, a few inches in front of you on the floor, keeping your neck in a long and neutral position. Figure 9-3d gives you a visual of this step.

5. **As you exhale, step your left foot back beside the right and hold a push-up position; if your arms tire, bend your knees to the floor and pause on your hands and knees (see Figure 9-3e).**

6. **Inhale and then, as you exhale, lower your knees (from the push-up), chest, and chin to the floor, keeping your buttocks up in the air (see Figure 9-3f).**

7. **As you inhale, slide your chest forward along the floor, and then arch back into cobra II, as in Figure 9-3g.**

8. **As you exhale, turn your toes under, raise your hips, extend your legs, and bring your chest down, keeping both hands on the floor (see Figure 9-3h).**

   This pose is the same downward-facing dog position from Book II, Chapter 3.

9. **As you inhale, step your right foot forward between your hands and, again, point your gaze toward the floor a few inches ahead of you (see Figure 9-3i).**

10. **As you exhale, step your left foot forward, parallel to and even with your right foot; soften your knees and fold into a forward bend, as in Step 3 (see Figure 9-3j).**

11. **As you inhale, raise your arms either forward and overhead from the front, or out and up from the sides like wings; then arch back and look up, as in Step 2 (see Figure 9-3k).**

If you have back problems, lifting up from the forward bend with your arms to the front or sides may cause you some discomfort. If so, you can try the roll-up: Keep your chin on your chest and roll up, stacking the vertebrae one at a time, with your arms hanging at your sides and your head coming up last. When you're fully upright, bring your arms forward, up, and overhead from the front; arch your back just a little; and look up.

12. **As you exhale, return your hands to the prayer position, as in Step 1 (see Figure 9-3l).**

Repeat the entire sequence 3 to 12 times. First lead with the right foot, and then alternate with the left foot for an equal number of repetitions (each side counts as half a sequence).

If you're ready for greater challenges, consider Power Yoga's advanced sun salutations (Book IV, Chapter 5), or check the Internet for the Iyengar sun salutation or various "flow" sequences.

Book II

Basic Yoga Techniques and Postures

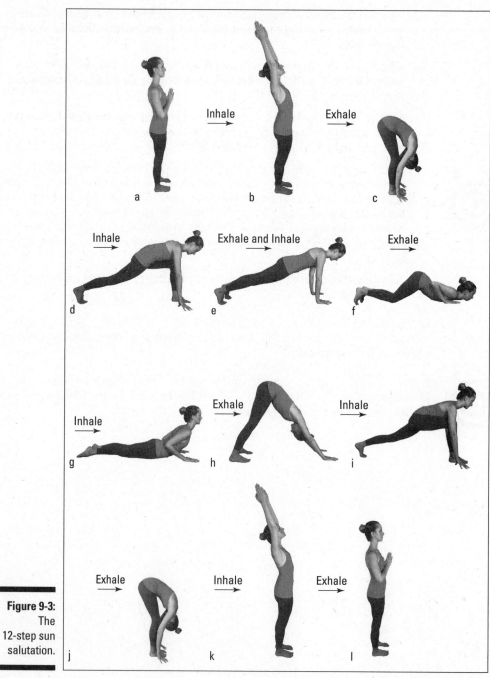

Figure 9-3:
The 12-step sun salutation.

Chapter 10

Basic Preparation, Compensation, and Rest Poses

The art and science of sequencing in yoga, called *vinyasa-krama* (pronounced veen-yah-sah-krah-mah), is often referred to as *flow*. Paying attention to proper sequencing can help you achieve the best possible flow of postures and derive maximum benefit from your yoga session.

Although sequencing has many approaches, you can't go wrong when you bear in mind the following four basic categories:

✔ Warm-up or preparation

✔ Main postures

✔ Compensation

✔ Rest

Chapters 2 through 9 of Book II outline a variety of main postures. This chapter explains common warm-up, compensation, and rest postures that you're likely to perform in your yoga sessions.

Getting Started with Warm-Ups

Any physical exercise requires adequate warm-up, and yoga is no exception. Warm-up exercises increase circulation to the parts of your body you're about to use and make you more aware of those areas of your physical self. What's different about the yoga warm-up (called *preparation postures*) is that you do it slowly and deliberately, with conscious breathing and awareness.

You typically perform warm-up postures *dynamically,* which means you move in and out of them. In general, the safest yoga warm-ups are simple forward bends and easy sequences that fold and unfold the body. Figure 10-1 shows some recommended warm-up exercises. You may select from the various

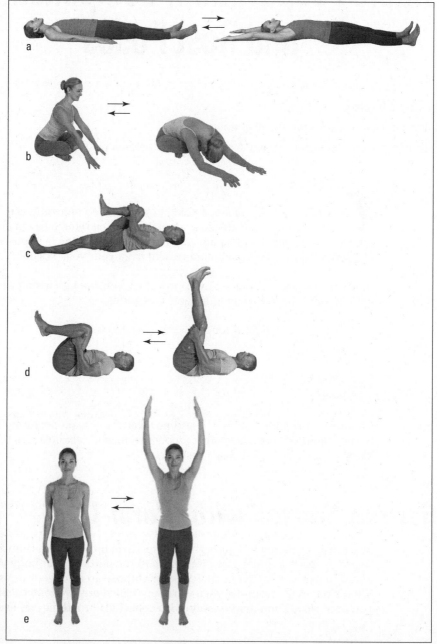

Figure 10-1: Warm-ups usually include gentle bending and extending.

Photographs by Adam Latham

reclining, sitting, and standing positions in this chapter. Normally, two or three postures make for an adequate warm-up.

If you have disc problems in your lower back, forward bends may not be a good way to warm up. Check with your medical or chiropractic doctor.

Warm-up or preparation postures are also used throughout a given routine to precede and enhance the effect of the main postures. For example, you do the leg lift just before a seated forward bend to stretch the hamstrings; you do the bridge posture just before a shoulder stand.

Reclining warm-up postures

Most yoga practitioners enjoy reclining *(supine)* exercises because the postures are intrinsically relaxing. When you pair them with warm-ups, the combination effectively allows you to warm up specific muscles or muscle groups while keeping the other muscles at rest.

The following warm-up exercises require you to start with the corpse posture, described in Book VII, Chapter 2. These exercises help revive you even when you start your yoga session dead tired.

Lying arm raise

Many of the muscles that go to the neck start between your shoulder blades. Raising the arms brings circulation to frequent sites of tension (see Figure 10-1a).

1. **Lie flat on your back, with your arms relaxed at your sides and your palms turned down.**
2. **As you inhale, slowly raise your arms over your head and touch the floor.**
3. **As you exhale, bring your arms back to your sides, as in Step 1.**
4. **Repeat Steps 1 through 3 six to eight times.**

The double breath

If you want to double your pleasure, the double breath enhances tension release in your body and prepares your muscles for the main postures.

1. **Repeat Steps 1 and 2 of the lying arm raise in the preceding section.**
2. **After you raise your arms overhead on the inhalation, leave them on the floor above your head and fully exhale.**

   Your arms remain where they are for another inhalation while you deeply stretch your entire body from the tips of your toes to your fingertips.

3. **On the next exhalation, return your arms to your sides and relax your legs; repeat three to four times.**

Knee-to-chest posture

Use this exercise for either warm-up or compensation. The knee-to-chest posture, shown in Figure 10-1c, is also a classic in lower back programs.

1. **Lie on your back, with your knees bent and your feet flat on the floor.**

2. **As you exhale, bring your right knee into your chest and hold your shin just below your knee.**

   If you have knee problems, hold the back of your thigh instead of your shin.

3. **If you can do so comfortably, straighten your left leg on the floor.**

   If you have back problems, though, keep your left knee bent.

4. **Repeat Steps 1 through 3 on the other side, holding each side for 6 to 8 breaths.**

Double leg extension

This exercise, shown in Figure 10-1c, uses both legs simultaneously and prepares the lower back and gently stretches the hamstrings.

1. **Lie on your back, and bring your bent knees toward your chest.**

2. **Hold the backs of your thighs at arm's length.**

3. **As you inhale, straighten both legs perpendicular to the floor; as you exhale, bend both legs again.**

4. **Repeat Steps 2 and 3 six to eight times.**

Hamstring stretch

You can injure the hamstrings quite easily, especially if you overwork them, so you want to prepare them properly for exercise. Refer to Figure 10-2 for a visual.

1. **Lying on your back with your legs straight, place your arms along your sides, with your palms down.**

2. **Bend just your left knee, and put that foot on the floor (see Figure 10-2a).**

3. **As you exhale, bring your right leg up as straight as possible (see Figure 10-2b); as you inhale, return your right leg to the floor.**

   Keep your head and your hips on the floor.

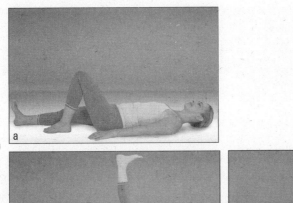
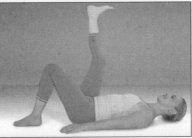
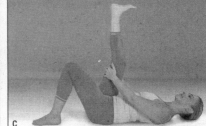

Figure 10-2:
Unlock your
hamstrings,
and you
open the
door to
many yoga
postures.

Photographs by Adam Latham

Book II

**Basic Yoga
Techniques
and
Postures**

4. **Repeat Steps 3 and 4 three times, and then, with your hands interlocked on the back of your raised thigh just above your knee, hold your leg in place for 6 to 8 breaths (see Figure 10-2c).**

5. **Repeat Steps 1 through 4 on the other side.**

Support your head with a pillow or folded blanket if the back of your neck or your throat tenses when you raise or lower your leg.

Dynamic bridge: Dvipada pitha

You can use this exercise, shown in Figure 10-3, for warm-up, compensation, and as a main posture.

1. **Lie on your back, with your knees bent, your feet flat on the floor at hip width, and your arms at your sides, with your palms turned down (see Figure 10-3a).**

2. **As you inhale, raise your hips to a comfortable height (see Figure 10-3b).**

3. **As you exhale, return your hips to the floor.**

4. **Repeat Steps 3 and 4 six to eight times.**

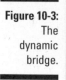
Figure 10-3:
The dynamic bridge.

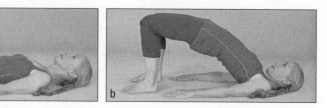

Photographs by Adam Latham

Bridge variation with arm raise

This posture is another good candidate for both warm-up and compensation.

1. **Lie on your back, with your knees bent, your feet flat on the floor at hip width, and your arms at your sides, with your palms turned down (refer to Figure 10-3a).**

2. **As you inhale, raise your hips to a comfortable height and, at the same time, raise your arms overhead to touch the floor (see Figure 10-4).**

Figure 10-4:
Bridge variation with arm raise.

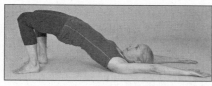

Photograph by Adam Latham

3. **As you exhale, return your hips to the floor and your arms to your sides.**

4. **Repeat Steps 3 and 4 six to eight times.**

Dynamic head-to-knee

The dynamic head-to-knee posture is a nice warm-up before a slightly more physical routine. Because it is a little more vigorous, don't perform this sequence if you're having neck problems.

1. **Lie flat on your back, with your arms relaxed at your sides and your palms turned down, as in Figure 10-1a earlier in the chapter.**

2. **As you inhale, raise your arms slowly overhead and touch the floor.**

3. **As you exhale, draw your right knee toward your chest, lift your head off the floor, and then grasp your right knee with your hands.**

   Keep your hips on the floor. Bring your head as close to your knee as possible, but don't force it. Figure 10-5 shows you what this position looks like.

Book II

Basic Yoga Techniques and Postures

Figure 10-5:
The dynamic head-to-knee.

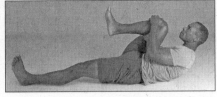

Photograph by Adam Latham

4. **As you inhale, release your knee and return your head, arms, and straightened right leg to the floor as they are in Step 2.**

5. **Repeat Steps 2 through 4 six to eight times on each side, alternating right and left.**

To make the sequence a little easier, keep your head on the floor in Step 3.

Standing warm-up postures

The standing postures are probably the most versatile of all the groups. Use them for warm-up/preparation, for compensation, or as main postures. As a warm-up, use standing postures when you also plan to perform the next part of your routine from a standing position.

Standing arm raise

You can perform this versatile warm-up (see Figure 10-1e) almost anywhere you want to enjoy a complete break from sitting.

1. **Stand tall but relaxed, with your feet at hip width.**

2. **Hang your arms at your sides, with your palms facing in; look straight ahead.**

3. **As you inhale, raise your arms forward and then up overhead.**

4. **As you exhale, bring your arms down and back to your sides.**

5. **Repeat Steps 3 and 4 six to eight times.**

The head-turner

Sequences like the head-turner combine breath and movement in parts of the upper body to stretch, strengthen, and heal your entire wingspan. This breath and movement sequence for the upper back and neck is great for minor stiff necks.

1. **Stand tall but relaxed, with your feet at hip width.**

2. **Hang your arms at your sides, with your palms turned back; look straight ahead.**

3. **As you inhale, raise your right arm forward and overhead as you turn your head to the left, as Figure 10-6 illustrates.**

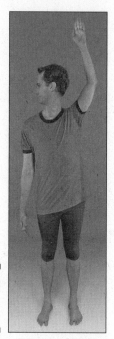

Figure 10-6:
The head-
turner.

Photograph by Adam Latham

4. **As you exhale, bring your arm down and turn your head forward.**

5. **As you inhale, raise your left arm forward and overhead while turning your head to the right.**

6. **Repeat Steps 3 through 5 six to eight times on each side, alternating right and left.**

Shoulder rolls

Shoulder rolls crop up in many types of exercise routines. When you do them in yoga, you move slowly and with awareness, coordinating with the breath.

1. **Stand tall but relaxed, with your feet at hip width.**

2. **Hang your arms at your sides, with your palms turned back; look straight ahead.**

3. **As you inhale, roll your shoulders up and back, as in Figure 10-7; as you exhale, drop your shoulders.**

4. **Repeat Step 3 six to eight times, reversing the direction of the rolls.**

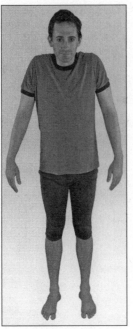

Figure 10-7:
Move
slowly in the
shoulder
rolls,
coordinating
breath and
movement.

Photograph by Adam Latham

Dynamic standing forward bend

As with many other warm-ups, you can also use this exercise for compensation.

1. **Stand tall but relaxed, with your feet at hip width.**

2. **Hang your arms at your sides, with your palms turned back.**

3. **As you inhale, raise your arms forward and overhead (see Figure 10-8a).**

4. **As you exhale, bend forward; when you feel a pull in the back of your legs, bend your legs and arms slightly (see Figure 10-8b).**

   This position is called Forgiving Limbs, covered in Book I, Chapter 3.

5. **As you inhale, roll up slowly, stacking the bones of your spine one at a time from bottom to top; then raise your arms overhead and, finally, release your arms back to your sides.**

6. **Repeat Steps 3 through 5 six to eight times.**

Rolling up is the safest way to come up in Step 5. If you don't have back problems, you may want to try two more advanced techniques after a few weeks: As you come up, sweep your arms out and up from the sides like wings, then overhead. Alternately, as you inhale, extend your slightly bent arms forward and up until they're parallel with your ears. Then raise your upper back, your midback, and then your lower back until you're all the way up and your arms are overhead.

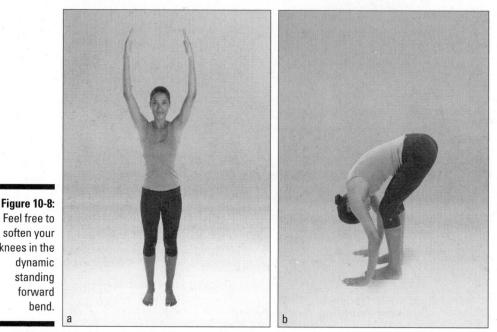

Figure 10-8: Feel free to soften your knees in the dynamic standing forward bend.

Photographs by Adam Latham

Seated warm-up postures

You can do an entire routine from a seated position, including forward bends, back bends, side bends, and twists. This section shows you how to prepare for main postures from a seated position. (***Note:*** Most of the postures here utilize the easy posture, *sukhasana.* Check out that discussion in Book II, Chapter 2.)

Seated fold

The seated fold is a simple way to warm up your back for forward bends or to compensate after seated twists.

1. **Sit on the floor with your legs crossed in the easy posture, and place your hands on the floor in front of you, with your palms down (refer to Figure 10-1b for a visual).**

2. **As you exhale, slide your hands out along the floor and bend forward at the hips.**

   If possible, bring your head down to the floor; otherwise, just come as close as you comfortably can.

3. **As you inhale, roll your torso and head up and return to the starting position in Step 1.**

4. **Repeat Steps 2 and 3 four to six times; then switch your legs and repeat four to six times.**

If you have a disc-related back problem, exercise caution with forward bends.

Rock the baby

This series prepares you for advanced sitting postures and forward bends.

1. **Sit on the floor, with your legs stretched out in front of you.**

   Press your hands on the floor behind you for support.

2. **Shake out your legs.**

3. **Bend your right knee and place your right foot just above your left knee, with your right ankle to the outside of the left knee (see Figure 10-9a).**

4. **Stabilize your right foot with your left hand and your right knee with your right hand; swing your right knee up and down six to eight times by gently pressing and then releasing your inner right thigh.**

5. **Carefully lift your right foot, and cradle it in the crook of your left elbow or support it with your left hand; cradle your right knee in the crook of your right elbow or cradle it with your right hand and, if you can, interlock your fingers (see Figure 10-9b).**

6. **Lift your spine and rock your right leg gently side to side six to eight times.**

7. **Repeat Steps 1 through 6 with your left leg.**

8. **Shake out your legs to finish.**

If you can't do this sequence without pain, don't try the more advanced seated postures in Book II, Chapter 2. Moreover, avoid the rock the baby sequence if you have knee or hip problems.

Book II

Basic Yoga Techniques and Postures

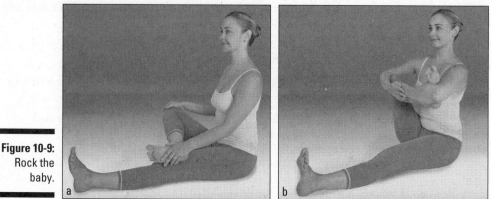

Figure 10-9:
Rock the
baby.

Photographs by Adam Latham

Selecting Your Compensation Poses

The main postures are the standard *asanas* you find featured in the classical yoga texts and modern manuals. These *asanas* are the stars of your routine, requiring you to work a little harder. Chapters 2 through 9 of Book II describe many of the main postures recommended for beginners. Interspersed among the main postures of a routine are *compensation postures.* These postures allow your body to come back into balance after each main posture and prevent discomfort and injury.

Figure 10-10 shows you some examples of compensation poses. Whichever *asanas* you select, remember to match them with your specific goals.

Whenever possible, a warm-up posture precedes and a compensation posture follows each category of main postures. Some basic guidelines are useful with compensation postures:

✔ Use one or two simple compensation postures to neutralize tension you feel in any area of the body after a yoga posture or sequence.

✔ Always use the conscious breathing described in Book II, Chapter 1.

✔ Perform compensating postures that are simpler or less difficult than the main posture right after the main posture. Do them dynamically.

✔ Don't follow a strenuous posture with another strenuous posture in the opposite direction. Some yoga instructors teach the fish posture as compensating for the shoulder stand. However, this combination can cause problems, especially for beginners, so opt for the less strenuous cobra posture instead.

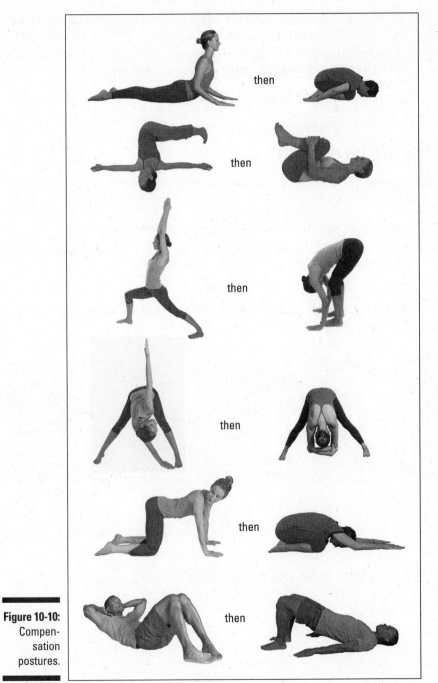

then

then

then

then

then

then

Book II

Basic Yoga Techniques and Postures

Figure 10-10: Compensation postures.

Photographs by Adam Latham

✔ Use compensation postures even when you feel no immediate need for them, especially after deep back bends, twists, and inverted postures.

✔ Rest after strenuous postures, such as inverted postures or deep back bends, before beginning the compensation postures.

Following are some great compensation postures.

The dynamic cat

The dynamic cat is a nice compensation posture for twists, but you can also use it as a warm-up.

1. **Starting on your hands and knees, look straight ahead.**

2. **Place your knees at hip width, with your hands below your shoulders (see Figure 10-11a).**

   Straighten but don't lock your elbows.

3. **As you exhale, sit back on your heels and look at the floor (see Figure 10-11b).**

Figure 10-11:
Dynamic
cat.

 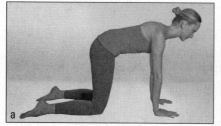 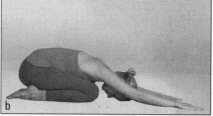

Photographs by Adam Latham

4. **As you inhale, slowly return to the starting position in Step 1.**

   Again, look straight ahead.

5. **Repeat Steps 3 and 4 six to eight times.**

Dynamic knees-to-chest

You can find many variations of knees-to-chest (including the regular version later in this chapter), but this variation is especially good after back bends.

1. **Lie on your back, and bend your knees toward your chest.**

2. **Hold your legs just below your knees, with one hand on each leg (see Figure 10-12a).**

   If you have any knee problems, be sure to hold the backs of your thighs.

3. **As you exhale, draw your knees toward your chest (see Figure 10-12b).**

Book II

Basic Yoga Techniques and Postures

Figure 10-12: Dynamic knees-to-chest.

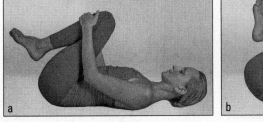 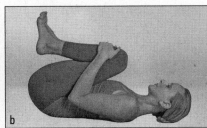

Photographs by Adam Latham

4. **As you inhale, move your knees away from your chest.**

5. **Repeat Steps 3 and 4 six to eight times.**

Thunderbolt posture: Vajrasana

This exercise is useful for compensation or warm-up. *Vajra* (pronounced vahj-rah) means both "diamond/adamantine" and "thunderbolt."

1. **Kneel on the floor, with your knees and feet at hip width.**

2. **Sit back on your heels, and bring your back up nice and tall. Hang your arms close to your sides.**

3. **As you inhale, lift your hips up and sweep your arms up over your head (see Figure 10-13a); lean back and look up.**

4. **As you exhale, sit on your heels again, fold your chest to your thighs, and bring your arms behind your back (see Figure 10-13b).**

   Get into a nice flow: Inhale when you open, exhale when you fold.

5. **Repeat Steps 3 and 4 six to eight times.**

WARNING!

Don't perform the thunderbolt if you have knee problems.

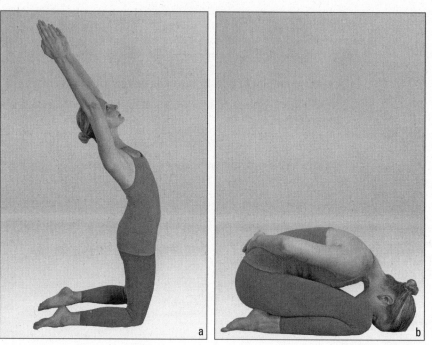

Photographs by Adam Latham

Figure 10-13: The thunderbolt posture.

Mastering Rest Postures

The two best indicators of your need to rest are your breath and your energy level. Monitor yours throughout the session: If your breath is loud and uneven, rest. If you feel a little tired after a posture, rest. No formula can prescribe how long you need to rest. Simply rest as needed until you're ready for the next posture. Don't cheat yourself out of well-deserved rest periods between the postures and at the end of a session.

Figure 10-14 shows you some recommended rest postures; read on for descriptions of each of these postures.

Stay in any rest posture for 6 to 12 breaths or as long as you take to feel rested, which may depend on how much time you have and where you are in the sequence of the routine. Yoga must never feel like you're in a hurry.

> ✔ **Corpse posture (shavasana):** The word *shava* (pronounced shah-vah) means "corpse," and *asana* means "posture." Refer to Figure 10-14a and Book VII, Chapter 2 for a full description of the posture.

Book II

Basic Yoga
Techniques
and
Postures

Figure 10-14:
You can
rest in many
different
positions.

Photographs by Adam Latham

- **Shavasana variation with bent legs:** Follow the steps for *shavasana* in Book VII, Chapter 2, but keep your knees bent, with your feet on the floor at hip width, as in Figure 10-14b.

  If your back is uncomfortable, place a pillow or blanket roll under your knees. If your neck or throat is tense, place a folded blanket or small pillow under your head.

✔ **Easy posture (sukhasana):** The word *sukha* means "easy" or "pleasant" — indeed, this posture is as its name suggests. You can keep your eyes open or closed in this posture. Check out Figure 10-14c and Book II, Chapter 2 for more details.

✔ **Mountain posture (tadasana):** The Sanskrit word *tada* (pronounced tah-dah) actually means "palm tree"; hence, this exercise is also called the palm tree posture. Check out 10-14d and Book II, Chapter 3 for details on this posture.

✔ **Child's posture (balasana):** The Sanskrit word *bala* (pronounced bah-lah) means "child." This classic version of the child's posture is a nurturing pose.

1. **Start on your hands and knees.**

2. **Place your knees about hip width, with your hands just below your shoulders.**

   Keep your elbows straight but not locked.

3. **As you exhale, sit back on your heels; rest your torso on your thighs and your forehead on the floor.**

4. **Lay your arms on the floor beside your torso, with your palms up, as in Figure 10-14e.**

5. **Close your eyes and breathe easily.**

✔ **Child's posture with arms in front:** This variation of the child's posture gives you more stretch in your upper back. Follow the steps for the child's posture in the preceding list item, but extend your arms forward at Step 4, spreading your palms on the floor, as Figure 10-14f illustrates.

✔ **Knees-to-chest posture (apanasana):** The Sanskrit word *apana* (pronounced ah-pah-nah) refers to the downward-going life force or exhalation. In this posture, you lie on your back and bend your knees in toward your chest, holding your shins just below the knees, as in Figure 10-14g. If you have any knee problems, hold the backs of your thighs instead.

Book III
Yoga for Life

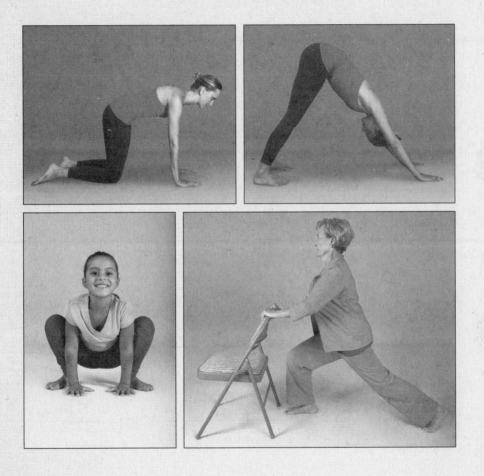

Contents at a Glance

Chapter 1

A Recommended Beginners' Routine for Men and Women

In This Chapter

▶ Keeping current on basic yoga principles

▶ Presenting a basic yoga routine for beginners

*T*he yoga routine in this chapter is a tried-and-true sequence from Larry Payne's Prime of Life Yoga and is an excellent way for a beginner to get started. Taught around the world, this routine is safe and doable and includes segments that reduce stress and increase strength, flexibility, and overall pep and vitality. To see someone do an abbreviated sequence of this beginning-level routine, go to www.dummies.com/go/yogaaiofd.

The short *asana* routine in this chapter takes only about 15 to 20 minutes — an optimum length for jump-starting your yoga practice. If you practice this routine three to six times per week, you'll notice improvements in your flexibility, muscle tone and strength, and concentration. You'll likely notice a number of other benefits as well, such as better stamina, digestion, and sleep.

When practicing the postures described in this chapter, keep these points in mind:

✔ **If this is your first yoga experience — you may have turned directly to this chapter — take a quick peek at Book I.** The chapters there introduce some basic yoga principles that help you get the most benefit from your yoga practice.

✔ **Move slowly into and out of the postures.** Never rush your yoga session. Remember that coming into a posture and moving out of a posture are integral parts of the posture itself.

✔ **Use yogic breathing throughout the routine, and pause briefly after each inhalation and exhalation.** Book II, Chapter 1 gives you more info on yogic breathing.

✔ **Move smoothly into and out of a posture several times before holding the posture.** Doing so prepares your body for a deeper stretch and helps you concentrate on linking the body, breath, and mind.

✔ **Don't change the order of the sequence and just randomly pick the postures you want.** All the routines have a special order or sequence, to give you the maximum benefits. (For details on why sequencing is important, see Book II, Chapter 10.)

Trying out a Fun Beginner Routine

As you perform the postures in this short routine, notice how you start by giving your body and mind a chance to transition from your previous activity, how you move your body in several different directions, and how you end the routine with rest. These activities are some of the fundamental elements of a well-balanced yoga routine, regardless of its length. Use focus breathing (which is covered in Book II, Chapter 1) throughout the routine.

Corpse posture

1. **Lie flat on your back, with your arms relaxed along the sides of your torso, your palms up, and your feet open out toward the sides of the room (see Figure 1-1).**

2. **Inhale and exhale through your nose slowly for 8 to 10 breaths.**

   Pause briefly after each inhalation and exhalation.

Figure 1-1:
Corpse
posture.

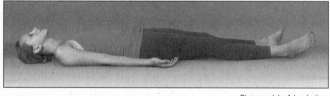

Photograph by Adam Latham

Lying arm raise

1. **Lie in the corpse posture (see the preceding section), with your arms relaxed at your sides and your palms down (see Figure 1-2a).**

2. **As you inhale, slowly raise your arms overhead and touch the floor behind you, as in Figure 1-2b; pause briefly.**

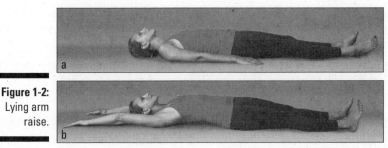

Figure 1-2:
Lying arm
raise.

Photographs by Adam Latham

3. **As you exhale, bring your arms back to your sides, as in Step 1.**

4. **Repeat Steps 2 and 3 six to eight times.**

Knees-to-chest posture

1. **Lie on your back with your knees bent and your feet flat on the floor.**

2. **As you exhale, bring your right knee into your chest and extend your left leg down; hold your shin just below your knee (see Figure 1-3).**

   If you have knee problems, hold the back of your thigh instead.

3. **Stay in Step 2 for 6 to 8 breaths, and then repeat on the left side.**

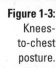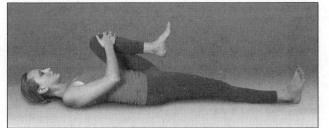

Figure 1-3:
Knees-
to-chest
posture.

Photograph by Adam Latham

Downward-facing dog

1. **Beginning on your hands and knees, place your hands directly under your shoulders, with your palms spread on the floor and your knees directly under your hips.**

   Straighten your arms, but don't lock your elbows. Figure 1-4a shows an example.

2. **As you exhale, lift and straighten (but don't lock) your knees; as your hips lift, bring your head down to a neutral position so that your ears are between your arms (see Figure 1-4b).**

   If possible, press your heels to the floor and your head toward your feet (stop if doing so strains your neck).

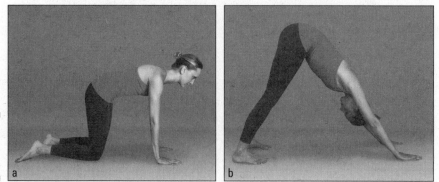

Figure 1-4: Downward-facing dog.

Photographs by Adam Latham

3. **As you inhale, come back down to your hands and knees, as in Step 1.**

4. **Repeat Steps 1 through 3 three times, and then stay in Step 2 for 6 to 8 breaths.**

Child's posture

1. **Starting on your hands and knees, place your knees about hip width apart, with your hands just below your shoulders.**

   Keep your elbows straight but not locked.

2. **As you exhale, sit back on your heels; rest your torso on your thighs and your forehead on the floor.**

   You don't have to sit all the way back.

3. **Lay your arms back on the floor beside your torso, with your palms up, or reach your relaxed arms forward, with your palms on the floor.**

4. **Close your eyes and stay in the folded position for 6 to 8 breaths (see Figure 1-5).**

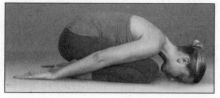

Figure 1-5:
Child's
posture.

Photograph by Adam Latham

Warrior 1

1. **Stand in the mountain posture (see Book II, Chapter 3 for this pose). Turn your left foot out to about 45 degrees, and raise your right arm out in front of your right shoulder. Take a big step forward (about 3 to 3½ feet, or the length of your arm) with your right foot as you exhale.**

   To watch a video of how to prepare for and move into the warrior pose, go to www.dummies.com/go/yogaaiofd.

2. **Place your hands on the top of your hips, and square the front of your pelvis; release your hands and hang your arms.**

3. **As you inhale, raise your arms forward and overhead, and bend your right knee to a right angle so that it's directly over your ankle and, ideally, your thigh is parallel to the floor (see Figure 1-6).**

Book III

Yoga for Life

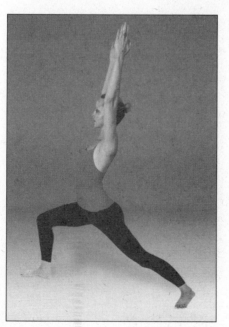

Figure 1-6:
Warrior I.

Photograph by Adam Latham

4. **Soften your arms (see Book I, Chapter 3 for a description of Forgiving Limbs) and face your palms toward each other; look straight ahead.**

   If your lower back is uncomfortable, lean your torso slightly over the forward leg until your back releases any tension that may be present.

5. **Repeat Steps 3 and 4 three times, and then hold once on the right side for 6 to 8 breaths.**

6. **Repeat Steps 1 through 5 on the other (left) side.**

Standing forward bend

1. **Start in the mountain posture (refer to Book II, Chapter 3), and raise your arms forward and then up overhead as you inhale (see Figure 1-7a).**

2. **As you exhale, bend forward from the hips; when you feel a pull in the back of your legs, soften your knees (see Book I, Chapter 3 for more on Forgiving Limbs) and hang your arms as in Figure 1-7b, and relax your head and neck downward.**

   If your head isn't close to your knees, bend your knees more. If you have the flexibility, straighten your knees while keeping them soft.

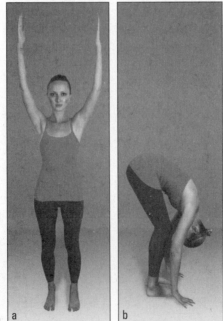

Figure 1-7:
Standing
forward
bend.

a

b

Photographs by Adam Latham

3. **Exhaling, roll your body up like a rag doll, stacking your vertebrae one at a time.**

   Flip to Book II, Chapter 4 for more advanced ways to come up from a forward bend.

4. **Repeat Steps 1 through 3 three times, and then stay down in Step 2 for 6 to 8 breaths.**

Reverse triangle posture variation

1. **Stand in the mountain posture (check out Book II, Chapter 3 for a description), and step out to the right about 3 to 3½ feet (or the length of one leg) with your right foot as you exhale.**

2. **As you inhale, raise your arms out to the sides, parallel to the line of your shoulders (and the floor), so that your shoulders form a *T* with your torso (see Figure 1-8a).**

3. **As you exhale, bend forward from your hips and place your right hand on the floor near the inside of your left foot.**

4. **Raise your left arm toward the ceiling and look up at your left hand (see Figure 1-8b).**

   Soften your knees and arms. Bend your left knee or, if you experience strain or discomfort, move your right hand away from your left foot and more directly under your torso.

Book III

Yoga for Life

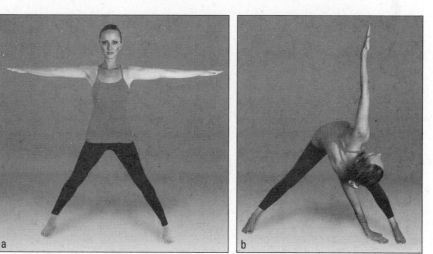

Figure 1-8:
Reverse triangle posture.

Photographs by Adam Latham

5. **Repeat Steps 2 through 4 on the same side three times, and then stay down in Step 4 for 6 to 8 breaths.**

6. **Repeat Steps 1 through 5 on the right side.**

You can strengthen or strain your neck in this posture, so turn your neck down if you're uncomfortable.

Standing wide-legged forward bend

1. **Stand in the mountain posture (see Book II, Chapter 3), and step out to the right about 3 to 3½ feet (or the length of one leg) with your right foot as you exhale.**

2. **As you inhale, raise your arms out to the sides, parallel to the line of your shoulders (and the floor), so that your shoulders form a *T* with your torso (see Figure 1-9a).**

3. **As you exhale, bend forward from the hips and soften your knees.**

4. **Hold your bent elbows with the opposite-side hands, and hang your torso and arms (see Figure 1-9b).**

5. **Stay folded in this posture for 6 to 8 breaths.**

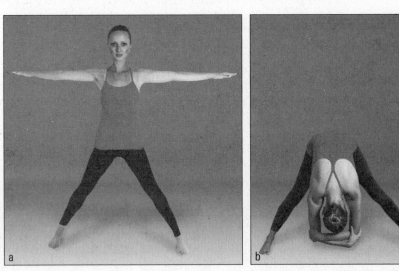

Figure 1-9:
Standing wide-legged forward bend.

Photographs by Adam Latham

The karate kid

1. **Stand in the mountain posture (see Book II, Chapter 3), and raise your arms out to the sides, parallel to the line of your shoulders (and the floor), so that your shoulders form a *T* with your torso as you inhale.**

2. **Steady yourself and focus on a spot on the floor 10 to 12 feet in front of you.**

3. **As you exhale, bend and raise your left knee toward your chest, keeping your right leg straight (see Figure 1-10); hold for 6 to 8 breaths.**

4. **Repeat Steps 1 through 3 with your legs reversed.**

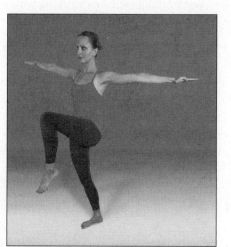

Figure 1-10:
The karate
kid.

Photograph by Adam Latham

When you become stable in the karate kid posture, try extending your bent left leg forward and up. Gradually work toward fully extending your left leg parallel to the floor — take your time! Try this added step on both sides.

Corpse posture redux

Repeat the corpse posture exercise as the earlier section "Corpse posture" describes (see Figure 1-1 for an illustration). Stay in this posture for 8 to 12 breaths, or choose one of the relaxation techniques in Book VII, Chapter 2.

Book III

Yoga for Life

Reaching beyond the Beginning

When you become comfortable with the beginners' routine in this chapter, you can expand it and add variety. If you're young and fit, you may want to try the routines in Book III, Chapter 2. If you're midlife or older, or if you haven't exercised for a while, Book III, Chapter 3 provides less strenuous (but equally beneficial) routines.

Of course, with a taste of Hatha Yoga, you may want to take private lessons or go to a group class for feedback, to boost your morale, or simply to practice — with new confidence — in the company of others.

Practicing on your own is fine, but nothing replaces working with a teacher. Before you get into too much of a yoga groove, ask a yoga teacher to check for any bad postural habits and, if you like, to give you some suggestions for taking the next step. Book I, Chapter 3 has advice on finding a yoga class.

Chapter 2

Yoga for Kids and Teens

Young people have a natural affinity for yoga. You can introduce even the youngest children to yoga through play. As the names of common yoga postures reveal, the postures were inspired by animals — the cat, the cow, the dog, the bear, and so on. The focused coordination of movement and breath that makes these movements yoga and not just physical exercise easily lends itself to child's play. When you combine these elements with play — for example, imitation of animal sounds, a magic box of plush animal toys, balls of various sizes — you have the beginnings of kid-friendly yoga.

For teens, yoga offers tools to cultivate health in body, mind, and spirit. It provides a noncompetitive way for young people to develop strength and confidence and to manage stress — a plague of the times.

This chapter offers pointers, sample postures, and kid-friendly ways for parents or caregivers to introduce yoga to children. Teens and adults with energy to spare also get a guide to a classical routine that challenges the body while focusing the mind.

Making Yoga Fun for Youngsters

The sense of calm, focus, and balance that draws adults to the practice of yoga is also available to children, even ones as young as 3, as long as you introduce them to it in a playful, child-friendly fashion. When guided with a developmentally appropriate approach, preschoolers and the primary school set alike can reap yoga's numerous benefits, such as improved concentration skills, an ability to calm and center themselves, and greater self-esteem and self-confidence. The following sections give you some tips on engaging your child in yoga, as well as several poses to try.

Approaching poses in a child-friendly way

Child's play, when slowed and joined with consciousness, can provide a platform for kid-friendly yoga practice. As you introduce your child to yoga, keep these pointers in mind:

- ✔ **Make it fun.** Yoga postures (originally derived from and often named for animals) and concepts lend themselves to play in a variety of ways. For example, you can have your child vocalize a posture's animal's call to draw attention to the breath, and you can incorporate balance into any number of children's games that involve running and stopping at a specified moment by directing your child to be still and balance on one leg after stopping.

- ✔ **Shorter is better than longer.** Short, happy practice sessions that your child wants to come back to are better than a longer session that loses her attention.

- ✔ **Be willing to adjust the yoga session to your child's mood.** A tired child may enjoy sitting poses. Cooling breathing exercises help a cranky child calm down. On a rainy day, active poses bring physical release of pent-up energy.

- ✔ **No matter how short your child's yoga session, be sure to include a period of final relaxation, or *shavasana*.** Shavasana allows a child to relax her body without forcing it. It can be as simple as counting 5 breaths.

- ✔ **Find a special spot to practice yoga with your child.** Does he gravitate to a certain spot in your home for play? That area may be the perfect place to begin to share your love of yoga.

Finding yoga postures kids love

The postures in the following sections were designed to be kid-friendly, and the accompanying text is intended to be parent-friendly to help you guide your child. You can find more detail about each of the postures in the chapters in Book II.

When done in sequence, this set of postures forms a well-balanced routine. In addition to providing you with instructions to give your child as he gets into the posture, the sections suggest sounds he can make while in the pose. The sounds serve a dual purpose: They inspire your child's imagination while he's holding the pose (keeping him engaged) and also guide him to breathe rather than hold his breath. But if your child is reluctant to make the animal sounds, don't try to force it.

Children need to skip the headstand and shoulder stand. Although their bodies are flexible, they lack the strength and stability to do those postures safely.

Note: In these sections, you see references to *yummy poses*. The term *yummy pose* is just a kid-friendly description of a resting pose, in which you allow your body and mind to release. Afi Kobari, a specialist in yoga for children, coined the phrase.

Children have short attention spans. You know your child best, so do only as many postures as he has attention for. In time, he'll be able to do more. Also, ask your child to hold the position only as long as you feel she will be comfortable. If she starts to get squirmy, have her come out of the position.

The mountain posture

Figure 2-1 gives you and your child a visual of this kiddie posture; flip to Book II, Chapter 3 for more info on the adult version. Give your child the following instructions:

1. **Stand tall like a mountain.**

2. **Breathe through your nose, and imagine you're in a very, very quiet place.**

Book III

Yoga for Life

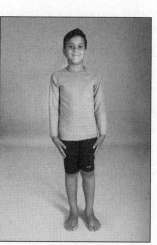

Figure 2-1: The mountain posture for kids.

Photograph by Adam Latham

Warrior I

See the preceding section for instructions to get your child into mountain posture. Figure 2-2 and Book II, Chapter 3 give you more guidance on warrior I. You can also find general information about preparing for and moving into the warrior pose in at www.dummies.com/go/yogaaiofd.

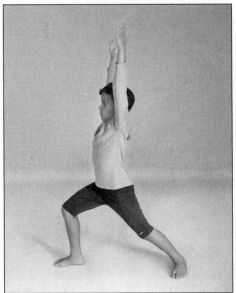

Figure 2-2:
Warrior I for
kids.

Photograph by Adam Latham

1. **Start in the mountain posture, and take a big step forward with one leg.**

   If your child's knee bends so much that you see it extending farther than the ankle, tell him to bend the knee a little bit less.

2. **Bend your front knee and raise your arms overhead by your ears.**

3. **Feel how powerful and strong you are in this posture; next time, as you bend your knee and raise your arms, say, "Yes! I can!"**

4. **Keeping your knee bent and your arms raised, stay in this position and really feel like a warrior.**

5. **Try the same movements on the other side.**

Bear posture

Check out Figure 2-3 and the following instructions to direct your child into bear posture.

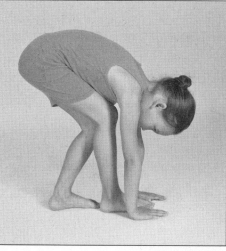

Figure 2-3:
Bear
posture for
kids.

Photograph by Adam Latham

1. **Start in the mountain posture, and then bend forward and hang down.**

2. **Staying bent, walk around, dragging your arms and hands as you growl and imagine you're a bear.**

Cat and cow

The following directions help you walk your child through cat and cow; kids usually have a lot fun with this sequence, especially when you do it with them.

1. **Get down on your hands and knees as if you're going to crawl, but stay in one place.**

2. **Make your back round so you can look down and back at your legs (see Figure 2-4a).**

3. **Imagine you're a cat, and make the sound of a cat: meow.**

4. **Move your back so that your belly goes down toward the floor, your chest goes up, and you look ahead.**

   Show your child Figure 2-4b for help in visualizing this step.

5. **Imagine you're a cow, and make the sound of a cow: mooo, mooo.**

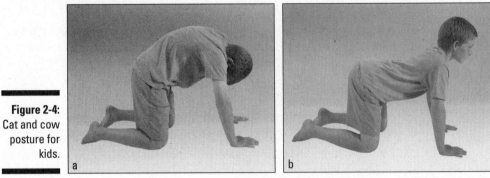

Figure 2-4:
Cat and cow
posture for
kids.

a   b

Photographs by Adam Latham

Jumping frog

Use these instructions to lead your tot through jumping frog.

1. Stand with your feet wide apart, and squat low (see Figure 2-5).

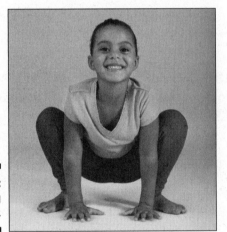

Figure 2-5:
Jumping
frog for kids.

Photograph by Adam Latham

2. Place your hands on the ground, and then jump and raise your arms.

3. Imagine you're a frog, and make the sound of a frog: ribbit, ribbit.

Tree posture

Work your child through tree posture by using the following instructions, and check out Figure 2-6 for an illustration. Flip to Book II, Chapter 3 for more information on the adult version.

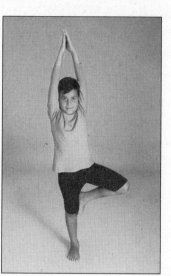

Figure 2-6:
Tree
posture for
kids.

Photograph by Adam Latham

Book III

Yoga for Life

1. **Start in the mountain posture, standing tall and still.**

2. **Bend one of your legs, and place the bottom of that foot high on the inside of your other thigh.**

3. **Bring your hands together high above your head, and imagine that you're a tree as you make the sound of the wind blowing through your leaves: shhhhhhhh.**

4. **Now try the same movements on the other side.**

PLAY THIS!

Cobra II

Book II, Chapter 7 gives you more information on the adult version of cobra II, as does the video at www.dummies.com/go/yogaaiofd; the following instructions and Figure 2-7 help you lead your child through this version.

1. **Lie flat on your belly, and place your hands on the floor near your armpits, with your fingers going forward.**

2. **Raise your head, shoulders, and back as you press down on your hands, keeping your hips on the ground.**

3. **Imagine that you're a cobra, and make the cobra's sound: sssssss.**

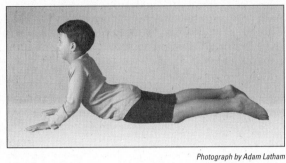

Figure 2-7:
Cobra II for
kids.

Photograph by Adam Latham

Lion posture

With the help of these instructions and Figure 2-8, your youngster can take pride in the lion posture. Book II, Chapter 2 provides additional information on the adult version.

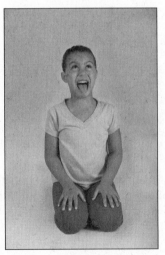

Figure 2-8:
Lion posture
for kids.

Photograph by Adam Latham

1. **Sit on your heels, and place your hands on your knees.**

2. **Open your mouth wide, stick your tongue way out, and roll your eyes upward as though you're trying to see something high above you.**

3. **Imagine you're a mighty lion, and roar: ahhaahh!**

Downward-facing dog

You can find the adult version of this posture in Book II, Chapter 3, but the following steps and Figure 2-9 lay out a child-friendly variety.

1. **Start on your hands and knees.**

2. **Press through your arms, pushing down on your hands; straighten your legs and look down.**

3. **Imagine that you're a dog, and bark: woof, woof.**

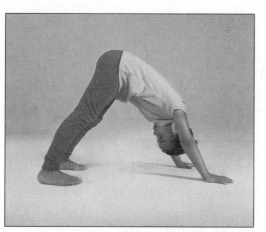

Figure 2-9:
Downward-facing dog for kids.

Photograph by Adam Latham

Child's posture

This pose (one of the yummy poses) even has *child* in the name! Use the following instructions and Figure 2-10 to guide your tyke through the child's posture.

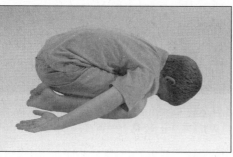

Figure 2-10:
Child's posture for kids.

Photograph by Adam Latham

1. Kneel on the ground and fold up like a ball.

2. Place your hands at your sides, with your palms up.

3. Relax and think good thoughts.

The bridge

Figure 2-11 illustrates this easy posture. Give your child the following instructions to help him through the pose, and check out Book III, Chapter 1 for the adult bridge.

Figure 2-11:
Bridge for
kids.

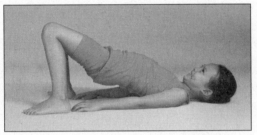

Photograph by Adam Latham

1. Lie on your back, bending your knees and letting your feet be firm on the ground.

2. Place your arms at your sides, with your palms down.

3. Raise your hips and become a bridge.

4. Imagine that you're a bridge, and make the sound of the cars traveling over you: chuga chuga chuga.

The wheel

The following directions and Figure 2-12 help your child get rolling with the wheel posture.

This advanced posture requires a fair amount of strength and flexibility. If your child isn't ready for it, come back to it when he's stronger and more flexible.

1. Lie on your back with your knees bent and your feet on the ground.

2. Place your arms over your head, and turn your hands so that they're flat and your fingers are facing back toward the top of your shoulders.

3. Press up into the wheel.

4. Smile from the inside out.

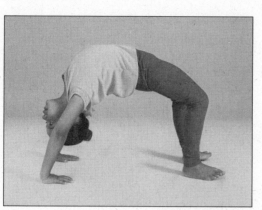

Figure 2-12:
Wheel for
kids.

Photograph by Adam Latham

Knee-hugger

Knee-hugger is another of the yummy poses. These steps and Figure 2-13 show you how to help your child do it. You can find the adult version in Book III, Chapter 1 (there it's called knees-to-chest posture).

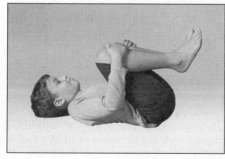

Figure 2-13:
Knee-
hugger for
kids.

Photograph by Adam Latham

For an added benefit, have your child rock his knees from side to side while he's hugging them — it gently massages the back.

1. **Lie on your back, and then bend and hug your knees.**

2. **Just relax and think good thoughts.**

Easy posture

These instructions help you walk (sit?) your young yogini through the easy posture; check out Figure 2-14 for the proper sitting posture. (The adult version is covered in Book II, Chapter 2.)

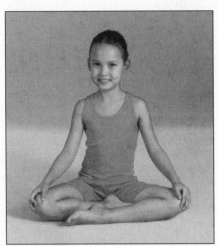

Figure 2-14: Easy posture for kids.

Photograph by Adam Latham

Your child may be more comfortable with a blanket under her hips.

1. **Sit on the floor and cross your legs comfortably.**

2. **Keep your back and head tall, without straining.**

3. **Imagine a big balloon in your belly: When you breathe in, fill the balloon, and when you breathe out, let the air out of the balloon.**

The big yummy posture: Shavasana

Use the following instructions to help your child relax at the end of the session. Figure 2-15 illustrates the pose, and you can read more about the adult version in Book VII, Chapter 2.

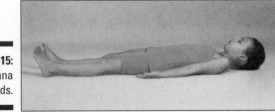

Figure 2-15: Shavasana for kids.

Photograph by Adam Latham

1. **Lie flat on your back, turning your palms up and letting your feet flop out.**

2. **Close your eyes gently, or keep them open and soft — whichever feels best.**

3. **Relax and think good thoughts.**

Easing the Transition into Adulthood: Yoga for Teens

Yoga practice in the teenage years is so much more than an exercise program. Yes, it provides an energy outlet and a way to build muscle and flexibility — both important in their own right. But yoga practice also provides an entry point for a healthful and balanced perspective on life and self that can remain for a lifetime. Here are some of the benefits yoga can offer teens:

- ✔ **The antidote to stress in an overscheduled life:** Yoga, a union of mind and body, can make weathering the demands of daily life easier. With regular practice, you may find that you have a greater ability to think for yourself and trust yourself — important at a time of life when peer pressure can feel overwhelming, when shifting hormone levels leave you feeling like a different person from day to day (or hour to hour!), and poor judgment and bad decisions can impact your health, your well-being, and your future.

- ✔ **A way to develop a lifelong friendship with your body and more:** Yoga helps you tune in to your body; develop the focus, concentration, and discipline you need to study well and pursue your dreams; and become self-confident and courageous without competing.

- ✔ **A great way to become and stay fit:** Both the USDA and Health Canada rank having an adequate level of physical activity as a high health priority. At ChooseMyPlate.gov, the United States Department of Agriculture (USDA) puts physical activity on par with eating a balanced diet for a healthful life.

The routines in this section have been specifically designed for teens, and they're meant to be challenging. However, always keep in mind yoga's fundamental principle: "Do no harm." Trust your inner teacher. If your body says it's time to rest, rest (even if others are still in their poses). Trusting yourself in this way is an important step toward becoming a balanced adult.

Can yoga help you maintain a healthy weight?

According to Robert M. Sapolsky's *Why Zebras Don't Get Ulcers* (Henry Holt and Company), modern garden-variety stressors can lead to overeating — in particular, choosing the wrong kinds of food to overeat. Stress floods your body with hormones that affect your appetite. If the stress is intense but short-lived, most people usually experience a loss of appetite — the way you feel when you're too nervous to eat. But when you experience frequent on-and-off stress throughout the course of the day, day in and day out, the hormonal levels in the body increase appetite — and not for the healthy stuff. What helps? Engaging in regular exercise that you look forward to doing, meditating, and cultivating a self-accepting, nonperfectionist approach to life are a few practices that have been shown to help. How handy to be able to find all that in yoga!

When done carefully, these routines also work for men and women well into their 30s, but they're not recommended for the typical middle-aged person over 40. A lot of what group yoga classes across America (especially in health clubs) offer today was originally designed for lightweight teenage boys in India whose lifestyles involved a lot of squatting. Middle-aged beginners often jump into that kind of yoga in a competitive way and end up with injuries to show for it because it's just not built for them (or they for it). If you're middle-aged or older and just beginning yoga, check out Chapter 1 or Chapter 3 of Book III.

Headstands, shoulder stands, and the lotus position may look like the popular idea of yoga, but in fact, they can be dangerous. Young people are still growing and generally don't yet have the necessary musculature and stability to tackle these postures safely, so stay away from them for now.

Standing routine

This routine takes about 15 to 20 minutes. Before you begin, here are some general tips and instructions to keep in mind:

- ✔ Choose either focus or chest-to-belly breathing from Book II, Chapter 1.
- ✔ With the exception of the jumps, move slowly and stay in the moment.
- ✔ Stay and breathe in each posture for 8 to 10 breaths.
- ✔ Do the whole routine twice on both sides.
- ✔ Refer to Book II, Chapter 3 for detailed instruction on all the postures in this routine (although note that some postures here are variations on Chapter 3's postures).

When you're ready, follow these steps to complete the standing routine:

1. **Start in the mountain posture (see Figure 2-16a).**

   Initiate the yoga breathing style of your choice from the list earlier in this section.

2. **As you exhale, jump or step out into a wide stance with your arms in a *T* parallel to the floor, as in Figure 2-16b.**

3. **As you inhale, raise your arms from the sides and overhead as you rotate your feet and torso to the right (see Figure 2-16c).**

4. **As you exhale, sink into warrior I position, with your right knee bent in a 90-degree angle (as in Figure 2-16d).**

5. **As you inhale, rotate your shoulders to the left and drop your arms into a *T*, with your palms down, for the warrior II position; open your back (left) hip to the left as far as it can go, and tuck your tail under comfortably.**

   Figure 2-16e gives you a visual.

6. **As you exhale, rotate your shoulders to the right, and reach forward with your left arm and back with your right arm so they're parallel to the floor (as in Figure 2-16f), for the reverse triangle variation I.**

7. **Inhale and then, as you exhale, drop your left hand to the floor and bring your right arm straight up for the reverse triangle variation II; keep your right leg bent and rotate your head up to the right (see Figure 2-16g).**

   If your neck gets tired, turn your head down.

8. **As you exhale, roll down with your arms, trunk, and head; turn your feet forward and parallel, and then hang down the middle, holding your elbows for the standing wide-legged forward bend (see Figure 2-16h).**

9. **Roll your body up, and then jump or step back into the mountain posture in Step 1.**

10. **Repeat Steps 1 through 9 on the left side.**

Floor routine

Some people call this routine the Lifetime Sequence because getting into wide-legged seated forward bend postures takes a lifetime if you aren't naturally flexible in the hips. And if you happen to believe in reincarnation, you have the luxury of another lifetime to work on it.

Book III

Yoga for Life

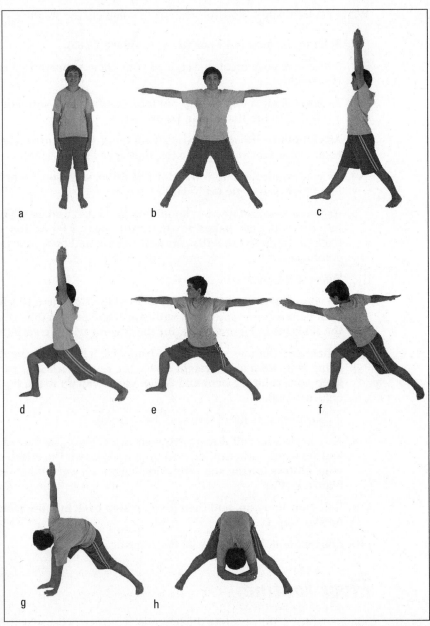

Figure 2-16:
Sequence
of poses for
the standing
routine for
teens.

Photographs by Adam Latham

This routine takes 20 to 25 minutes. Before you begin, here are some tips to keep in mind:

✔ Choose focus or chest-to-belly breathing from Book II, Chapter 1.

✔ Stay in each posture (including each time you raise your arms) for 6 to 8 breaths.

✔ Do the whole sequence twice.

✔ Feel free to soften your knees in all the forward bends.

✔ Challenge yourself, but don't strain yourself.

This routine isn't recommended for people with lower back problems aggravated by rounding.

When you're ready, follow these steps to complete the floor routine:

1. **Start with your arms in the air and with a straight back, as in Figure 2-17a.**

2. **As you exhale, bend forward and down to the seated forward bend pose in Figure 2-17b.**

3. **As you inhale, raise your trunk and arms to a straight back, and separate your legs wide, as in Figure 2-17c.**

4. **As you exhale, bend forward and down to a spread-legged forward bend, as Figure 2-17d illustrates.**

5. **As you inhale, raise your trunk and arms up to a straight back position, as you did in Step 3 (see Figure 2-17c).**

6. **As you exhale, rotate to the right, as in Figure 2-17e, and bend forward and down, as in Figure 2-17f.**

7. **As you inhale, raise your trunk and arms to a straight back position, as you did in Step 5 (see Figure 2-17c).**

8. **As you exhale, rotate to the left as in Figure 2-17g, and bend forward and down (see Figure 2-17h).**

9. **As you inhale, raise your trunk and arms to a straight back position and bend your legs halfway, with your toes up (see Figure 2-17i).**

10. **As you exhale, bend forward and down, and try to move your toes down, as in Figure 2-17j.**

11. **As you inhale, raise your trunk and arms to a straight back position, drop your knees to the sides, and join the soles of your feet together, as Figure 2-17k illustrates.**

12. **As you exhale, bend forward and down and hold your feet (see Figure 2-17l).**

Book III

Yoga for Life

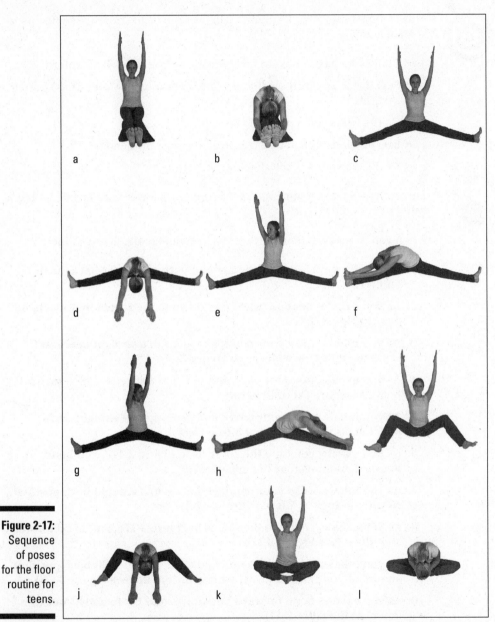

Figure 2-17:
Sequence
of poses
for the floor
routine for
teens.

If you have back problems lifting up from the forward bends in this routine, try the roll-up: Keep your chin on your chest and roll up, stacking your vertebrae one at a time, with your arms hanging at your sides. When you're fully upright, bring your arms up and overhead from the front, and look forward.

Chapter 3

It's Never Too Late: Yoga for Midlifers and Older Adults

*I*f you're on the senior side of the life curve and you're considering taking up yoga, you're not alone. A 2012 *Yoga Journal* study reported that approximately a third of the 20.4 million adults in America who practice yoga are older than age 45.

This chapter presents safe yoga routines for people in their middle-aged and senior years. The Prime of Life Yoga discussion addresses folks who fall within the vast expanse of the middle years — generally between 40-something and 70-something. The "Cherishing the Chair" section addresses the needs of folks who are generally older than 70; however, people of any age can follow these routines.

Reaping the Benefits of Yoga through Midlife and Beyond

Midlife, as the word suggests, refers to the middle of life. It's not, as some people think, "The End," but rather a new beginning. Yoga helps you navigate the physical and emotional changes associated with midlife and allows you to age gracefully, healthfully, and actively. Consider these benefits:

 ✔ **Working through menopause:** Regular yoga practice can help alleviate the physiological side effects of menopause and help you cultivate a forgiving, accepting, and positive attitude important for your emotional well-being. Inversions (see Book II, Chapter 6), which have a profound effect on the glands and inner organs and (both literally and figuratively) allow you to view things from a new perspective, are especially helpful. For soothing rest and whole-person recovery, cultivate the corpse posture described in Book II, Chapter 10.

✔ **Navigating andropause:** Men experience something similar to menopause called *andropause*. When they see their vitality and hairline recede a little, men are often thrown into an existential crisis. Regular yoga practice can buffer the unpleasant physiological side effects of andropause and stabilize the emotions triggered during this period.

✔ **Promoting bone health:** With regular exercise, you can prevent the bone loss *(osteoporosis)* associated with midlife and old age.

Developing User-Friendly Routines for Midlifers

As you age, mobility is the new flexibility. So although you may have been able to do the most acrobatic postures in your youth, the important goal now is to maintain the mobility to remain fit and active. In the Prime of Life approach to yoga postures, spinal freedom and movement take precedence over form. Adjustments to the posture, such as bending the knees *a lot* if necessary, encourage movement of the spine. This section presents routines for two different skill levels, both of which are equally ideal for men and women.

The attitude you bring to your practice is critical. The right attitude on the mat allows you to practice postures safely and spills over to your life off the mat. For key yoga principles that ensure a safe and fulfilling practice, refer to Book I, Chapter 3.

Prime of Life Yoga routine: Level 1

This routine is a nice general-conditioning routine for midlifers and even younger folks who want to ease back into physical activity. This user-friendly sequence strings together a series of safe postures that work each side of the body separately, helping to achieve greater balance. This routine takes about 30 to 35 minutes. You can see an abbreviated version at www.dummies.com/go/yogaaiofd.

You can find detailed instructions for each of these poses or their variations in Chapters 3, 4, and 10 of Book II as well as Chapter 2 of Book VII. Choose a breathing technique from Book II, Chapter 1. Hold each posture and its variation for 6 to 8 breaths, with the exception of warrior I (Steps 2 and 3) and revolved triangle variation (Steps 9 and 10). For each of these postures, move into and out of the postures three times, and then hold for 6 to 8 breaths.

1. **Start in the mountain posture (see Figure 3-1a); initiate the yoga breathing style of your choice for 6 to 8 breaths (see Book II, Chapter 1).**

2. **As you exhale, step forward with the right foot about 3 to 3½ feet (or the length of one leg). Your left foot turns out naturally; turn it out more to increase stability. Place your hands on the tops of your hips, and square the front of your pelvis; release your hands and hang your arms (see Figure 3-1b).**

3. **As you inhale, raise your arms from the front up and overhead, and bend your right leg into a right angle for warrior I, as Figure 3-1c illustrates.**

4. **Repeat Steps 2 and 3 three times, and then stay in warrior I for 6 to 8 breaths.**

5. **As you exhale, bend both arms downward and draw your elbows back, as you turn your palms up and lift your chest (see Figure 3-1d); hold this proud warrior posture for 6 to 8 breaths.**

6. **As you inhale, keep your right leg bent, and join your palms together in front of you and bring them up and overhead as you look up and back (see Figure 3-1e); stay in the exalted warrior posture for 6 to 8 breaths.**

7. **As you exhale, come down over your bent right leg and place your hands on the floor for the standing asymmetrical forward bend (see Figure 3-1f); stay in the posture for 6 to 8 breaths.**

   Work on straightening your right leg based on your flexibility in the moment. A soft or bent leg is okay.

   If you want to feel the stretch more, square your hips by pulling your right hip back and putting your left hip forward. A more challenging option is to rotate the back foot inward, called *paralleling the feet*.

8. **As you inhale, roll your body up vertebra by vertebra, and then step your feet together back into the mountain posture from Step 1.**

9. **Repeat Steps 1 through 8 on the left side.**

10. **From the mountain posture, step out with your right foot about 3 to 3½ feet (or the length of one leg); as you exhale, bend forward from the hips, hang down, and place the palms of both hands on the floor directly below your shoulders, as in Figure 3-1g.**

11. **As you inhale, raise your right arm toward the ceiling and look up at your right hand for the reverse triangle variation, as Figure 3-1h illustrates.**

12. **Repeat Steps 10 and 11 three times, and then remain with your right arm up for 6 to 8 breaths; repeat on your left side.**

    Soften your knees and arms. Turn your head down if your neck gets sore.

13. **As you exhale, hang your torso, head, and arms down, holding your bent elbows with opposite-side hands for the standing spread-legged forward bend (see Figure 3-1i); stay for 6 to 8 breaths.**

14. **Transition to your hands and knees, and slide your right hand forward and your left leg back as you exhale, keeping your hand and your toes on the floor; as you inhale, raise your right arm and left leg to a comfortable height for the balancing cat posture (see Figure 3-1j).**

    Stay up for 4 to 8 breaths, and then repeat with opposite pairs, lifting your left hand and your right leg.

    If you want a bigger challenge in this posture, raise your bottom foot just off the floor.

15. **As you exhale, come back to all fours and fold down into the child's posture variation (with your arms in front of you), as in Figure 3-1k; hold for 6 to 8 breaths.**

16. **Lie flat on your back, with your arms along the sides of your torso, your palms up, and your eyes closed for the corpse posture, as in Figure 3-1l.**

17. **To finish, use belly breathing from Book II, Chapter 1 or a relaxation technique from Book VII, Chapter 2 for 3 to 5 minutes.**

Prime of Life Yoga routine: Level II

After you master the level I sequence in the preceding section, enjoy the challenge of this section's level II sequence. It's a little longer and more physically demanding. Like the other routine, it brings balance by working each side of the body separately.

Plan to spend approximately 45 minutes to complete this sequence, which has two parts: standing postures and postures on the floor.

For detailed information on the postures in this section or their variations, head to Book II, Chapters 3, 4, 7, 8, and 10. Select a breathing technique from Book II, Chapter 1. Hold each posture and variation for 6 to 8 breaths, with the exception of the warrior II posture (Steps 3 and 4) and the seated forward

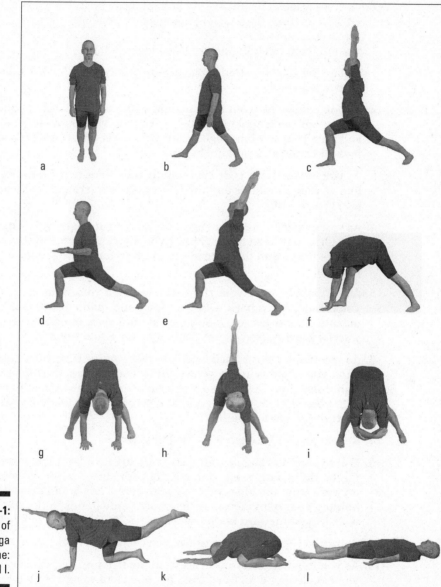

Figure 3-1:
Prime of
Life Yoga
routine:
Level I.

Photographs by Adam Latham

bend posture (Steps 12 and 13) — in both of those postures, you move into and out of them three times before holding for 6 to 8 breaths.

1. **Start in the mountain posture (see Figure 3-2a).**

   Initiate the yoga breathing style of your choice from Book II, Chapter 1 for 6 to 8 breaths.

2. **As you exhale, step out to your right with your right foot about 3 to 3½ feet (or the length of one leg); turn your right foot out 90 degrees, and turn your left foot slightly inward, or keep it straight if a slight inward turn isn't available to you.**

3. **As you inhale, raise your arms out to your sides in a *T* parallel to the line of your shoulders and the floor, for the warrior II ready posture (see Figure 3-2b).**

4. **As you exhale, bend your right knee to a right angle with the floor, and turn your head to the right, as in Figure 3-2c; repeat Steps 3 and 4 three times, and then remain in the warrior II posture for 6 to 8 breaths.**

5. **As you inhale, raise your right arm and turn your right palm up; as you exhale, reach back with your left hand (palm down) and hold the outside of your left leg, looking up at your right hand for the reverse warrior posture (see Figure 3-2d). Stay for 6 to 8 breaths.**

6. **As you inhale, move back briefly to the warrior II position, and then bend your right arm, lay your right forearm across the top of your right thigh, and extend your left arm over your head in alignment with your left ear, as in Figure 3-2e; stay in this extended right angle posture for 6 to 8 breaths.**

7. **Repeat Steps 1 through 6 on the left side.**

8. **From your wide stance, roll your body up, turn both feet forward (to the right), and hang your arms at your sides; as you exhale, bend forward from the hips and hang your torso, head, and arms down, holding your bent elbows with opposite-side hands in the standing wide-legged forward bend (see Figure 3-2f). Hold for 6 to 8 breaths.**

9. **Return to the mountain posture (refer to Figure 3-2a.)**

10. **As you inhale, raise your arms from the front up and overhead; as you exhale, bend forward from the hips, and raise your left leg back and up until your arms, torso, and left leg are all parallel to the floor and you're balancing on your right leg in the warrior III posture (see Figure 3-2g). Hold for 6 to 8 breaths.**

11. **Repeat Steps 9 and 10, balancing on the other side with your left leg.**

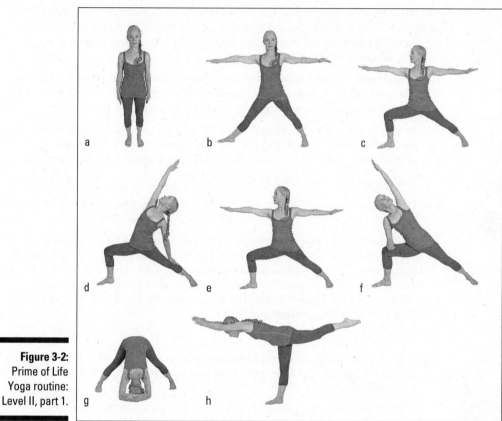

Figure 3-2:
Prime of Life
Yoga routine:
Level II, part 1.

Photographs by Adam Latham

12. Lie on your back, with your knees bent and feet flat on the floor at hip width, and place your hands at your sides palms down; as you inhale, raise your hips and your arms overhead to touch the floor behind you in the bridge variation with arm raise posture (see Figure 3-3a). Hold for 6 to 8 breaths.

13. Lie on your abdomen with your left arm forward (palm down) and your right arm back at your right side (palm up), and then bend your right knee and hold your right foot with your right hand; lift your chest, left arm, and right foot to a comfortable level as you inhale into the half bow posture (see Figure 3-3b). Stay up for 6 to 8 breaths, and then repeat with opposite pairs, holding your left foot with your left hand and extending your right arm forward.

14. **Move to your hands and knees, with both at hip width; as you exhale, sit back on your heels and fold your head and hips down into a comfortable position for the child's posture variation (see Figure 3-3c). Stay folded for 6 to 8 breaths.**

15. **Transition to a seated position, with your legs stretched out in front of you, and bring your back up nice and tall, moving your arms forward and up alongside your ears as you inhale (see Figure 3-3d).**

16. **As you exhale, bend forward from your hips, bringing your hands, chest, and head toward the floor, as in Figure 3-3e; repeat Steps 15 and 16 three times, and then stay down and folded for 6 to 8 breaths.**

Soften your legs and arms as needed.

Take extra caution or avoid seated straight-legged forward bends if you have back problems that rounding the back may exacerbate.

17. **Lie flat on your back, with your legs stretched out and your arms extended into a _T_, with your palms up; as you exhale, bring your right leg up and across your torso to the opposite side, slide your left arm overhead, and turn your head to the right until you're in the Swiss army knife (see Figure 3-3f). Stay in the posture for 6 to 8 breaths, and then repeat with opposite pairs.**

Soften your limbs as needed.

18. **Stay on your back, and hug both knees to your chest with your hands as you exhale for the knees-to-chest posture (see Figure 3-3g); hold for 6 to 8 breaths.**

Hold under your thighs if you have knee problems. As an alternative, rock gently from side to side.

19. **Lie flat on your back in the corpse posture (refer to Figure 3-3h), with your arms along the sides of your torso, your palms up, and your eyes closed to finish; use belly breathing from Book II, Chapter 1 or a relaxation technique from Book VII, Chapter 2 for 3 to 5 minutes.**

a b

c d e

f g h

Figure 3-3:
Prime of Life
Yoga routine:
Level II, part 2.

Photographs by Adam Latham

Cherishing the Chair: A Safe Routine for Older Adults

As a form of exercise, yoga has many benefits specific to seniors. Improved balance and flexibility reduce the risk for (and fear of) injury and increase mobility. Yoga also improves circulation and your ability to sleep, and adding even light weights to the postures increases bone density and lowers the risk of fracture. Plus, group practice promotes social interaction and a sense of connectedness.

If you're hesitant to try yoga because you're not as limber as you used to be, keep in mind that you don't have to practice yoga on the floor. If getting down to the floor or getting up and down is difficult, chair yoga offers spinal freedom while allowing you to remain in your comfort zone. The postures in the seated yoga routine offered in this section give you the same main benefits of a regular yoga class, including stress reduction, improved circulation, better concentration, and an overall sense of well-being. This routine takes about 15 to 20 minutes. Choose one of the yoga breathing techniques in Book II, Chapter 1, and use it for this entire routine.

Before you begin your journey into yoga, first check with your physician. After you get the green light, seek out a class that focuses on your age group, both for the social benefits and to be guided by a teacher who can adapt postures to your needs and abilities. (Book I, Chapter 3 offers advice on picking a teacher and a class.)

You're in charge of whether you do a particular posture. If it doesn't feel right for you, don't do it. The National Institute of Aging provides a wealth of information to help guide you on what may be safe for you and what you may want to avoid. Educate yourself, and enjoy the benefits of breath and movement.

Place blankets or a block under your feet if they don't sit flat on the floor in any of the chair postures.

Seated mountain posture

Check out Figure 3-4 and the following steps for a visual of this posture.

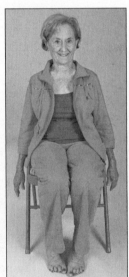

Figure 3-4: Seated mountain posture.

Photograph by Adam Latham

1. Sit comfortably in a chair, with your back extended and your eyes either open or closed.

2. Hang your arms at your sides, and visualize a vertical line down the middle of your ears, shoulders, hips, and backs of your hands; stay for 8 to 10 breaths.

Seated mountain arm variation

You can see how to do this posture in Figure 3-5. Just follow these steps.

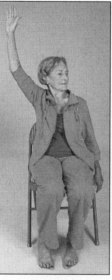

Figure 3-5:
Seated
mountain
posture
variation.

Photograph by Adam Latham

Book III

Yoga for
Life

1. Start in the seated mountain posture from the preceding section; raise your right arm and turn your head to the left as you inhale.

2. As you exhale, return to the seated mountain posture.

3. Repeat Steps 1 and 2 with your left arm and a right head turn, alternating right and left sides slowly for a total of 4 to 6 repetitions on each side.

Seated karate kid variation

Figure 3-6 illustrates this posture. Executing it is easy.

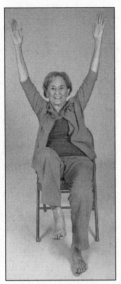

Figure 3-6:
Seated
karate kid
variation.

Photograph by Adam Latham

1. **Start in the seated mountain posture, and raise your arms forward and up alongside your ears as you inhale.**

2. **As you exhale, bend your right knee and raise it toward your chest to a comfortable level.**

3. **Take another breath and then, as you exhale, lower your right knee and your arms back to the seated mountain posture.**

4. **Repeat Steps 1 through 3 with both arms and your left knee, alternating both your knees slowly as you raise your arms, for a total of 4 to 6 repetitions on each side.**

Be careful with this posture if you've have a hip replacement. If you aren't sure whether your hips can handle it, check with your doctor first.

Seated wing-and-prayer

PLAY THIS!
▶

Figure 3-7 shows you this posture. You can also see a demonstration of the seated wing-and-prayer posture at www.dummies.com/go/yogaaiofd. Here's how you do it.

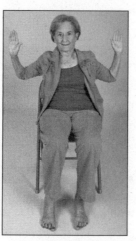

Figure 3-7:
Seated
wing-and-
prayer.

Photograph by Adam Latham

Book III

**Yoga for
Life**

1. **Start in the seated mountain posture, with your hands together in prayer position and your thumbs at your breastbone.**

2. **As you inhale, open your hands outward and lift your chest like wings.**

3. **As you exhale, bring your hands and arms back together into the prayer position.**

4. **Repeat Steps 1 through 3 slowly for 4 to 6 repetitions.**

Seated butterfly posture

Check out the seated butterfly in Figure 3-8, and then follow these steps to try it on your own.

1. **Start in the seated mountain posture, with your arms extended fully to the sides and parallel to the floor, and your palms facing forward.**

2. **Inhale and then, as you exhale, bring your right hand toward the inside of your left arm in a twisting motion.**

3. **Repeat Steps 1 and 2 slowly for 4 to 6 repetitions, and then do the same with your left hand and right arm.**

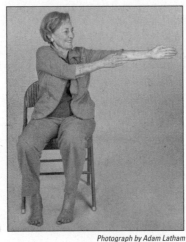

Figure 3-8:
Seated
butterfly
posture.

Photograph by Adam Latham

Standing warrior I chair variation

Use Figure 3-9 and the following steps to guide you through this posture.

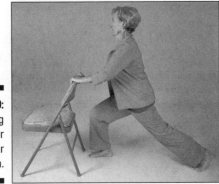

Figure 3-9:
Standing
warrior
I chair
variation.

Photograph by Adam Latham

1. **Stand in the mountain posture (see Figure 3-2a earlier in the chapter), facing the back of your chair from about 3 to 3½ feet away.**

2. **As you exhale, step forward with your right leg, place your hands on the back of the chair, and bend your forward leg into approximately a right angle.**

   You can keep your back foot flat or pivot on the ball of your back foot. Don't be tempted to force the angle.

3. **Stay in Step 2 for 4 to 6 breaths, and then repeat with your left leg forward for 4 to 6 breaths.**

Seated sage twist

Check out Figure 3-10 and the following steps for the seated sage twist.

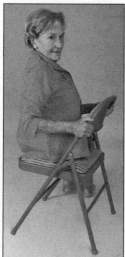

Photograph by Adam Latham

Figure 3-10:
Seated sage
twist.

1. **Sit in your chair sideways, with the back of the chair to your right and your feet flat on the floor.**

2. **As you exhale, turn to your right and grasp the sides of the chair back with your hands.**

3. **As you inhale, bring your back and head up nice and tall; as you exhale, twist deeper.**

4. **Continue this sequence three times, or until you reach your comfortable maximum, and then stay for 4 to 6 breaths; repeat Steps 1 through 4 on the left side.**

Seated forward bend

These steps help you achieve this bend; see Figure 3-11 for an illustration.

1. **Start in the seated mountain posture.**

2. **As you exhale, bend forward from your hips and slide your hands forward and down your legs.**

3. **Let your head and arms hang down, and relax in the folded position for 4 to 6 breaths.**

4. **For a nice ending, use the seated mountain posture; close your eyes and choose focus breathing (Book II, Chapter 1) or a relaxation technique (Book VII, Chapter 2) for 2 to 5 minutes.**

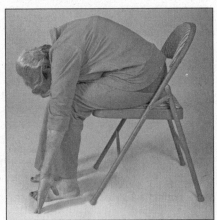

Figure 3-11: Seated forward bend.

Photograph by Adam Latham

Book IV

Powering Your Way to Fitness: Power Yoga

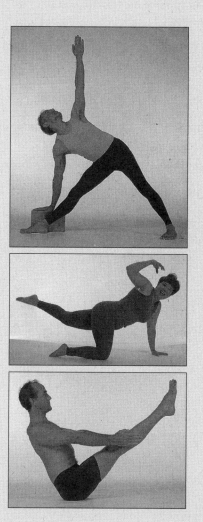

Contents at a Glance

Chapter 1

Key Principles of Power Yoga

In This Chapter

▶ Recognizing the difference between Traditional and Power Yoga breathing

▶ Picking up the soft, graceful dance of Power Yoga

▶ Understanding and using energy locks

▶ Maintaining your focus

▶ Setting your internal thermostat

▶ Taking on a pose that lets you practice important Power Yoga principles

As yoga gained popularity in the United States, the different types of yoga began to separate into two major categories — soft and hard. Soft-form yoga practice emphasizes meditation, relaxation, and separate, distinct postures. Hard-form yoga emphasizes attaining physical strength, improving muscle action, and building physical vitality and endurance. Ashtanga Yoga (see Book I, Chapter 1) is a prime example of hard-form yoga, because it involves nonstop, high-energy routines that increase the circulation, raise body heat, and get your heart and lungs working. *Power Yoga* is a general name for any yoga style that closely follows Ashtanga Yoga.

To really enjoy (and benefit from) your Power Yoga practice, you need to utilize some power tools of your own: your natural powers of breathing, muscle control, movement, focus, and body heat. In this chapter, you discover how to concentrate on each of these tools and develop it into the Power Yoga techniques of connecting poses, focused gazing, muscle locks, and managed body heat. After taking a quick tour through your natural power tools' "user's manual" provided in this chapter, you'll be ready to launch into some basic Power Yoga routines.

Power Yoga Breathing versus Traditional Yoga Breathing

All forms of yoga breathing are similar, but they have subtle differences. If you're a practitioner of traditional soft-form yoga, you need to note a few critical differences between the Power Yoga breathing techniques covered here and those of your current yoga practice. With traditional yoga breathing, you use the same complete yoga breathing technique explained in Book II, Chapter 1. But in traditional yoga breathing, you expand the lower abdominal muscles on inhalations and contract those muscles on exhalation.

Incorporate proper yoga breathing, called *ujjayi,* in every Power Yoga pose. You know you have it down when you make a slight purring or hissing sound as you inhale and exhale. Follow these steps to become familiar with proper yoga breathing and refer to Book II, Chapter 1 for more information:

1. **Sit comfortably.**

2. **Close your eyes and inhale slowly through your nose, fully expanding your lungs.**

3. **Exhale just as slowly through your nose.**

4. **Keep breathing through your nose and tighten your throat muscles a bit as you whisper "haaaaa" through your mouth.**

5. **Continue breathing deeply and slowly, feeling and hearing the air passing through your slightly tightened throat and over the roof of your mouth.**

In Power Yoga breathing, you keep your abdominal muscles firm and slightly contracted. When you inhale, you expand your chest and lift your rib cage. As you exhale, your chest sinks and your lungs contract. Your abdominal muscles remain engaged throughout the breathing cycle. The Power Yoga breathing technique is best for giving you strength and stability as you practice your poses, and this added stability can help you avoid injuries.

Making the Most of Vinyasas: Mastering Movement in Power Yoga

Vinyasas, or connecting movements, link the power of your Power Yoga poses like electrical lines that carry power between generating stations. As you use a vinyasa to move from one pose to the next, you build upon the body heat and life-force energy that your exercises generate, and you maintain the power of your routine's momentum. The powerful conditioning and aerobic boost of the vinyasa connecting movements are what put the power in Power Yoga.

Moving with your breathing

Your breathing brings strength, vitality, and life to your vinyasa. As you move through your Power Yoga routines, always remember to move *with* your breathing. You can use your breathing to set the speed at which you move from one pose to the next. Use these guidelines for coordinating your breathing and movement during Power Yoga practice:

- ✔ As a general rule, exhale as you move into a yoga posture, and inhale as you move out.
- ✔ Inhale when you're going against gravity, and exhale when you're going with gravity.
- ✔ Expand your chest as you inhale, and contract your chest as you exhale.
- ✔ Inhale before you move into a strength vinyasa, and then relax into the movement.

Using connecting links

In Power Yoga, you use connecting poses, or vinyasas, to enter and exit each posture, or *asana*. These connecting movements help you maintain the energy flow of your routine. For example, if you're in a seated posture and you need to go into a standing pose, you can scramble to your feet, tug at your workout clothes, and slowly shake yourself into position. The calm, gently flowing movement of a vinyasa, however, can transport you from one posture to the other with no break in energy, keeping the natural rhythm you've developed in your routine. Well-formed vinyasas make up the dance of Power Yoga. Do them correctly, and you're in *Swan Lake;* ignore them, and your routine is Funky Chicken all the way.

Some vinyasas are very strenuous. Because one function of the vinyasas is to generate body heat, strenuous vinyasas are referred to as *hot. Cool vinyasas* are less strenuous movements that you use to connect poses in the warm-up and cool-down phases of your Power Yoga routine.

Book IV

Powering Your Way to Fitness: Power Yoga

Combining grace with power in your movements

As you move from one pose to the next during your Power Yoga workout, try to enter and exit each posture with grace and elegance. In all forms of yoga, you develop power by developing softness. The smoother, gentler, and more controlled your movements are, the more they strengthen your body. And don't forget that the way you move has a big impact on your state of mind. When your body's jumping and jerking, your mind is twitchy and unsettled. But when you move smoothly and softly, your mind is calm, relaxed, and in control.

If you're new to yoga, you may be a bit awkward and uncoordinated, moving between poses like a clumsy bull. Many beginners to Power Yoga move into vinyasas in spurts of speed. As you work to refine your technique, think of each posture as a delicate flower and, as you move between the postures, try to float like a butterfly so as not to disturb the calm beauty of the pose after you land. As you gain experience, your Power Yoga practice will improve in many ways; careful, controlled movement is just one of the improvements you'll notice over time.

Time teaches you to go with the flow of your practice. Your practice becomes smooth and fluid and, ultimately, takes on the quality of a slow, soft dance. As you combine this gentle yet powerful movement with your deep breathing and mental focus, you gain the maximum Power Yoga benefit.

Controlling the Gateways of Internal Power (Energy Locks)

One of the important natural tools your body makes use of during Power Yoga practice is the *bandha,* or energy lock. You engage an energy lock by contracting certain muscles in your body; these contractions, or locks, direct through your body the flow of energy (the *prana*) that you create during Power Yoga exercises. Not only do energy locks help direct the flow of energy to high-demand areas during your Power Yoga practice, but they also can give you energy boosts and added stability and tone your stomach and cleanse your internal organs.

Understanding how energy locks work

To better understand the way energy locks work, visualize the workings of your circulatory system for a moment. Your heart pumps blood throughout your body, using your veins and arteries as the delivery system. When you practice Power Yoga, you create an enormous amount of life-force energy. This energy travels throughout your body through unseen channels called *nadis.* The energy locks act as valves to regulate the flow of life energy through the *nadis* in your body. In this respect, your bandhas work much like your heart, to control the flow of essential forces through your system.

Using muscle locks for a powerful practice

You should engage your energy locks each time you hold a yoga asana or pose. You should release the bandha as you leave a pose, but often you reengage the energy locks during your vinyasa, or connecting movements.

Unlike the nadis (which you can't see), energy locks are made up of muscle groups in your body. To engage a bandha, you physically contract muscles in one of three areas of your body. Each of these three energy locks has a special name (see Figure 1-1):

- ✔ **Mula bandha:** The *Mula bandha* is called the *root lock,* and it's located in the perineal muscles between your genitals and anus. To identify these muscles, imagine that you need to make an emergency trip to the bathroom and the nearest one is w-a-a-y down the hall. As you take that long walk, you engage your Mula bandha to fend off an unfortunate accident. Isn't that a great energy lock to have available?

- ✔ **Uddiyana bandha:** The name *Uddiyana* means "flying up." This bandha is located about three fingers' width below your navel. In this bandha, you lift your stomach, drawing up your diaphragm. This bandha helps flatten your stomach. In your Power Yoga practice, however, this bandha firms your abdominal muscles; you use it in conjunction with the Mula bandha.

- ✔ **Jalandhara bandha:** The *Jalandhara bandha* is called a *chin lock.* You engage this bandha by stretching the back of the neck as you lower your chin into the notch in your breastbone. You engage this bandha in a few poses and in some yoga breathing exercises, but you don't use it nearly as often as you use the Mula bandha or the Uddiyana bandha.

Book IV

Powering Your Way to Fitness: Power Yoga

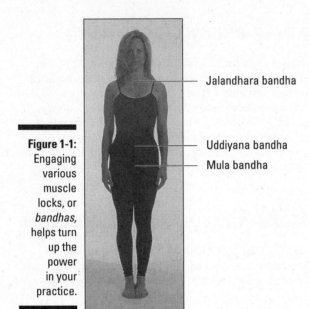

Jalandhara bandha

Uddiyana bandha

Mula bandha

Figure 1-1:
Engaging various muscle locks, or *bandhas,* helps turn up the power in your practice.

Photograph by Raul Marroquin

Keeping Your Eyes on the Power Yoga Prize: Directing Your Gaze

"Looking good" during Power Yoga isn't about wearing the right clothes, having the right hairstyle, or sporting the right genetic background. Nope, it refers to the way you direct your gaze as you move into and hold each Power Yoga posture. The way you direct and hold your gaze during Power Yoga practice has an impact on your mental state, your posture, and your ability to remain focused and energized.

In yoga, the gazing point for each posture is called a *drishti,* which means both "looking out" and "looking in." The purpose of the drishti isn't to get your vision fixed on a particular place or part of your body; it's actually an exercise in turning your gaze inward. When you gaze inward, you can check to make sure that you're breathing properly, that your posture alignment is accurate, and that your energy lock is engaged. Gazing inward is a form of sense withdrawal, so your gaze is a tool to help you in this important part of Power Yoga practice. When you're "doing the drishti," you're focused.

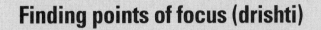

Finding points of focus (drishti)

This list includes the classic drishti used in traditional yoga; the name of each drishti is followed by the place or thing on which you should focus your eyes when assuming this gazing point:

✔ **Nasagrai:** Tip of nose

✔ **Ajna chakra:** Between the eyebrows

✔ **Nabi chakra:** Your navel

✔ **Hastagrai:** Your hand

✔ **Padhayoragrai:** Your toes

✔ **Parsva drishti:** Far to the side (either right or left)

✔ **Angustha Ma Dyai:** Your thumbs

✔ **Urvhva or Antara drishti:** Up to the sky

In most Power Yoga postures, you gaze in the direction of the posture's stretch. If you want to get technical about it, you can memorize the focus or drishti gazing points listed in the "Finding points of focus (drishti)" sidebar in this chapter.

Benefiting from Body Heat

Power Yoga practice generates body heat. This body heat comes from the inside out, sort of like the heat that forms in a microwave oven. Your body heat is an important natural tool in Power Yoga. Body heat makes your muscles, tendons, and joints more pliable.

Body heat is a tool that you really need to use correctly, or it can hurt you. Follow these guidelines to get the most benefit from the body heat that you generate during your Power Yoga workouts:

✔ As you sweat, you lose fluids, so drink lots of water before and after your Power Yoga practice.

✔ Try to work out in a warm (but not hot) room.

✔ If possible, have fresh air entering the room, but try to avoid blasts of cold air. Your muscles are most flexible in a warm environment, but quick changes in temperature can be damaging to them (and your entire body, for that matter).

Book IV

Powering Your Way to Fitness: Power Yoga

Putting All Your Power Tools to Work

Reading about how to practice yoga breathing, energy locks, and points of gaze is one thing. But the real trick is figuring out how to put them all to use while you're practicing a Power Yoga pose — especially one that requires lots of balance. But you can do it! To boost your confidence in your ability to perform Power Yoga, try the asana in this section. This asana requires you to pay special attention to balance. The extended foot one leg stand posture (*utthita hasta padangusthasana*) trains you to incorporate all your natural tools into your Power Yoga practice.

In Sanskrit, the word *utthita* means "extended," *hasta* means "hand," and *padangustha* loosely translates to "big toe." In this posture, you stand on one leg while extending your other leg forward and grabbing your big toe with your hand.

The extended foot one leg stand posture stretches and strengthens muscles in your legs, expands your chest, and opens those tight hips. In addition, this posture is wonderful for teaching balance and coordination. Follow these steps to perform this posture:

1. **Stand with your spine straight and your shoulders back, and extend your arms down the sides of your torso; keep your vision forward.**

   This is mountain pose. (Refer to Book II, Chapter 3 for more on the mountain pose.)

2. **Close your eyes for a few slow, deep yoga breaths while you maintain good posture.**

   Ground yourself firmly onto the floor, and be conscious and aware of your breathing.

3. **Open your eyes, and place your left hand on your left hip.**

4. **Pick your right foot up off the floor and, balancing on your left foot, bend your right knee and place your right hand around the outside of your right knee.**

   You should now be balancing on your left foot, holding your right knee with your right hand.

5. **Pull your right knee 90 degrees toward your right side as you open your hip.**

6. **Keep your torso and chest facing forward, and pull your right leg to your right side, turning your head to your left side and looking over your left shoulder (see Figure 1-2).**

   If you have trouble balancing, place your left hand on a wall for support.

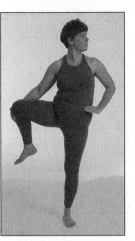

Figure 1-2:
This version of the extended foot one leg stand posture is a great beginner's pose.

Photograph by Raul Marroquin

7. **Put your power tools to work:**

   • Listen to the sound of your slow, deep breaths.

   • Engage your Mula bandha by tightening your perineal muscles.

   • Engage your Uddiyana bandha by firming and lifting your stomach.

   • Direct your gaze (drishti) by looking over your left shoulder, parallel to the floor.

8. **Hold this position for 5 to 10 slow, deep breaths.**

9. **Release your energy locks, turn your head back to the center, and exhale as you bring your right leg back to the center and lower your foot to the floor.**

10. **Repeat these steps, but this time balance on your right leg, lift your left leg off the floor, and direct your drishti to the right.**

Book IV

Powering Your Way to Fitness: Power Yoga

If you're an advanced student, you can do a full version of this posture. Follow the same series of steps, but instead of holding onto your knee, grab your right big toe with the first two fingers of your right hand and fully extend your leg out to the front and off to the side, as illustrated in Figure 1-3.

Figure 1-3:
Advanced
students
can try this
version
of the
extended
foot one
leg stand
posture.

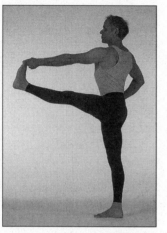

Photograph by Raul Marroquin

Chapter 2

Preparing with Powerful Warm-Ups

*E*ver driven your car without first warming up the engine? Everyone knows that a cold engine is a poor performer, subject to backfiring and stalling out. Well, the wonderful machine that you call your body doesn't run smoothly without a warm-up, either. If you want your body to function at full capacity, with limber joints, flexible muscles, and energy to spare, you need to take time to warm 'er up before any strenuous activity — and that definitely includes your Power Yoga workouts. Even the most advanced Power Yoga practitioners take time to warm up before launching into a fast-paced Power Yoga session.

In this chapter, you find a series of warm-up routines. They're divided into two categories: warm-ups practiced on the floor (lying down, sitting, or kneeling) and standing warm-ups.

Getting Down with Warm-Ups on the Floor

These gentle warm-ups are designed to gradually speed up the circulation of your whole body, through balanced stretches and counter-stretches. (A *counter-stretch* stretches the opposite side of the body or muscle, as the case may be. For example, the counter-stretch for a forward bend is a backward bend.)

As an added bonus, these warm-ups help you develop coordination and balance as they take you through twists, turns, and stretches.

Twisting with the spine toner

The spine toner is relaxing, easy to practice, and a great way to flex your spine. Your everyday routines — work, play, even sitting — can deliver lots of abuse to your spine. This simple warm-up helps your spine recuperate from its long, hard days.

The spine toner invigorates your entire spine with gentle twisting movements that stretch the muscles in your back and hips. To get the most from this warm-up, be sure to combine it with the Power Yoga breathing techniques described in Book IV, Chapter 1.

Follow these steps to tone your spine:

1. **Lie down on the floor on your back, with your legs straight and your feet about 12 inches apart (a position known as the corpse posture; refer to Book III, Chapter 1), and extend your arms straight out from your shoulders at a 90-degree angle from your torso.**

2. **On an inhalation, bend your right knee and lift your right leg toward the ceiling; exhale, lower your right leg over your left leg toward the floor on the left side of your body, and then extend your leg fully to the side.**

   Keep your legs straight, but not rigid. If you find this posture uncomfortable, keep your right knee bent.

3. **Your right hip will automatically rise off the floor, and your whole torso will twist, but try to keep your shoulders flat on the floor as you turn your head and gaze to the right.**

   Figure 2-1 illustrates what this pose looks like.

4. **Hold this position for 5 to 15 slow, deep breaths, and then slowly lift your right leg and return it to its original position (see Step 1).**

5. **Repeat Steps 1 through 4, this time using your left leg and gazing toward the left in Step 3.**

6. **Relax in the corpse posture for 5 to 10 slow, deep breaths.**

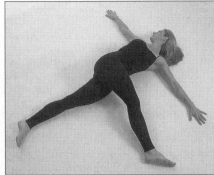

Figure 2-1:
The spine toner gently twists your spine.

Photograph by Raul Marroquin

Walking upside-down

Even for a complete novice, this exercise is easy and fun. In this pose, you look like someone who's walking upside-down — and you don't require a zero-gravity chamber! This exercise delivers many of the same benefits to your body that you get from walking right-side up. The upside-down walker is an excellent warm-up exercise; it speeds up your circulation, stretches your arms and legs, and helps send a fresh supply of blood to the brain.

Follow these steps to walk upside-down:

1. **Lie flat on your back, with your arms and legs straight but not rigid.**

2. **Stretch your arms and legs upward, pointing toward the ceiling, like a bug stuck on its back.**

3. **Now swing your arms and legs as though you're walking in the air (see Figure 2-2).**

   Swing your left arm forward (toward your face), when your right leg is forward; then swing your right arm forward when your left leg is forward.

   If you have stiff leg muscles and tight hips, bend your knees more to protect your lower back from overstrain.

4. **Take 15 to 30 strides.**

5. **Return your arms and legs to the floor, and relax in your original position.**

Make sure to move your limbs in opposite directions — move your right arm and left leg at the same time and your left arm and right leg together.

Book IV

Powering Your Way to Fitness: Power Yoga

Figure 2-2:
The upside-
down
walker
can make
you feel
like you're
walking on
the moon.

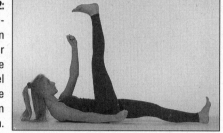

Photograph by Raul Marroquin

Hugging those knees

Your knees are responsible for lots of work and some of your most important moves; here's your chance to thank them for all their effort! In this exercise, you pay tribute to your knees by giving them a big hug.

This exercise relieves tension in your lower back, expands your chest, and tones up your stomach muscles. And as an added bonus, these knee hugs can also help relieve your system of excessive gas — something for which everyone can be grateful.

Hug your knees close to you with these steps:

1. **Assume the corpse position: Lie down on your back, with arms by your sides, palms facing up, and legs extended.**

   Leave your feet about one foot apart.

2. **Calm your mind, and relax for a few slow, deep breaths.**

3. **On an inhalation, stretch your whole body in both directions, lifting your arms above your head and stretching your legs out from your feet; keep your head on the floor and gaze upward.**

4. **Exhale, and lower your arms toward your waist while bending your right knee into your torso, wrapping your arms around your shin, and hugging your right knee.**

   If you have a weak lower back, bend your extended left leg, knee raised upward and place your left foot on the floor about 2 feet from your seat.

5. **On an exhalation, lift your head off the floor and try to touch your nose to your knee.**

6. **Inhale, and release your knee, again stretching your whole body in both directions.**

   Lift your arms over your head, and stretch your legs toward your feet.

7. **Repeat Steps 1 through 6, this time hugging your left knee to your chest.**

8. **You can repeat this knee-hugging exercise three to five times.**

9. **Relax as you lower your arms to your sides and melt softly into the floor, returning to the corpse position.**

Another way to ease the strain on your lower back is to bend your downward knee — point your knee toward the ceiling with your foot 12 to 18 inches from your seat. Keeping your knee bent reduces the intensity of the effort required and is gentler on your lower back.

Releasing shoulder and neck tension

Who can resist a nice shoulder and neck massage? All day, you build tension and stress in your neck and shoulders, and by the end of the day you need a massage in the worst way! The problem is that you also need a willing masseuse. Well, these two exercises let you give *yourself* a massage to roll the tension right out of those tight neck and shoulder muscles.

These exercises are also terrific warm-ups for your Power Yoga routines. Give them a try before your Power Yoga workout or anytime you need to roll the weight of the world off your shoulders.

Rolling the boulders off your shoulders

"Row, row, row your boat, gently down the stream," goes the song. Wouldn't that hurt with your shoulders feeling as tight as they do right now? You need strong, healthy shoulders to excel in Power Yoga, so this shoulder roll exercise can be an important preamble to your workout.

In this exercise, you lift and lower your shoulders while rotating them in forward and backward circles. These shoulder rolls help you release tension from your shoulders and upper back, and get your rotator cuff (where your arm connects into your torso) warmed up and ready for action.

Follow these steps to get your shoulders rolling:

1. **Sit on the floor, with your spine straight and shoulders back (see the seated angle pose in Figure 2-3).**

   If sitting on the floor is uncomfortable for you, you also can sit on the edge of a sturdy chair.

2. **On an inhalation, rotate your shoulders backward as you lift them up toward your ears.**

Book IV

Powering Your Way to Fitness: Power Yoga

3. **As you exhale, finish the backward rotation as you lower your shoulders to their original position.**

4. **Repeat Steps 2 and 3, reversing the direction of your shoulder rotation.**

5. **Repeat each rotation three or four times, and then relax your shoulders.**

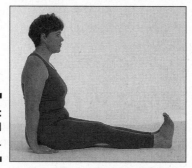

Figure 2-3:
The seated
angle pose.

Photograph by Raul Marroquin

Getting rid of that pain in the neck

When the muscles in your neck get tight and stiff, they can interfere with all your upper body movements. This exercise knocks the kinks out of stiff necks to get you warmed up and ready for action.

This simple but powerful exercise helps you to release stress and tension from your neck, stimulating the nerves in your upper spine and the base of your skull. It's also a great way to build strength and flexibility in all the muscles in your neck, leaving you less prone to future attacks of neck stiffness and pain. Best of all, this exercise is very relaxing.

Follow these steps to warm up your neck muscles:

1. **Sit on the floor (or on the edge of a sturdy chair) with your spine straight and your shoulders back; relax your arms and rest your hands in your lap.**

2. **On an exhalation, tilt your head forward and let your chin drop to your chest.**

   You feel the muscles in the back of your neck stretch.

3. **Inhale, and lift your head back to its upright position.**

4. **Exhale, and tilt your head back as far as you can without hurting anything.**

   You feel the muscles in the front of your neck and under your chin stretch.

5. Again, inhale and return your head to its upright position.

6. Repeat Steps 1 through 5 four times, and then return to your original posture.

7. Exhale, and lower your head to your right shoulder; inhale, and raise your head to its original position.

8. Repeat Step 7, lowering your head to the left side on an exhalation and back to center on an inhalation.

9. Relax for 3 complete breaths.

   Use your yoga breathing technique for maximum benefit.

10. On an exhalation, turn your head to the right, keeping your head level as you gaze over your right shoulder; inhale, and turn your head to look straight ahead.

11. Repeat Step 10, turning your head and gazing to the left on an exhalation and back to center on an inhalation.

12. Finish by closing your eyes and relaxing for 3 complete breaths.

Playing with the kitty (cat stretch)

The movements of the cat stretch resemble a cat stretching out the kinks after a good long sleep. An excellent exercise for almost anyone, the cat stretch tones up your back muscles and can make your entire spine feel stronger and more flexible. If you suffer from minor back pain brought on by stress, over-activity, or bad posture, this exercise can help relieve that pain.

Follow these steps to imitate a cat:

1. Start from a kneeling position; sit back on your heels with your toes pointed backward, your back straight, your neck lengthened, and your head facing forward.

2. Lift your hips, and place your hands on the floor so that you're resting on your hands and knees.

3. Keep your back straight but not rigid, and relax as you take 3 slow, deep breaths.

   Your body forms a table in this pose, as shown in Figure 2-4.

4. On an exhalation, arch your back like a cat.

5. Relax your neck as you drop your head downward and gaze toward your knees, as illustrated in Figure 2-5.

Book IV

Powering Your Way to Fitness: Power Yoga

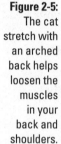

Figure 2-4:
The table
pose.

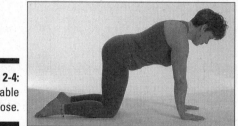

Photograph by Raul Marroquin

Figure 2-5:
The cat
stretch with
an arched
back helps
loosen the
muscles
in your
back and
shoulders.

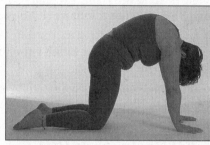

Photograph by Raul Marroquin

6. **On an inhalation, lower your back, expanding your chest, and let your back arch downward as you bend your arms to lower your chest and bring your chin to rest on the floor between your hands, as shown in Figure 2-6.**

7. **Exhale, and slowly draw your body up to return to the arched-back position you entered in Step 4.**

Figure 2-6:
The cat
stretch with
a swayed
back helps
relieve
tension in
your spine.

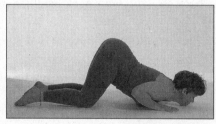

Photograph by Raul Marroquin

8. **On an inhalation, sway your back downward again, but keep your arms straight and lift your head up as you extend your right leg back and up.**

   If your back is arched properly and your leg and head are extended up, your body forms a smile in this phase of the cat stretch, as shown in Figure 2-7.

   Don't swing or jerk into this posture: Try to keep your movements fluid and soft as you lift your head and extend your leg back and up.

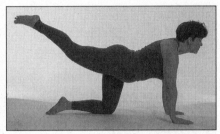

Figure 2-7:
The cat stretch with the right leg back.

Photograph by Raul Marroquin

9. **On an exhalation, reverse the stretch; arch your back again and drop your head, bending your right knee into your chest**

   Try to touch your nose with your knee, as illustrated in Figure 2-8.

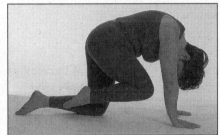

Figure 2-8:
The cat stretch with nose to knee.

Photograph by Raul Marroquin

10. **Repeat Steps 8 and 9, extending your left leg back.**

    Beginners should practice one or two repetitions with each leg; more experienced students can practice three or four rounds.

Book IV

Powering Your Way to Fitness: Power Yoga

11. **Sit back on your heels, and relax your torso onto your thighs; extend your arms by your sides, and rest your forehead on the floor, as illustrated in Figure 2-9.**

    This posture, called the child's posture, is a good resting posture.

Figure 2-9: The child's posture allows your muscles to rest after a good stretch.

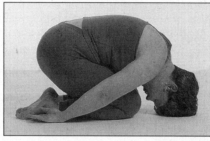

Photograph by Raul Marroquin

Chasing the wild alley cat

Alley cats tend to be a bit sassy and wild, and as the name of this exercise implies, you have to try a bit harder to catch this cat. The alley cat begins with the cat stretch (see the preceding section), and it delivers all the benefits of that stretch. It also gives your arms and shoulders an energizing stretch, and it promotes flexibility in your hips and thighs.

A soft exercise mat is an important prop for this exercise to pad your knees from the floor and increase your stability.

This exercise is definitely for those with healthy lower backs. If you have a weak back or have had problems with your back, the alley cat isn't for you.

These steps help you tame the alley cat:

1. **Follow Steps 1 through 4 for the cat stretch; as you complete Step 4, you're on your hands and knees, with your back arched and your head and hips tucked down (refer to Figure 2-5).**

2. **Inhale, and open your chest by pulling your shoulders back, arching your back, and expanding your chest as you lift your right arm up and forward in front of your head.**

3. **Lengthen your right arm upward on an inhalation.**

4. **At the same time, lift and extend your left leg behind your back, keeping your knee bent (see Figure 2-10).**

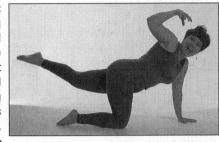

Figure 2-10:
Scratching (and yowling) like an alley cat is a fun and energizing part of this exercise.

Photograph by Raul Marroquin

5. Lower your extended hand and leg to the floor; reach behind your back with your left hand and grasp your right ankle.

6. Stretch your leg back and up as you hold this position for 2 complete breaths (see Figure 2-11).

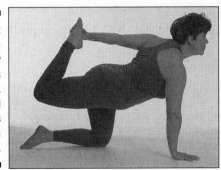

Figure 2-11:
This phase of the alley cat gives your torso, hips, and thighs an extra stretch.

Photograph by Raul Marroquin

7. On an inhalation, release and lower your leg, and then lower your back; let your back sway downward as you bend your arms to lower your chest and bring your chin to rest on the floor between your hands, gazing in front of you.

8. Exhale, and slowly draw your body up to return to the arched-back position you entered in Step 1.

9. Repeat Steps 2 through 8, using your right arm and left leg in Steps 4 and 5.

10. Finish by sitting back on your heels and relaxing your torso onto your thighs; extend your arms by your sides, and rest your forehead on the floor in the child's posture (refer to Figure 2-9).

Book IV

Powering Your Way to Fitness: Power Yoga

Strengthening with push-ups

Power cat push-ups are quite a bit easier than traditional push-ups and have a yogic flavor. You practice traditional push-ups with your legs straight, but power cat push-ups let you rest on your knees, making them a little easier.

Power cat push-ups work to strengthen your shoulders, arms, and pectoral muscles. This exercise is a great way to prepare you for the Power Yoga vinyasas. The core of Power Yoga is these flowing movements that keep your muscles working and your energy flowing between yoga postures.

Use these steps to get the most out of your cat push-ups:

1. **Form a "table" by supporting your body on your hands and knees, keeping your back straight but relaxed and your abdominal muscles firm to help support your back.**

2. **Move your arms forward about 6 inches, bend your elbows, interlace your fingers, and, on an exhalation, flatten your chin and entire torso down on to your extended hands (refer to Figure 2-6).**

3. **Inhale, and push your torso up to the arched-back cat position (refer to Figure 2-5).**

4. **Repeat this exercise three to ten times.**

5. **When you're done, relax into the child's posture, shown in Figure 2-9.**

Standing Up, Warming Up

Standing warm-ups are every bit as invigorating and useful as the floor-based models. Those explained here help limber up your body to give you more freedom of movement and stability. And these warm-ups also help heat up your body's "engine" to keep it running strongly and smoothly.

Spinning with the windmill

In the windmill, you swing the upper part of your body, down, around, and up, moving in a circular motion like a windmill. You can get some real mental relaxation in this exercise if you imagine that you're a windmill turning softly in the breeze of a warm summer's day.

The windmill helps to open the upper part of your body with gentle, flowing stretches. The spine is flexed and stimulated as you stretch the muscles of your back, stomach, and chest. This exercise brings a fresh supply of oxygenated blood to the brain, leaving you refreshed and invigorated.

Make like Don Quixote and chase windmills, using these steps:

1. **Begin in a standing position with your feet a little more than shoulder-width apart.**

2. **On an inhalation, raise your arms to reach up and over your head and expand your chest.**

3. **As you exhale, move your outstretched arms and torso down and to the left in a circular motion.**

4. **On an inhalation, lift your arms and torso up and to the right to complete the circle, as illustrated in Figure 2-12.**

   At the end of this exercise, you end up where you started, with your arms stretched over your head.

5. **Repeat Steps 1 through 4, circling your arms and torso in the opposite direction and performing two repetitions in each direction.**

   To get the most out of this exercise, make sure to time your movement with your breath.

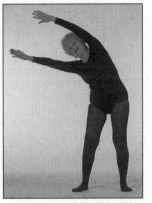

Figure 2-12: The windmill stretches your back, flexes your spine, and gets your blood pumping.

Photograph by Raul Marroquin

Book IV

Powering Your Way to Fitness: Power Yoga

Going into the deep lunge

The deep lunge *(sirsangusthasana)* creates great strength in your legs and, at the same time, opens and expands your chest. This exercise also increases the mobility of your ankles and helps release tension from your neck. You'll notice that this posture gives you a sense of strength and self-confidence as your balance improves.

You can easily see where this pose gets its name; in Sanskrit, *sirsa* means "head" and *angustha* relates to your big toe.

Lunge into this warm-up by following these steps:

1. **Start from a standing position with your legs firmly planted slightly more than shoulder-width apart.**

2. **Place your arms behind your back, interlock your fingers, and turn your left foot to the left.**

3. **Lift your arms up and behind you on an inhalation, expand your chest, and then exhale as you bend your left knee down, lowering your head and torso toward the toes of your left foot as shown in Figure 2-13.**

   Try to keep your back straight, shoulders back, fingers interlaced, and arms lifted off your back. If you're a beginner, you can rest your torso on your left thigh.

   Listen to your body. If this stretch is very painful or just too much for you, you can just lower your nose toward your knee. This modification puts less strain on your back and legs.

Figure 2-13:
The deep lunge stretches your back and legs.

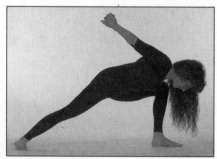

Photograph by Raul Marroquin

4. **Hold this position for 3 complete breaths, and then lift up to the center on an inhalation.**

5. **Repeat Steps 1 through 4, lunging to the right.**

Expanding the toe touch

This exercise expands your chest and stretches your arm and leg muscles. This simple warm-up is excellent for toning and strengthening your back, as well as warming up your body.

Reach for your toes, not the stars, following these steps:

1. **Start in the expanded mountain posture.**

   Stand up straight, with your shoulders back and your feet about 4 feet apart. Turn your toes slightly inward and heels outward, grounding yourself into the earth. Then rest your arms by your sides and relax.

2. **Bend your left elbow, and place your hand on your hip; inhale as you lift your right arm up straight over your right shoulder.**

3. **Exhale, and lower your right arm as you fold forward at your waist, trying to touch your left toes with your right hand.**

   If you aren't very flexible, bend your knees slightly. If you're more flexible, keep your legs straight.

4. **Inhale, and come to a standing position as you lift your arm over your right shoulder and stretch toward the ceiling.**

5. **Repeat Steps 1 through 4 five times, and then lower your arms to your sides and return to the expanded mountain pose in Step 1.**

6. **Repeat Steps 1 through 5, lifting your left arm and touching your right toes.**

Chapter 3

Taking a Walk in the Park: A Minimum Power Routine

In This Chapter

▶ Getting ready for an introductory Power Yoga workout

▶ Taking that walk in the park

This routine, named Just a Walk in the Park, is fairly easy and makes a good introduction to Power Yoga. This workout is perfect if you have just under an hour for your practice. You can complete it in 30 to 45 minutes.

In this chapter, you find some background information about the postures of this short, well-balanced workout, and the instructions show you when to incorporate a linking movement, or *vinyasa,* to move from one posture to the next. Because this routine takes relatively little time, you get a full dose of Power Yoga benefits in a small package; that's a good deal from all angles. So grab your yoga mat, put on those Power Yoga togs, and get moving!

Talking before Walking

Just a Walk in the Park gives you a gentle introduction to a full Power Yoga workout. This routine leaves you feeling energized and refreshed. To get the most from this walk, keep these tips in mind:

✔ **Prepare your space.** Make sure that your workout room is warm and has a good supply of fresh air. Have a good, soft yoga mat ready, along with some pillows, towels, and blocks. (If you're a beginner or you have physical limitations, you may want to use yoga props.)

✔ **Follow the instructions.** Following the instructions as written is the key to reaping the benefits of this routine.

✔ **Take your time.** If you rush just to get through this — or any — Power Yoga routine, you miss out on many of the mental and physical benefits.

✔ **Incorporate yoga breathing techniques.** Keeping your breathing going is crucial during every phase of your workout. For specific information about breathing the Power Yoga way, refer to Book IV, Chapter 1; for general information about yoga breathing, head to Book II, Chapter 1.

One of the most important concepts in Power Yoga is to practice a routine that's appropriate for your present level of yoga fitness. "Yoga fitness" is different from fitness in general because even the most fit individuals can find the stretching and strengthening exercises of Power Yoga to be a challenge in the beginning. If you're out of shape, take it easy and move through this routine slowly and without putting undue strain on your muscles (or your good humor).

The Beginner's Routine: Just a Walk in the Park

This routine starts you off with some Power Yoga breathing techniques, moves you softly into a few warm-ups, and then gives you a mild vinyasa to take you to a standing pose. After you get a taste of some powerful standing poses, you move softly back to the floor and practice the traditional, whole-body finishing poses, or *asanas*. You complete your journey with breathing and deep relaxation.

Starting well is breathing well

Always start your Power Yoga practice with yoga breathing to find your center and quiet your mind. Check out Book IV, Chapter 1 for a reminder of how to do this.

Follow these steps to begin your walk in the park:

1. **Sit cross-legged on the floor with your spine straight and your shoulders back.**

   If you find this position uncomfortable, experiment with placing a small but firm pillow or rolled blanket under just the bony part of your seat (leave those cheeks behind!). If you still feel uncomfortable or if your knees just hang high in space, place a small, supportive pillow under each thigh just above the knee.

TIP

If you're a beginning Power Yoga student, you may find it more comfortable to sit on the edge of a small pillow or on the edge of a chair until you gain more flexibility.

2. **Extend your arms over your knees, resting your wrists on your knees, with your palms facing upward.**

3. **Form jnana mudra with your hands by bending your index finger in to touch the tip of your thumb; your remaining fingers should be straight but not stiff or tense (see Figure 3-1).**

Figure 3-1:
The jnana mudra hand gesture is part of many Power Yoga seated postures.

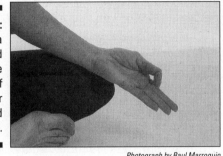

Photograph by Raul Marroquin

4. **Practice your yoga breathing.**

   Allow your breathing to calm your mind and body and help center your thoughts on your practice. Continue your yoga breathing for 5 to 10 slow, deep breaths.

5. **Open your eyes, and go on to the neck and shoulder exercise listed in the next section.**

Working the kinks out of your shoulders and neck

REMEMBER

The steps in this section walk you through these powerful neck and shoulder exercises. If you need more background information, refer to Book IV, Chapter 2.

Follow these steps to warm up your neck and shoulders:

1. **Sit on the floor, with your spine straight and shoulders back; keep your arms relaxed and your hands resting in your lap.**

   If sitting on the floor is uncomfortable, sit on the edge of a heavy chair.

2. On an inhalation, rotate your shoulders back as you lift them toward your ears; then, as you exhale, finish the backward rotation as you lower your shoulders to their original position.

3. Repeat Step 2, reversing the direction of your shoulder rotation.

   Repeat each rotation three or four times, and then relax your shoulders.

4. Maintain your erect, relaxed sitting position; on an exhalation, tilt your head forward and let your chin drop to your chest.

   You'll feel the muscles in the back of your neck stretch.

5. Inhale, and lift your head back to its upright position.

6. Exhale, and tilt your head back as far as you can without hurting anything.

   You'll feel the muscles in the front of your neck and under your chin stretch.

7. Inhale again, and lift your head back to the center.

8. Repeat Steps 4 through 7 four times, and then return to your original upright posture.

9. Exhale, and lower your head to your right shoulder; inhale, and raise your head to its original position.

10. Exhale, lower your head to the left side, and then go back to the center on an inhalation.

11. Relax for 3 complete breaths, using your yoga breathing technique.

12. On an exhalation, turn your head to the right, keeping your head level as you gaze over your right shoulder; inhale and turn your head back to look straight ahead.

13. Repeat Step 12, turning your head and gazing to the left on an exhalation and back to the center on an inhalation.

14. Finish by closing your eyes and relaxing for 3 complete breaths.

Moving into the cat stretch

The cat stretch is a wonderful warm-up exercise because it affects almost every part of your body. Book IV, Chapter 2 covers the details of this posture, so if you need a refresher, you can refer to that chapter.

Follow these steps to stretch like a cat (see Figure 3-2):

1. **Start from a kneeling position; sit back on your heels, with your toes pointed backward.**

   Your back should be straight, and you should feel your neck lengthen.

2. **Lift your hips, and place your hands on the floor so that you're resting on your hands and knees.**

3. **Keep your back straight, but not rigid, and relax as you take 3 slow, deep breaths.**

   Have your hands right under your shoulders and your knees right under your hips — this is the table pose (Figure 3-2a).

4. **On an exhalation, arch your back like a cat; relax your neck as you drop your head downward and gaze toward your knees (Figure 3-2b).**

5. **On an inhalation, lower your back and let it sway downward as you bend your arms to lower your chest and bring your chin to rest on the floor between your hands (Figure 3-2c).**

6. **Exhale, and slowly draw your body up and return to the arched-back position you reached in Step 4 (Figure 3-2b).**

   Time your moves with your breathing. Take your time, and try to flow from one position to the next.

7. **On an inhalation, sway your back downward again, but keep your arms straight and lift your head upward as you extend your right leg back and upward (Figure 3-2d).**

   Your body should form a smile. Don't swing or jerk into this posture: Try to keep your movements fluid and soft as you lift your head and extend your leg back and up at the same time.

8. **On an exhalation, reverse the stretch by arching your back again, dropping your head, and bending your right knee toward your chest; try to touch your nose with your knee (Figure 3-2e).**

9. **Repeat Steps 7 and 8, but extend your left leg this time.**

10. **Practice two to four repetitions of Steps 1 through 9, and then relax into the child's posture with arms in front, shown in Figure 3-2f.**

11. **Relax for 2 breaths, and then push your torso off the floor and come to rest on your hands and knees.**

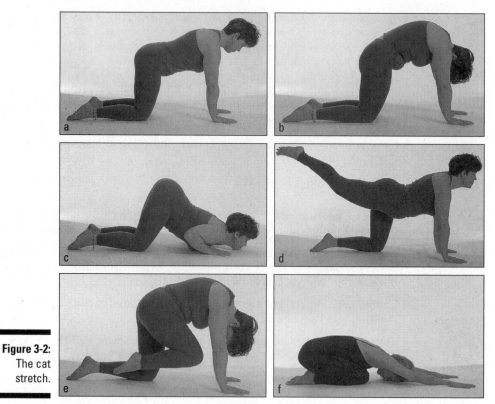

Photographs by Raul Marroquin

Figure 3-2:
The cat stretch.

Strengthening with power cat push-ups

The power cat push-ups strengthen the shoulder, arm, and pectoral muscles. Follow these steps to perform the power cat push-ups:

1. **Form a table by supporting your body on your hands and knees, with back straight but relaxed (see Figure 3-3a).**

   This is the table pose.

2. **Move your arms forward slightly, bend your elbows, and on an exhalation, lower your whole torso flat to the floor (see Figure 3-3b).**

   If you can't get all the way down at first, lower as far as you can and still push yourself up again. You'll soon be doing the full power cat push-up!

3. **Inhale, and push your torso up to the starting position on your hands and knees (as in Figure 3-3a again).**

4. **Repeat Steps 1 through 3 three to ten times, and then relax into the child's posture with arms in front (refer to Figure 3-2f).**

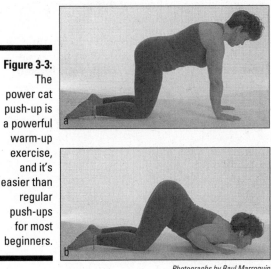

Figure 3-3: The power cat push-up is a powerful warm-up exercise, and it's easier than regular push-ups for most beginners.

Photographs by Raul Marroquin

Stretching into the downward-facing dog

The downward-facing dog *(adhomukha shvanasana)* position resembles a dog stretching after awakening from his nap. As the dog awakens, he stretches his hips high in the air while he lengthens his entire spine and stretches his back. If you've ever been around a dog, you've seen this posture, and you may have thought "Oh, that looks like it feels so good."

Follow these steps to find out how good Fido feels when he stretches:

1. **Move into the table pose: Rest on your hands and knees, with your hips, back, neck, and head forming a straight line.**

   Your knees should be directly under your hips and your hands directly under your shoulders.

2. **Roll up on your toes, *slowly* straighten your legs to push your hips upward, and drop your head toward the ground; keep your arms straight and elbows relaxed.**

   Keep your shoulders wide and away from your ears, and your feet about a foot apart.

TIP

Book IV

Powering Your Way to Fitness: Power Yoga

3. **Try to flatten your soles on the ground as your legs straighten; your feet should be about 1 foot apart.**

If you can't comfortably straighten your legs, don't force it! Don't worry if you can't straighten your legs when you first try this posture. Power Yoga is supposed to feel good, so don't push too hard.

4. **Without straining or locking your elbows or knees, try to create a 90-degree angle with your body as you make a straight line from your heels to your hips and another straight line from your hips to your hands (see Figure 3-4).**

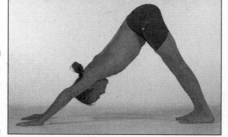

Figure 3-4:
The
downward-
facing dog.

Photograph by Raul Marroquin

5. **Gaze toward your toes, and begin taking slow breaths; try to hold this position for 3 to 5 complete breaths.**

6. **Relax, lower your knees to the ground, and fold your body in half, so that your seat rests near your heels and your forehead reaches all the way to the floor.**

Again, don't force yourself. Just relax.

7. **Stretch your arms in front of you, with palms facing downward.**

Keeping a relaxed and extended neck and throat, get as close to the floor as you can. This is called the child's pose with arms in front (head to Book II, Chapter 10 for details on this pose).

8. **Remain in this position as you take a few slow, deep breaths, and then slowly lift your torso and return to sitting on your knees in preparation for the next exercise.**

Moving with the missing link upward

The missing link upward pose is a movement that lets you connect seated poses to standing poses. In the missing link, you stretch and counter-stretch your back and neck, and you invigorate your spine with the movement's wavelike motion. This vinyasa teaches balance, grace, and self-confidence. The brain receives a gentle, peaceful vibration from the vinyasa's fluid movement and quiet transition. This cooler vinyasa requires minimum amounts of energy and is poetry in motion.

Follow these steps to achieve the missing link upward:

1. **Start from the seated angle pose.**

   Sit on the floor with your legs stretched straight before you and your arms at your sides (refer to Book IV, Chapter 2 to see what this posture looks like); engage your Mula bandha and Uddiyana bandha now (see Book IV, Chapter 1 for the location of these muscle locks).

2. **Exhale completely, and then inhale as you expand your chest and lift your arms out to your sides and over your head.**

3. **Start your exhalation, and slowly bend your elbows as you fold your arms over your chest in prayer fashion; as you fold your arms, bend your knees and bring your feet toward your torso (see Figure 3-5a).**

4. **When your knees are drawn up to your hands, separate your hands and lower your arms to your sides (see Figure 3-5b).**

   You should now be sitting in a compact ball, with your knees tucked into your body, your arms by your sides, and your hands resting on the floor.

5. **Still exhaling, push against your hands to raise your hips from the floor as you roll your torso forward and drop your head.**

   These movements help you flow into a standing forward bend, shown in Figure 3-5c.

    You should do Steps 3, 4, and 5 all in one exhalation, but if you can't quite handle that yet, take extra breaths as necessary. As your Power Yoga skills build, so will your ability to match your breathing to the ideal in this posture.

6. **Expand your chest as you lift your arms out to your sides, and come to a full standing position; stretch your arms straight up over your head, and gaze up toward your hands (Figure 3-5d).**

7. **Stand up straight as you lower your arms toward your sides and gaze forward in the mountain pose.**

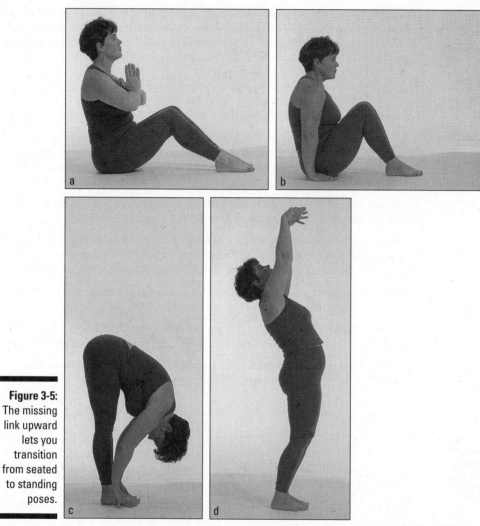

Figure 3-5:
The missing link upward lets you transition from seated to standing poses.

Photographs by Raul Marroquin

Building stability with the powerful chair

In the powerful chair posture *(utkatasana)*, you strengthen and firm the muscles of your legs, expand your chest, and release tension from your shoulders. In this posture, you take on the characteristics of a strong and powerful chair.

Follow these steps to achieve the powerful chair pose:

1. **Stand up straight, with shoulders back, spine straight, and vision forward; keep your feet together, and stand strong, yet relaxed.**

2. **Start taking slow, deep inhalations and exhalations, and practice your yoga breathing throughout this exercise.**

3. **On an inhalation, lift your arms out to your sides and over your head, bringing your palms together.**

4. **At the same time, bend your knees and come to a half sitting position, as if you were preparing to sit in a chair; gaze up toward your hands, and keep your lower back flat, tucking your tailbone forward. Feel your abdominal muscles engage (see Figure 3-6).**

5. **Hold this position for 5 to 10 slow, deep breaths.**

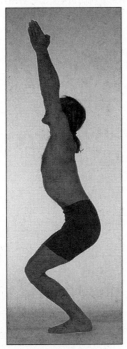

Figure 3-6:
The powerful chair pose.

Photograph by Raul Marroquin

Strengthening your upper body with wall push-ups and the standing dog stretch

Wall push-ups strengthen the muscles of your arms and shoulders and give your upper-body muscles a great stretch. In this exercise, you do some modified push-ups against a wall, and you finish with a standing dog stretch.

1. **With your arms extended, your hands should be about 1 to 2 feet from the wall.**

   Stand facing a wall, and extend your arms in front of you, toward the wall.

2. **From your standing position, lean forward and support yourself against the wall with your hands.**

3. **Exhale, and bend your arms to lower your chest to the wall; inhale, and push yourself away from the wall by straightening your arms, as shown in Figure 3-7.**

4. **Repeat Steps 1 through 3 five to ten times.**

Figure 3-7: Move fluidly through your wall push-ups without jerking or locking your elbows.

Photograph by Raul Marroquin

To make your wall push-ups more difficult, move out away from the wall; to make them easier, move closer to the wall.

5. **When you finish your push-ups, place your hands on the wall at about head level; keeping your arms straight, lean toward the wall, drop your head and shoulders downward, and extend your hips backward as if you were pushing a heavy load.**

   This exercise, called the standing dog stretch, gives your shoulders a great stretch and releases tension.

6. **Relax and return to a standing position.**

Building balance with the warrior I

In Power Yoga, you use three variations of the warrior pose *(virabhadrasana)*. In warrior I, used in this exercise, your arms come together pointed toward the sky.

The warrior I pose opens your chest and shoulders and works to stimulate the nerves in your spine and to correct its alignment. This pose strengthens the muscles of your legs, opens your hips, and builds flexibility in your back and ankles. The warrior I posture improves your balance and can leave you feeling refreshed and confident. To see how to prepare for and move into the warrior pose, check out the video at www.dummies.com/go/yogaaiofd.

Follow these steps to be a warrior, or at least feel like one:

1. **Start this posture from the expanded mountain pose (see Figure 3-8a).**

   Stand with your spine straight, shoulders back, arms at your sides, and feet about 4 feet apart.

2. **Pivot on your feet to turn your body to the right until your right foot points straight to your right and your left foot is at a 45-degree angle from your right.**

   Your hips, shoulders, and torso should be squarely aligned to your right and your feet firmly planted on the ground.

3. **Lunge forward by bending your right knee until it forms a 90-degree angle from your hamstring to calf muscle.**

   Your knee should be over your heel and your thigh parallel to the floor.

4. **On an inhalation, lift your arms out to your sides and over your head; straighten your arms, touch your palms together, and point toward the sky.**

   Tilt your head back only as far as necessary to see your thumbs. Remember to keep your shoulders broad and down from your ears.

Book IV

Powering Your Way to Fitness: Power Yoga

TIP

5. **Drop your head back and stretch your torso upward, as shown in Figure 3-8b, keeping your back foot flat on the floor.**

If this move is too difficult or uncomfortable, turn your toes downward on your left leg and rest on your toes.

Figure 3-8:
From the expanded mountain pose (a), you pivot to the right, and then lower your body into the warrior I posture (b).

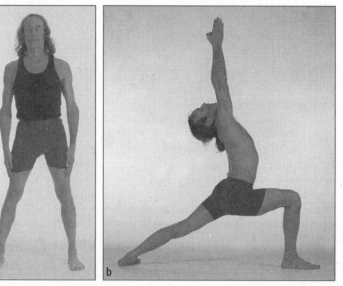

Photographs by Raul Marroquin

6. **Hold this position for 5 to 10 complete breaths, and then inhale and straighten your right leg.**

7. **Drop your arms to your sides, return to the expanded mountain pose (as described in Step 1), and relax.**

8. **Repeat Steps 3 through 7, but lunge on your left leg this time.**

Finding the missing link downward

It's time to take the missing link in the opposite direction to return you to the floor for your seated asanas.

Follow these steps to achieve the missing link downward:

1. **Start from the mountain I pose: Stand up straight, with your shoulders back and your arms down by your sides.**

2. **On an inhalation, lift your arms out to your sides and over your head, and touch your palms together in the mountain III pose as seen in Figure 3-9a.**

3. **Exhale, and fold forward at your hips, moving into a standing forward bend as you lower your arms toward your feet (Figure 3-9b).**

   Rest your hands on the floor beside your feet.

4. **Inhale, and bend your knees as if you were preparing to sit in a chair.**

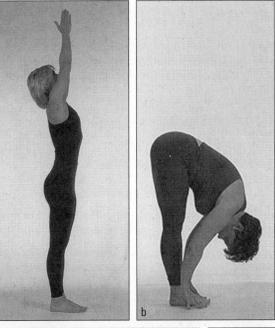

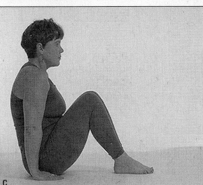
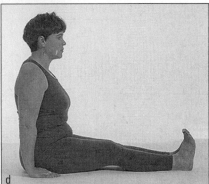

Figure 3-9:
The missing link downward lets you transition from standing to sitting poses.

Photographs by Raul Marroquin

5. **Lift your head upward, and continue lowering your body until your hips touch the floor; support your hips with your hands on the floor in the beach ball pose, as shown in Figure 3-9c.**

6. **Exhale, and straighten your legs in front of you, resting into the seated angle pose and forming a 90-degree angle from head to hips and hips to feet (Figure 3-9d).**

Stretching your leg and back muscles with the seated forward bend

The seated forward bend (*paschimottanasana*) stretches muscles on the back of your body — the back of your legs, the muscles along your spine, and your shoulders and upper back — and therefore is named for the direction that those muscles belong to.

The Sanskrit word *paschima* translates as "west." As you face the east, your back is to the west.

Follow these steps to practice stretching your "west" side:

1. **Start from the seated angle pose; exhale completely.**

2. **With an inhalation, lift your arms in front of your body and over your head; keep your wrists soft as you completely fill your lungs with air.**

3. **On an exhalation, gently lower your arms outward in a circular motion, reaching toward your toes, as shown in Figure 3-10a.**

Figure 3-10:
The seated forward bend (a) and expanded seated forward bend (b) stretch the whole back of your body — neck to calves.

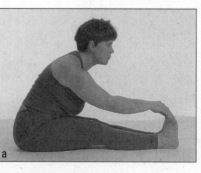 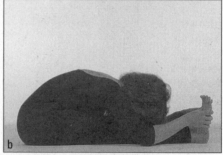

Photographs by Raul Marroquin

4. **If you're relatively flexible, try to rest your torso on your thighs and take hold of your toes with your hands, keeping your feet flexed upward; relax and hold this position for 5 slow, deep breaths.**

   This is the extended seated forward bend, as shown in Figure 3-10b.

   As an alternative, you can place a pillow under your knees for support and place your hands on your shins instead of reaching for your toes. You can also wrap a yoga strap around your feet and hold the ends of the strap rather than grasping your feet in your hands.

5. **On an inhalation, slowly return your torso to an upright position as you lift your arms over your head, keeping your wrists soft; exhale, and lower arms to your sides, returning to the seated angle pose.**

Working your stomach muscles in the boat pose

The boat pose *(navasana)* is a good alternative for a full-power vinyasa, and it strengthens many of the muscles necessary for a progressive Power Yoga practice. In this pose, you resemble a boat floating in the water.

Follow these steps to work your stomach muscles with the boat pose:

1. **Begin in the seated angle pose — hands by your sides and legs extended in front of you; bend your knees, and place your feet flat on the floor.**

2. **Rock back on your rear as you lift your feet off the floor and extend your arms to your sides parallel to the ground; balance in this position for 3 complete breaths.**

3. **Straighten your legs as you lift them to form a 45-degree angle with the floor, as shown in Figure 3-11.**

   This leg-lift gives your stomach and legs an even greater workout.

Figure 3-11:
In the boat pose, you strengthen the muscles of your stomach, legs, and arms.

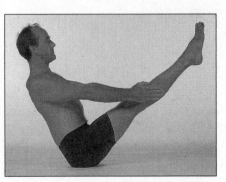

Photograph by Raul Marroquin

Counter-stretching with the cobra pose

In the cobra pose *(bhujangasana),* you resemble a snake slowly uncoiling as you roll back your vertebra one at a time. The cobra pose is an excellent counter-stretch for the seated forward bend because it stretches the muscles on the front of your body. For help with preparing for and moving into the cobra pose, watch the video at www.dummies.com/go/yogaaiofd.

Follow these steps to achieve the cobra pose:

1. **Lie on your stomach with your arms extended by your sides and your palms facing upward; turn your head to one side and then the other, and then close your eyes and relax for a few seconds.**

2. **Turn your face to the floor, and rest on your forehead; bend your elbows, and place your hands up under your shoulders.**

   Your feet should be pointed yet relaxed.

3. **On an inhalation, slowly lift your shoulders and torso off the floor, one vertebra at a time (see Figure 3-12).**

   Lift as high as is comfortable for you. If the lifting action becomes uncomfortable, rest on your elbows. If you're more flexible, lift your torso as you straighten your arms higher by extending your arms more.

   You can protect your lower back by pressing the tailbone down to engage the abdominal muscles. Keep the abs engaged as you lift your torso to prevent over-arching the lower back.

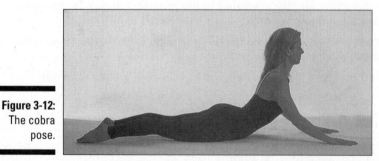

Figure 3-12:
The cobra
pose.

Photograph by Raul Marroquin

4. **When you reach your maximum comfortable stretch, remain in that position for 5 deep breaths.**

   If you have a stiff lower back, you can separate your legs a bit and allow your ankles to turn outward.

5. Exhale, and lower your torso and shoulders to the floor; take your hands out from under your shoulders, extend your arms to your sides, turn your head to the side, and relax.

Sitting and breathing in the easy posture

Before you go into a deep relaxation at the end of your Power Yoga workout, you can slow yourself down with some yogic breathing techniques. This gradual cooling off in your routine helps you to relax completely.

When you prepare for any breathing exercise, begin by finding your center and quieting your mind. You may be more comfortable and find holding a good posture easier if you sit on a small pillow rather than sitting directly on the floor or on your yoga mat. As always, you may sit on the edge of a chair if that is more comfortable to you. The object is to be able to concentrate on your breathing, not the pain in your backside!

Follow these steps to easy breathing:

1. **Repeat the yoga breathing exercise recommended at the beginning of this routine (refer to "Starting well is breathing well").**

2. **When you finish your yoga breathing, lie down on your back and prepare for a wonderful journey into deep relaxation.**

Enjoying a moment of deep relaxation with the corpse posture

In the corpse posture, you lie flat on the floor, completely relaxed and motionless. The corpse posture, shown in Figure 3-13, is a great way to experience the deep relaxation phase that caps off your Power Yoga session.

Figure 3-13: To get the most from the corpse posture, pay close attention to your yoga breathing techniques.

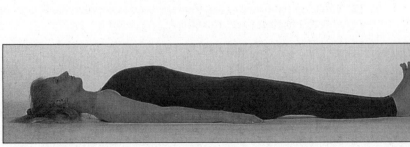

Photograph by Raul Marroquin

In the deep relaxation phase, you release stress and tension throughout your entire body and mind. Your blood pressure decreases, your heart rate slows, and you're rewarded with a euphoric feeling that can last for hours. You also relieve stress and tension and create total relaxation in every fiber of your body. The deep relaxation phase promotes complete physical and mental rejuvenation as it boosts your motivation and self-esteem.

1. **Lie on your back, with your arms at your sides and your legs extended (the corpse pose).**

2. **Close your eyes, relax, and begin taking slow, deep breaths.**

3. **Lift your right leg about 12 inches from the floor, tense every muscle in your leg for a few seconds, relax, and then gently lower your leg to the floor; repeat this step with your left leg.**

4. **Tighten the muscles in your hips and buttocks for a few seconds, and then relax and let your gluteus muscles melt into the floor.**

5. **Arch your back, pressing down with your elbows and shoulders as you expand your chest toward the ceiling; hold this position for a few seconds, gently lower your back to the floor, and then relax.**

6. **Press your lower back into the floor by tightening your buttocks and stomach muscles as you press against the floor; hold this position for a few seconds, and then relax completely.**

7. **Lift your right arm about 12 inches off the floor, tensing all the muscles; hold this position for a few seconds, relax and lower your arm to the floor, and repeat this step with your left arm.**

8. **Roll your head slowly to the right and then to the left; return your head to the center, and relax.**

9. **Fill your mouth with air, blowing your cheeks out like balloons; hold for a couple of seconds, and then relax and release the air.**

10. **Gently stretch all your facial muscles, and then relax them.**

11. **Close your eyes, take 5 slow, deep breaths, and clear your mind.**

12. **Working from your toes to your head, visualize each part of your body and tell each muscle to relax.**

13. **Visualize your heart, and mentally ask your heart to relax.**

14. **Visualize your brain, and calm it by releasing your thoughts.**

15. **Clear your mind of all but the most pleasant and positive thoughts.**

16. **After 5 to 30 minutes, slowly stretch your arms over your head on an inhalation and then roll over onto your right side, with your arms and legs slightly bent; remain in this position for a few breaths.**

17. Gradually return to a sitting position and try to preserve the positive uplifting thoughts you created.

You should feel calm, refreshed, relaxed, and ready to go! To keep the good feelings alive, consider taking a quiet walk in one of your favorite settings. Notice the world around you, and be happy that you're on the way to becoming a full-fledged power yogi or yogini.

Book IV

Powering
Your Way
to Fitness:
Power
Yoga

Chapter 4

Following Buddha's Way: A Moderate Power Routine

In This Chapter

▶ Getting ready for an intermediate-level workout

▶ Taking the middle road with Buddha's Way

Centuries ago, Buddha determined that the true path to enlightenment was the middle way — nothing radical or extreme, just consistent, persistent progress. This routine is named Buddha's Way because it's an intermediate-level Power Yoga routine that offers a moderate approach to building your Power Yoga fitness.

This routine is moderate in every way; it even takes a moderate amount of time to complete. Most folks can complete this routine in about 60 minutes. The Buddha's Way routine is a bit more challenging than the Just a Walk in the Park routine in Book IV, Chapter 3, but it's a good, strong intermediate workout when you're ready to move up to the next stage of your Power Yoga practice.

Progressing along Buddha's Way

The Buddha's Way routine helps you build the strength and stamina that you need to keep progressing in your Power Yoga practice.

As an intermediate-level student, you may want to concentrate some of your effort on developing the "flow" of your practice. Approach the workout with confidence, and move through it at your own pace, being sure to focus on your yoga breathing throughout the routine (see Book IV Chapter 1 for information specific to Power Yoga breathing and Book II, Chapter 1 for general yogic breathing techniques).

These tips may help you as you move through the Buddha's Way Power Yoga workout:

- ✔ **Practice at your own pace.** If you find that this routine is too strenuous for you, go back to the Just a Walk in the Park in Book IV, Chapter 3 until that routine feels too easy. You're on your own schedule, so choose the Power Yoga practice that's best for you.

- ✔ **Prepare your workout environment.** Before you begin this workout session, make sure that your workout space is ready. The room should be warm and, if possible, have a good supply of fresh air. Gather your props — a yoga mat, blocks, straps, or pillows — and have them nearby.

The Intermediate Routine: Buddha's Way

This routine starts off with some Power Yoga breathing techniques, moves softly into a few warm-ups, and then provides a mild *vinyasa* (linking movement) to standing. From the standing position, you get a taste of some powerful standing poses, and then move softly back to the floor for some traditional, finishing *asanas* (poses). Then your journey ends with breathing and deep relaxation.

Getting off to a good start with yoga breathing

Take a few minutes to practice your breathing before you start your yoga exercises. This routine is a bit more demanding than beginner-level routines, and you need to prepare your body and mind for the session ahead. In the course of this routine, you also use the yoga breathing and the jnana mudra hand position from Book IV, Chapter 3.

You may feel more comfortable sitting on the edge of a sturdy, non-rolling chair or on a pillow during this exercise. Either position is fine; just be certain to keep your back straight and your mind relaxed but alert.

Follow these steps to practice good yoga breathing:

1. **Sit on the floor in the seated posture of your choice.**

   Try out several seated poses and work on the ones you find the most difficult.

2. **Extend your arms over your knees, resting your wrists on your knees, with your palms facing upward; form jnana mudra with your hands.**

3. **Begin your yoga breathing; as you breathe, visualize your lungs expanding on inhalations and contracting on exhalations.**

   As an intermediate student, strive to lengthen the time of your inhalations and exhalations, so that you breathe more slowly and take in more oxygen.

4. **Hold this position for 10 to 15 slow, deep breaths.**

   Continue your yoga breathing throughout this session.

Letting the cat chase your dog

You begin this exercise with a little cat stretch, and then find your wild cat chasing your downward-facing dog up into the air. (If you need a brush-up on the downward-facing dog, check out Book IV, Chapter 3.)

The cat chases your dog stretch tones up your back muscles, strengthens your arms, and can make your entire spine feel stronger and more flexible. If you suffer from minor back pain brought on by stress, over-activity, or bad posture, this exercise can help relieve that pain and get you back in action.

Follow these steps to play cat-and-dog:

1. **Sit back on your heels, with your toes pointing back; your back should be straight, and you should feel your neck lengthen.**

2. **Lift your hips, and place your hands on the floor so that you're resting on your hands and knees (keep your shoulders over your hands). Keep your back straight, but not rigid, gaze toward the floor, and relax as you take 3 slow, deep breaths.**

3. **On an exhalation, arch your back like a cat; relax your neck as you drop your head and gaze toward your knees (see Figure 4-1a).**

4. **On an inhalation, lower your back and let it sway downward as you bend your arms to lower your chest and bring your chin to rest on the floor between your hands (see Figure 4-1b).**

Book IV

Powering
Your Way
to Fitness:
Power
Yoga

5. **Exhale, slowly draw your body upward, and return to the arched-back position you entered in Step 3.**

6. **Straighten your arms and legs, lifting your hips to form a 90-degree angle with your body; lengthen your torso from your hands to your hips, spread your fingers, and flatten your hands firmly onto the floor.**

   This position is the downward-facing dog pose (see Figure 4-1c).

7. **Roll your shoulders down toward your hips and open your chest.**

   Your feet should be about 12 inches apart, forming a solid base for this posture. Try to keep your feet flat on the floor, with your heels down. But if this position is uncomfortable for you, don't force it; bend your knees slightly and shorten the distance between your feet and your hands.

8. **Relax your mind, and gaze toward your toes; hold this position for 5 slow, deep breaths.**

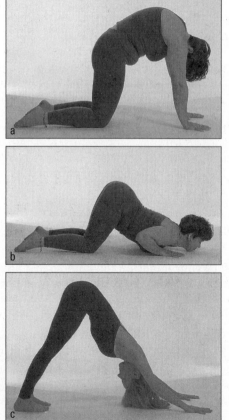

Figure 4-1:
The cat chases your dog stretch.

Photographs by Raul Marroquin

Warming your muscles with downward dog push-ups

Why not train your dog to do some push-ups and really turn up the heat? Downward dog push-ups help you to build strength in your arms and shoulders. This pose helps prepare you for headstands — some of the more demanding vinyasas — and arm-balance exercises.

Follow these steps to warm up your dog:

1. **From the downward-facing dog posture (refer to Figure 4-1c), bend your elbows so that they touch the floor; rest on your forearms, and interlace your fingers.**

2. **Keep your head off the floor, and gaze toward your hands (see Figure 4-2a).**

3. **On an exhalation, lower your chin over your interlocked hands as shown in Figure 4-2b, inhale, and push yourself back to the downward-facing dog posture.**

Figure 4-2:
You use the downward-facing dog posture to launch into these push-ups.

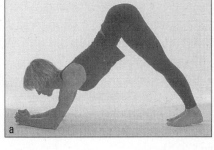 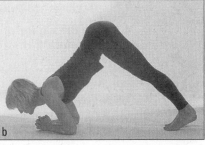

Photographs by Raul Marroquin

4. **Repeat Steps 1 through 3 five times and then lower your knees to the floor and bend forward at your waist, resting your torso on your thighs with your arms stretched in front of you, palms facing downward; relax in this child's pose for 1 to 2 breaths.**

5. **Sit up slowly.**

Book IV

Powering Your Way to Fitness: Power Yoga

Stretching into the extended triangle pose

In the extended triangle *(utthita trikonasana)* pose, you form an extended triangle with your body. This pose helps relieve backaches, tones your spine, and strengthens your back. It also helps strengthen your hamstrings, thigh muscles, and calf muscles.

Follow these steps to achieve the extended triangle pose:

1. **Begin in the mountain pose I (see Figure 4-3a).**

   Exhale completely, and on an inhalation, step your right foot out about 3½ to 4 feet from your left foot; at the same time, extend your arms out at your sides and parallel to the floor.

2. **On an exhalation, pivot your right foot to the right and turn your left foot in at about a 45-degree angle; try to keep your hips and shoulders facing forward.**

3. **Still exhaling, tilt your torso to your right and lower your right hand toward the toes of your right foot.**

   To keep your ribs extending evenly, roll your torso over the top of your thigh, creating a fold at the hip (not a rounding at the waist). It's much like folding the flap of an envelope over when sealing a letter.

4. **Grasp the big toe of your right foot with the first two fingers of your right hand.**

   If you aren't flexible enough to reach your toe, rest your elbow on your right knee or rest your right hand on a block at the outside of your right ankle.

5. **Lift your left arm straight into the air with your palm facing outward, making a 90-degree angle with your torso; direct your gaze toward your left hand (see Figure 4-3b).**

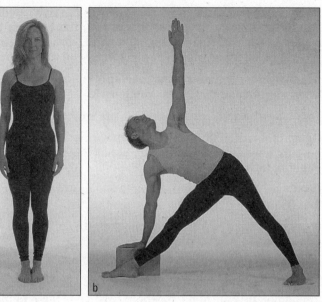

Figure 4-3:
The extended triangle pose is an excellent way to keep your back in shape, expand your chest, and improve your balance, even if you use a block.

Photographs by Raul Marroquin

6. **Continue your slow, deep yoga breathing, and hold this position for 5 complete breaths; keep your torso extended over your right leg, and try to keep your chest expanded and your back flat.**

7. **Inhale, and lift your torso to a standing position, extending your arms out to your sides so that they're parallel to the floor.**

8. **Exhale, and lower your arms by your sides.**

9. **Repeat Steps 2 through 8 on your left side.**

   Stand with your feet approximately 3½ to 4 feet apart.

10. **On an inhalation, turn both feet in to point forward; exhale, lower your arms to your sides, and then inhale, jumping or stepping your feet back together into the mountain pose I.**

Joining the two warriors

The warrior poses *(virabhadrasana)* get their names from their powerful, wide stance. Warrior pose I and warrior pose II tone and strengthen your leg muscles, expand your chest, and help you develop deep, powerful breathing and good balance. Follow these steps to achieve the warrior pose II:

1. **Begin in the expanded mountain pose.**

   Stand with your spine straight, your shoulders back, your feet about 4 feet apart, and your arms resting by your sides.

REMEMBER

Book IV

Powering
Your Way
to Fitness:
Power
Yoga

2. **Pivot on your feet, and turn your body to the right, with your right foot facing straight to your right and your left foot at a 45-degree angle to your right foot; square your hips, shoulders, and torso to your right side, and plant your feet firmly on the ground.**

3. **Lunge by bending your right knee until it forms a 90-degree angle from your hamstring to your calf muscle.**

   Your knee should be over your heel and your thigh parallel to the floor.

4. **On an inhalation, lift your arms out to your sides and over your head, keeping your arms straight, your palms together, and your fingers pointing toward the sky.**

5. **Drop your head, and stretch your torso upward, keeping your back foot flat on the floor.**

   If this position is too difficult or uncomfortable, turn the toes of your left foot down and rest on your toes.

6. **Hold this position for 5 breaths, and then lower your arms until they're parallel to the floor.**

7. **Remaining in your lunge position, twist your torso to the left as you extend your right arm over your right thigh and parallel to the floor; at the same time, extend your left arm behind you, over your left leg and parallel to the floor.**

8. **Square off your hips, shoulders, and torso to the front, in line with your arms (see Figure 4-4).**

   Your arms may form a slight incline as your right arm angles upward and your left arm angles down a bit.

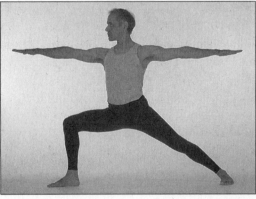

Figure 4-4:
The warrior
pose II.

Photograph by Raul Marroquin

9. Keep your gaze forward, along the line of your leading arm; anchor both feet firmly on the ground.

10. Hold this position for 5 complete breaths.

11. Straighten your right leg on an inhalation; drop your arms to your sides, return to the expanded mountain pose from Step 1, and relax.

12. Repeat Steps 1 through 11 on your left side.

Moving back down with the missing link downward

In this sequence, you take the missing link in the opposite direction, to return to the floor for your seated *asanas.* If you need a refresher on the movements for missing link downward, check out Book IV, Chapter 3.

1. Perform the missing link downward.

2. Continue your yoga breathing.

Stretching into the head-to-knee pose

The missing link downward *(janu sirsasana)* stretches your hamstrings and calf muscles, and it helps to keep your knees flexible and strong. This exercise can also enhance the functions of your prostate gland, spleen, and kidneys. In Sanskrit, *janu* means "knee" and *sirsa* means "head." So you won't be surprised that in this posture, you lower your head toward your knee.

Follow these steps:

1. Start from the seated angle pose (refer to Book IV, Chapter 3).

2. Keep your feet pointed upward and slightly flexed as you fold your hands in your lap.

3. Bend your right knee, placing your right foot against your left thigh and bringing the heel of your right foot toward your groin as you try to lower your right knee to the floor.

Don't push your knee past its endurance. If you can't lower your knee all the way to the ground, place a small pillow under it to provide support.

This pose depends on flexibility in your hips, not your knees. You should feel little, if any, tugging in your knees.

Book IV

Powering Your Way to Fitness: Power Yoga

4. **On an inhalation, expand your chest and lift your arms to your sides and over your head above your shoulders; let your eyes follow your hands as they rise above your head.**

   Your left leg should be extended and your foot flexed upward.

5. **Exhale, lowering your arms out and down toward your feet as you bend your torso forward and reach toward the toes of your extended left leg.**

   Keep your torso aligned with your extended left leg. If your flexibility is limited, try bending your left knee slightly and placing your hands on your left shin.

   Stay tuned into the sensations in your lower back and make sure you don't overstretch!

6. **Take the toes of your left foot in both hands, and gently pull back on your foot.**

   If you aren't feeling that flexible, use a yoga strap to extend your reach.

7. **Lift your elbows up; keeping them slightly bent, gaze toward your toes; hold the position for 5 deep breaths (see Figure 4-5).**

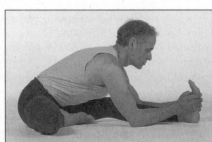

Figure 4-5: The seated angle pose gives your leg muscles a great stretch and opens your hips.

Photograph by Raul Marroquin

8. **Exhale completely; on an inhalation, return to the seated position by letting your hands slide up your leg and lifting your arms over your head.**

9. **Exhale, and lower your arms to your sides as you straighten out your bent right leg to return to the seated angle position.**

10. **Repeat Steps 1 through 9 on your other side.**

Flying on the incline plane (purvottanasana)

In this posture, the name relates to the front side of your body (which faces east during many Hindu practices). As you may guess from its name, in this posture you stretch the muscles on the front of your body. In the United States, you often hear this position called the incline plane.

1. **Start from the seated angle position (refer to Book IV, Chapter 3).**

2. **On an inhalation, expand your chest, lifting your arms out to your sides and over your head and keeping your wrists soft and your palms facing outward.**

3. **Exhale while lowering your arms to your sides — back to the starting position; place your hands on the floor behind your hips, and bend your knees to bring your feet toward your groin.**

4. **Inhale, and lift your hips into the air as you drop your head slightly backward and gaze toward the ceiling.**

   Your knees should be bent at a 90-degree angle and your feet flat on the floor; your arms and hands support your body, which is parallel to the floor from the knees to the shoulders. You're now in the beginner's incline plane (see Figure 4-6a).

5. **Hold this position for 3 complete, deep breaths, and then return to the seated angle position.**

   To do the advanced version of this position, try to straighten your legs completely to form a straight line with your body that inclines from the floor at a 45-degree angle, like a ramp.

6. **Place your feet as close together as possible with the soles of your feet flat on the ground, and try to maintain the line of your incline plane; drop your head backward, and continue with your slow, deep breathing for 5 complete breaths (see Figure 4-6b).**

Book IV

Powering Your Way to Fitness: Power Yoga

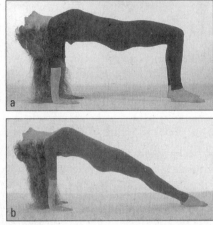

Photographs by Raul Marroquin

7. **Exhale, and bend at the waist to lower your hips to the floor and return to the seated angle position; exhale completely, relax, and prepare to move on to the next exercise.**

Rolling into the one-arm cobra pose

The cobra pose *(bhujangasana)* helps promote good posture, expand your chest, and open stiff shoulders. The cobra stretches all the muscles on the front of your body and builds flexibility in your spine.

1. **Lie on your stomach, with your arms along your sides and your palms facing upward; turn your head to one side, close your eyes, and relax for a few seconds.**

2. **Turn your face downward, and rest your forehead on the floor; bend your elbows, pulling them close to your body, and place your hands under your shoulders.**

   Your feet should be pointing straight behind you.

3. **On an inhalation, begin slowly lifting your shoulders and torso off the floor, one vertebra at a time, like a snake slowly uncoiling; lift as high as you comfortably can.**

   If you become uncomfortable, rest on your elbows. If you're feeling fairly flexible, lift your torso higher by extending your arms farther in front of you.

Keep your shoulders back and down, away from your ears. This position is the cobra pose.

4. **When you reach your maximum comfortable stretch, shift your weight to your right by pivoting your right forearm inward, parallel to your shoulders and extending your left arm across your lower back.**

5. **At the same time, bend your right knee and lift your right foot toward the ceiling; try to grasp your right ankle with your left hand, as shown in Figure 4-7.**

Figure 4-7: The one-arm cobra provides tension-releasing shoulder and thigh stretches.

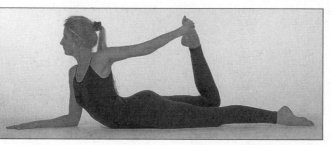

Photograph by Raul Marroquin

6. **Remain in this position for 5 deep breaths.**

   If you find this position too difficult, go back to Step 3 and remain in the cobra pose.

7. **Exhale, release your ankle, and return your torso and shoulders to the floor; as you do so, take your hands out from under your shoulders, and extend your arms back along your sides.**

8. **Turn your head to one side, and relax.**

9. **Repeat Steps 4 through 8 on the other side — reaching your right arm back behind your back and grasping your left ankle.**

Going all the way with the half vinyasa

This half vinyasa is just the right size to create a little heat as you move from a facedown resting pose to a sitting position.

Follow these steps to achieve a half vinyasa:

1. **As you lie facedown, bring your hands up under your shoulders, place your palms on the floor, and move your feet up onto your toes (see Figure 4-8a).**

   This pose is the four limb staff.

2. **On an inhalation, straighten your arms, lifting your torso, head, and shoulders upward in a big arch toward the ceiling; push forward with your toes, and look upward (see Figure 4-8b).**

   This position is upward-facing dog.

3. **Exhale; keeping your arms straight, drop your head toward the floor as you lift your hips upward to move into the downward-facing dog, forming a 90-degree angle with your legs and torso (see Figure 4-8c).**

4. **Bend your knees, and step or jump forward with your arms supporting your weight (see Figure 4-8d); then lower your hips to the floor, and come to a sitting position with your hands on the floor beside you (see Figure 4-8e).**

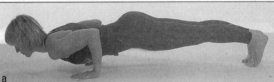

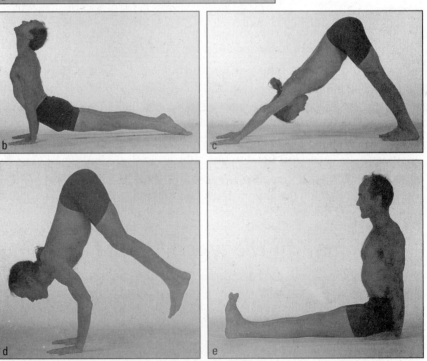

Figure 4-8: This half vinyasa jumps you from the downward-facing dog position (c) into the seated angle posture (e).

Photographs by Raul Marroquin

Cranking it up in the twist pose

The twist pose *(ardha matsyendrasana)* is a great stretching and flexing exercise for your spine, and it can help relieve backaches. The twist also stretches the muscles in your shoulders, around your ribs, and in your neck to relieve tension and leave you feeling invigorated.

In Hindu legend, Matsyendra was a fish that twisted around in order to hear the secrets of yoga from Lord Siva. Matsyendra was then incarnated in human form, in order to spread the knowledge of yoga. This posture is dedicated to Matsyendra, the twisted fish. The Sanskrit word *ardha,* meaning "half," refers to the half-twisting motion of the pose.

Follow these steps to twist the night away:

1. **Sit on the floor with both legs extended, your spine straight, and your shoulders back.**

   This position is the seated angle pose (refer to Book IV, Chapter 3).

2. **Bend your right knee, and place your right foot over and beside your left leg; then bend your left leg in to bring your left foot up toward your right hip.**

   Keep both cheeks on the floor. If this position isn't possible, add a little support under the side that rises up so that you can lengthen your back in comfort.

3. **Raise your arms, and twist your torso to the right; try to move your left elbow to the outside of your right knee.**

4. **Place your right hand on the floor behind your back for support.**

5. **Continue twisting your torso to the right and looking over your right shoulder; hold this position for 5 complete breaths.**

   If you're very flexible, move to Step 6; if you have limited flexibility, move to Step 7.

   Remember to lengthen, to keep both shoulders down, and to enjoy the sensation.

6. **Place your left hand and arm under the bridge that you form with your right leg; reach behind your back with your left hand and try to grasp your right wrist as you continue to gaze over your right shoulder (see Figure 4-9).**

   Hold this position for 5 complete breaths.

Book IV

Powering Your Way to Fitness: Power Yoga

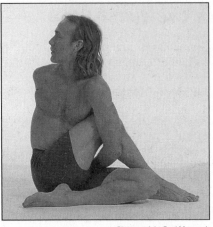

Figure 4-9:
The advanced twist pose gives your back and shoulder muscles a thorough stretch.

Photograph by Raul Marroquin

7. **Untwist your torso, and straighten your legs to return to the seated angle position; exhale and relax.**

   As you reverse the twist, release your head and neck first, your shoulders next, and finally your hips.

8. **Repeat Steps 3 through 7, this time twisting to the left (placing your left leg up and over your right leg, bending your right leg up, twisting your torso to the left, and so on).**

9. **After you return to the seated angle position, relax for a few breaths, and then lie on your back.**

Moving up to the shoulder stand

In the shoulder stand *(salamba sarvangasana),* you support your body with your hands and elbows, and balance on your shoulders. The shoulder stand is what's known in the yoga world as an *inverted pose;* inverted poses are powerful exercises that have positive effects on your entire body (refer to Book II, Chapter 6 for more on inversion poses).

The shoulder stand helps to create harmony and happiness throughout your body. In this inverted asana, your heart and brain receive a healthy rush of blood; the pose stimulates your endocrine system and gives your thyroid and parathyroid glands a tune-up. The shoulder stand can even help reverse the effects of varicose veins! Best of all, when you come out of the shoulder stand, you feel refreshed and rejuvenated.

Follow these steps to achieve the shoulder stand:

1. **Lie flat on your back, with your arms extended by your sides, your feet about 1 foot apart, your palms facing upward, and your mind calm and relaxed.**

   This pose is the corpse position (refer to Book IV, Chapter 3).

2. **Begin your yoga breathing, and bend your knees to pull your feet toward you, keeping them flat on the floor about 1 foot from your rear end.**

3. **Exhale completely, and on an inhalation, straighten your legs toward the ceiling; when your legs are straight, exhale and relax in that position.**

4. **On your next inhalation, place your hands under your hips and push down to lift your hips off the floor; tuck your elbows behind your back, and use your hands to support your elevated legs and hips.**

5. **Lift your feet toward the ceiling, tucking your chin down into your chest.**

   This position is the shoulder stand, as shown in Figure 4-10a.

6. **Extend your legs and torso as high as you comfortably can, supporting your back with your hands.**

   Hold this posture for 5 to 20 slow, deep breaths.

If your neck is stiff or if you have problems getting into or maintaining this pose, lower your legs and try the pose again. This time, use a folded blanket or towel as a prop to raise your shoulders a few inches off the floor. Your head should not rest on the prop, but should hang lower than your shoulders, as shown in Figure 4-10b. The key point is that your neck doesn't support the weight of your body.

Another alternative is to start your shoulder stand with your legs extended up a wall and your hips resting flush against the wall; doing so allows you to use the wall as a prop for support (see Figure 4-10c).

Book IV

Powering Your Way to Fitness: Power Yoga

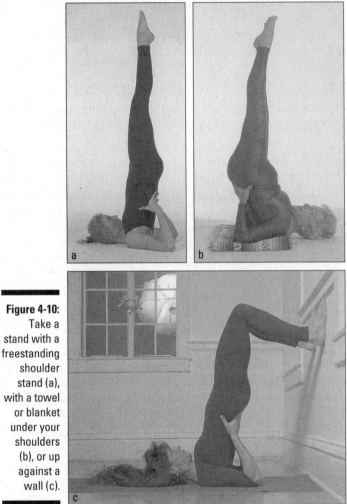

Figure 4-10:
Take a
stand with a
freestanding
shoulder
stand (a),
with a towel
or blanket
under your
shoulders
(b), or up
against a
wall (c).

Photographs by Raul Marroquin

Rising into the fish posture

The fish posture *(matsyasana)* stretches your neck and expands your chest
to help promote deep, healthy breathing. The posture also opens your hips,
rejuvenates your thyroid and parathyroid glands, and helps release tension
from your shoulders.

In Sanskrit, *matsya* means "fish." This posture is dedicated to Matsya, the fish incarnation of Visnu, the "source and maintainer of all things."

Follow these steps to achieve the fish posture:

1. **Lie flat on your back, with your feet about 1 foot apart and your arms extended by your sides.**

   This pose is the corpse position.

2. **Turn your palms downward, and arch your back to expand your chest.**

3. **Push down with your elbows, arms, and hands and place your hands under your hips; resting on your elbows, arch your back again to push your chest upward as you drop your head back (see Figure 4-11).**

Figure 4-11:
The object of the fish posture is to create a counter-stretch for the shoulder stand.

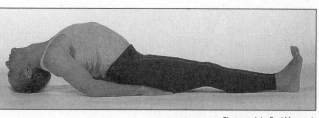

Photograph by Raul Marroquin

4. **Lower the top of your head to the floor.**

5. **Arch the front of your body as much as you can; hold this position for 5 slow, deep breaths.**

6. **Exhale, move your hands out from beneath you and straighten your legs; relax into the corpse position for 3 deep breaths.**

7. **Roll onto your right side, and come to a cross-legged sitting posture.**

Weighing in on the scale pose

The scale pose *(tolasana)* is an excellent posture for strengthening the muscles in your stomach, arms, and shoulders. Many Power Yoga routines incorporate this posture toward the end of the session to help practitioners prepare for deep relaxation. In Sanskrit, *tola* means a "pair of scales." In this asana, you balance your body's weight between your hands, using your shoulder muscles as the scales.

Book IV

Powering Your Way to Fitness: Power Yoga

These steps help you balance in the scale pose:

1. **Sit on the floor in the easy posture (legs crossed) or the lotus posture (legs crossed and feet on opposite thighs).**

2. **Place your hands on the floor beside your hips; push down with your hands to lift your torso off the floor, as shown in Figure 4-12.**

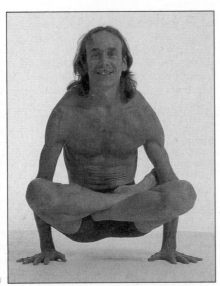

Figure 4-12:
The scale pose works almost all the muscles in your body and is traditionally used toward the end of a practice session, before deep relaxation.

Photograph by Raul Marroquin

If you have difficulty lifting your body with your hands, put some yoga blocks under your hands to give you some extra lift.

3. **While your body is suspended by your hands, lift your knees toward the ceiling and hold this position for 5 to 20 complete breaths.**

This movement works your stomach muscles.

4. **Lower your hips to the floor, straighten your legs, and relax.**

Congratulations! You've finished the intermediate-level Power Yoga routine with flying colors. You may want to extend the residual "good feeling" of this workout by taking a quiet walk in a favorite natural area. You'll find that the physical and mental benefits that you gained during this workout stay with you for a long time if you're aware of them (and the beauty of the world around you).

Chapter 5

Staying Young: Power Yoga for Seniors

Power Yoga can become your best friend as you hit the post-50 years. At any age, a moderate, regular Power Yoga practice can help you maintain good physical and mental health. But as you reach middle age and beyond, the Power Yoga benefits of increased strength, flexibility, and balance become even more critical. Power Yoga doesn't stop there, either, in helping you stay young as the years roll by. The strong cardiovascular workout of a good Power Yoga practice keeps your heart healthy and helps keep your blood pumping through strong, clean arteries. You'll be more alert and more comfortable in body and mind.

In this chapter, you discover how you can adapt Power Yoga routines to cater to your changing body, lifestyle, and fitness needs. This chapter also points out a few special considerations to ensure a safe and comfortable Power Yoga journey.

Embracing Power Yoga for All Ages

Beyond death and taxes, you can count on one other thing in life: change. Time passes, and everyone gets older (and that's the good scenario). But getting older doesn't mean that you have to be less active. In fact, after you jump that 50-year hurdle, a strong, active schedule of physical activity becomes more important than ever.

You don't need to be a mountain climber-in-training to require a good workout program in your later years; whether you plan to putter around the house or run marathons post-retirement, you need to work at maintaining good fitness, strength, and flexibility. Of all the forms of exercise practiced today, yoga has been proven to be one of the most beneficial exercises for your whole body and mind. Power Yoga has all the benefits of traditional soft-form yoga, with additional aerobic and muscle-strengthening aspects built in.

Of course, your body does change as it ages, and any fitness routine that you adopt needs to be designed to fit your body's current condition. No single "condition" describes every post-50 body. Countless people in their 60s, 70s, 80s, and even 90s are out climbing mountains and living active lives; other folks are learning to develop a fitness routine late in life, so their bodies need more foundation fitness building. Whatever your condition, the key to building good physical and mental health is to adopt a moderately active program that gets you up and moving regularly.

Power Yoga is such a diverse practice. Many Power Yoga exercises are appropriate for anyone of any age — and most of them have beginner's variations or can be modified to suit older students. If you aren't very active, you can use a beginning-level Power Yoga routine and modify it as necessary to fit your abilities. The key is to practice for short periods on a regular basis; that way, you'll make good progress and build your endurance, strength, and flexibility over time.

Understanding Power Yoga benefits for seniors

Seniors get many benefits, such as reduced prices at restaurants and hotels, and (usually) a prime seat on a crowded bus! But Power Yoga brings you better benefits: the benefits of mental and physical health. If you've been active all your life, you may not notice some of the typical changes of an aging body: Muscles get tighter, reaction times slow, and breathing can become shallower, limiting endurance. Power Yoga fights many signs of aging by offering these benefits:

✔ **Increased flexibility:** Power Yoga stretches muscles to increase flexibility and reduce stiffness.

✔ **Stronger respiratory and cardiovascular systems:** Regular practice strengthens your respiratory system; as you consume more oxygen during your workouts and yoga breathing exercises, your lung capacity goes up and your *prana* energy (vital life force) flourishes. By oxygenating your blood, you nourish your entire body — blood, muscles, and brain. You feel refreshed and can think more clearly.

✔ **Increased muscle strength:** Research touts the benefits of weightlifting for the elderly, including the prevention of osteoporosis. Power Yoga is a form of weightlifting. Your practice challenges you to lift, push, and pull the weight of your body as you move into one yoga posture after another.

✔ **Better endurance, balance, and coordination:** You grow stronger and build endurance to keep going longer. Power Yoga increases your coordination and balance, too. These are critical factors for leading an active, healthy life and avoiding painful, crippling falls and accidents.

✔ **Confidence and peace of mind:** With an energetic, strong, well-balanced, and vital body, you feel confident and at peace. You can think of Power Yoga as your ticket to a powerful and happy life throughout the years ahead.

If you think of Power Yoga as a full-throttle, no-holds-barred workout process, you may think that you're not interested in — or not capable of — doing it. Well, if Power Yoga is a wild beast, it's one you're perfectly capable of taming. Just as walking is the beginning phase of running, which is just another step down from marathon racing, Power Yoga can be as gentle or as demanding as you want it to be.

Considering some cautions

Most people (at any age) aren't in peak physical condition. If you've reached middle age or beyond and you're just beginning to think about getting in shape, you have a tougher road ahead than does someone who's been working out and watching his or her diet forever. But so what? Lots of people start working out when they're 60, 70, or 80; it's always a good idea, no matter what your age. But you have to keep the following realities of aging in mind as you build a safe practice program:

✔ **Take your time.** As you age, your bones become more brittle even as your joints and muscles become less flexible. With that in mind, be careful when you move in and out of poses. Slow your breathing, and move gently into and out of each yoga pose.

✔ **Use some props.** You're building balance as a Power Yoga student, but initially, your balance may be a bit off. To make sure that you can remain stable and secure during your yoga postures, use props during your Power Yoga workouts.

Props — things like pads, blocks, mats, straps, pillows, blankets, and other objects — help you build strength and stability faster than if you try to wobble through without them; you'll also enjoy your Power Yoga workouts more. When you first attempt certain Power Yoga postures, for example, you may have trouble keeping your balance or comfortably assuming or maintaining certain positions. With a pillow here or a block there, what had been a wobbly, unsatisfying perch becomes a comfortable, secure pose.

✔ **Grab a partner.** Practicing Power Yoga with a partner is fun! And having a partner to help you balance in some positions, hand you props, or just lend general moral support can make a big difference in your confidence — and safety. A partner is also great to have around if you're going to practice challenging balance postures, especially the upside-down postures such as headstands and handstands. For complete information on partnering in yoga, see Book VI, Chapter 1.

✔ **Balance your workouts with rest.** Your muscles may not recuperate from a brand-new workout as quickly as they did when you were younger. So use a low-level workout routine in the beginning, and if your muscles get sore, back off and rest between workouts. If you get sore and tired every time you do Power Yoga, you'll soon be discouraged by the whole process. If you feel yourself getting sore, take it easier.

✔ **Before you launch into becoming a student of Power Yoga, see your doctor for a general checkup.** Tell your doctor that you're thinking of doing some Power Yoga exercise, and ask whether that's okay, given your present condition. Your doctor or health clinic may even be able to recommend some good yoga programs in your area.

Many yoga studios ask all their students to bring in a doctor's permission for joining practice sessions. If you take medication of any kind, you should let your yoga instructor know.

Getting Acquainted with Power Yoga Poses for Seniors

After your doctor gives you the green light to begin Power Yoga exercises, you need to find a yoga class with which you feel comfortable. Ask your friends, look online (or in the phone book), check with your local senior citizens' action center, or ask at some local fitness centers. (Check out Book I, Chapter 3 to find info on locating and choosing a yoga center.) When you find a program that looks good to you, talk with the instructor to make sure that the class can accommodate your needs. Then try out a few sample classes to see whether everything feels like a good "fit."

No matter what your fitness level is, you should begin your Power Yoga work with some simple postures. Power Yoga makes demands on your body for which other types of exercises may not have prepared you. If you launch your practice by trying to put your feet behind your head while standing upside-down on one hand, you're unlikely to enjoy the experience and may even hurt yourself. Take it slow and work gradually toward building more complex postures into your beginning routines.

Power Yoga isn't a competitive sport. You're in it for you, and you determine what you want to do (or not do) with your practice. Follow your instincts and enjoy the process without feeling out of place, incapable, or silly. Life is an adventure, and developing a regular Power Yoga practice can be one of the most exciting and rewarding trips. Relax, explore, and enjoy.

The following sections describe some Power Yoga exercises that any beginner can enjoy. Check them out for a taste of power.

Developing shoulder relief and leg strength

Try the following gentle Power Yoga exercise routine working from a chair, and see how energized you feel. This exercise helps relieve stress and tension in your shoulders, it expands your chest, and it helps to loosen up tight joints as it strengthens your arms and legs.

You need two sturdy, straight-back chairs for the last part of this exercise. Place the chairs facing each other, and sit in one. Follow these steps to achieve the two-chair stretch and release tension:

1. **Sit in one chair, with your spine straight and shoulders back, hands folded in your lap (see Figure 5-1a).**

   Take a few slow, deep breaths, and relax.

2. **As you inhale, lift your arms out to your sides and over your head with palms touching, as if you're clapping your hands (see Figure 5-1b).**

3. **Exhale, and lower your arms to the starting position (hands in your lap).**

   Keep your shoulders away from your ears as you do.

4. **Repeat Steps 2 and 3 five times.**

   Remember to inhale as you lift your arms and expand your chest. Exhale as you lower your arms and relax.

Book IV

Powering Your Way to Fitness: Power Yoga

5. **Repeat Step 2, inhaling and lifting your arms over your head; exhale as you put weight on your feet and come to a full standing position, with your arms by your sides (see Figure 5-1c).**

6. **Sit back down in your chair, with your spine straight and shoulders back.**

7. **Repeat Step 5 for five repetitions.**

   Close your eyes and relax for 10 slow, deep breaths.

8. **Bend forward at the hips, resting your torso on your thighs, and place your arms on the chair in front of you (see Figure 5-1d).**

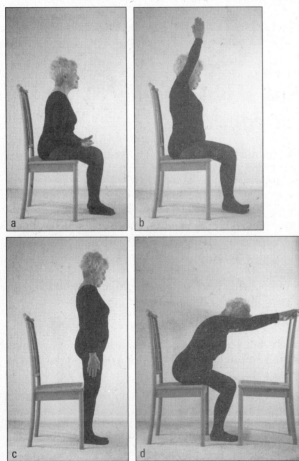

Figure 5-1:
This gentle Power Yoga exercise is easy to do, but it offers big benefits in flexibility, strength, and tension relief.

Photographs by Raul Marroquin

9. **Hold this position for 5 slow, deep breaths.**

   You're doing the two-chair stretch, which stretches your torso.

10. **Come back to a sitting position and relax.**

Propping up your extended side angle pose

This section provides an easy adaptation of a traditional Power Yoga posture. The traditional extended side angle pose, shown in Figure 5-2, requires you to lunge deep on your right leg with your left leg extended behind you and, at the same time, rest your right hand on the floor.

That's some pretty tricky stuff! If you're getting up there in years or you aren't in the greatest physical condition, you can do the same posture without lunging so deeply and with the benefit of some added support. The following version of the extended side angle pose strengthens legs and tones ankles, knees, and thighs. Using a chair as a prop makes this pose much easier to do, but it doesn't detract from the posture's ability to develop your chest and reduce fat around your waist and abdomen. Opening all the muscles of the rib cage also enhances your ability to breathe.

Have a sturdy chair ready to help you achieve the modified extended side angle pose:

1. **Start from the extended mountain pose.**

   Stand strong and firm with correct posture (refer to Book IV, Chapter 4).

2. **Turn your right foot outward 90 degrees, and turn your left foot in at a 45-degree angle.**

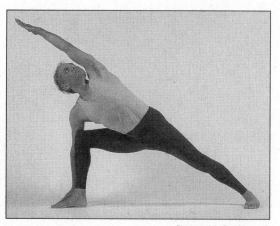

Figure 5-2:
The traditional extended side angle pose.

Photograph by Raul Marroquin

Book IV

Powering Your Way to Fitness: Power Yoga

3. **Inhale, lifting your arms to your sides and parallel to the floor.**

4. **Exhale as you lunge, bending your right knee so that your thigh and shin form a 90-degree angle.**

   Your right knee comes directly over your right heel, bringing your thigh parallel to the floor.

5. **Place your right forearm on the seat of the chair for support (see Figure 5-3).**

   Use your right hand to slide into position onto the chair close to your right knee.

6. **Form a 45-degree angle with your body, from your extended left leg (which is back behind you), through your torso, and all the way out to your fingertips.**

   Your left arm is extended up at a 45-degree angle on the same plane as your leg and your torso; your palm should be open, and your hand facing outward.

7. **Turn your head upward, looking up under your arm and toward the ceiling; hold this position for 5 slow, deep breaths.**

Figure 5-3:
A chair makes the extended side angle pose a bit easier to do, but it doesn't eliminate its stretching and strength-ening benefits.

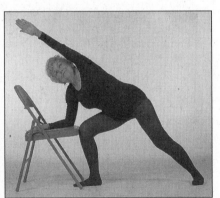

Photograph by Raul Marroquin

Using wall support for super shoulder stands

The shoulder stand (see Book IV, Chapter 4) helps to create harmony and happiness throughout your entire body. In this inverted *asana* (pose), your heart and brain receive a healthy rush of blood; the pose stimulates your endocrine system and gives your thyroid and parathyroid glands a tune-up. The shoulder stand can even help reverse the effects of varicose veins! Best of all, when you come out of the shoulder stand, you feel refreshed and rejuvenated.

You don't have to be a high-wire artist to pull off the shoulder stand. The version included in this section puts you up against the wall for a perfectly supported and stable experience. By putting your legs up against the wall, you feel more comfortable and less wobbly in this pose.

When you do this exercise, you should have a thick towel or blanket so you can use it to elevate your shoulders and protect your neck from too much tension. Move slowly and carefully, and ask someone to help stabilize your legs when they're in the air in this exercise.

1. **Position yourself near a wall, placing a folded blanket on the floor parallel to the wall.**

2. **Lie down in the corpse position (refer to Book IV, Chapter 3), with your shoulders on the blanket.**

   Keep your shoulders elevated and your head resting off the blanket. Lie on your back, arms extended by your sides, your feet about 1 foot apart. Make sure that your palms face upward and your mind is calm and relaxed. Bend your knees, and let your toes touch the wall.

   You don't want to use the blanket as a pillow, because that setup causes more harm than good. The object is to lift your shoulders and create less tension on your neck.

   Place your body so you have about 2 inches of blanket beyond the tops of your shoulders. Your body should roll back slightly as you lift up into this posture. When you're completely lifted up into the posture, your shoulders should still be entirely on the blanket, your neck should be free (that is, you can slip your fingers underneath your neck), and your head should be on the floor.

   The pose should feel comfortable. In fact, you may be surprised at how comfortable it does feel. If you feel a lot of pressure behind your eyes or in your head or if you feel pain in your neck or back, come on down and talk to your friendly yoga professional to see whether this pose can be right for you.

Book IV

Powering Your Way to Fitness: Power Yoga

3. **Exhale completely; on an inhalation, place your feet flat on the wall a couple of feet above the floor.**

4. **Push your weight into your feet as you lift your hips, supporting your hips with your hands.**

   Tuck in your elbows behind your back, and use your elbows and hands to support your lower back.

5. **Push up into a full wall-supported shoulder stand.**

   Hold this position for 5 to 20 complete breaths (see Figure 5-4).

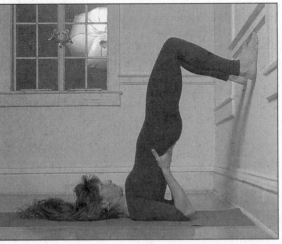

Figure 5-4:
Getting the benefits of a shoulder stand while using a wall for support.

Photograph by Raul Marroquin

6. **Inhale again, place your hands under your hips, and push down to lift your hips off the floor.**

7. **Tuck in your elbows behind your back, and use your elbows and hands to support your elevated legs and hips.**

   Ask your helper to steady you so you don't topple to the side.

8. **Extend your legs and torso as high as you comfortably can, remembering to support your back with your hands.**

9. **Hold this posture for 5 to 20 slow, deep breaths.**

10. **Come down slowly and relax on your back.**

If you have, or may have, osteoporosis, take care doing this pose. It's important not to put weight on your neck vertebrae.

Powering Up with a Post-50 Routine

The best way to make a productive start on your way to becoming a post-50 Power Yoga practitioner is to work with a beginning-level routine.

If you find that the routine in this section is too difficult using the postures as described in the referenced chapters, don't hesitate to use props and/or the modifications described in the preceding sections. And you don't need to work through the entire routine right off the bat. You can try practicing a half or a third of the routine, cutting down the number of recommended repetitions, and so on. In other words, make the workout work for you.

Just remember to do at least a 15-minute relaxation (and here, more is better) wherever and whenever you end!

Follow these steps:

1. **Move into the persuading posture (see Figure 5-5) and hold for 5 breaths.**

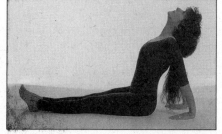

Figure 5-5:
The persuading posture.

Photograph by Raul Marroquin

2. **Perform five repetitions of the upside-down walker pose (see Figure 5-6).**

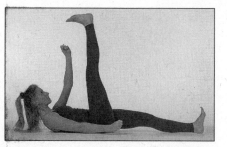

Figure 5-6:
The upside-down walker pose.

Photograph by Raul Marroquin

Book IV

Powering Your Way to Fitness: Power Yoga

3. Perform two repetitions of the cat stretch (see Figure 5-7).

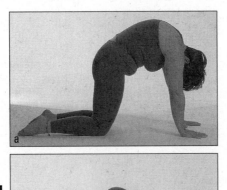

Figure 5-7:
The cat
stretch
pose.

Photographs by Raul Marroquin

4. Perform two repetitions of the seated forward bend (see Figure 5-8).

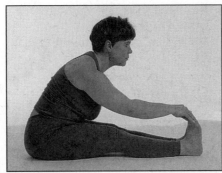

Figure 5-8:
The seated
forward
bend pose.

Photograph by Raul Marroquin

5. **Move into the cobra pose for two repetitions, holding each for 5 breaths (see Figure 5-9).**

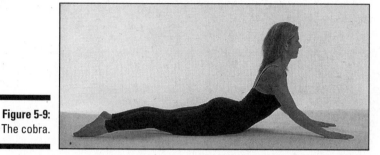

Figure 5-9:
The cobra.

Photograph by Raul Marroquin

6. **Assume the bridge pose and hold for 5 breaths (see Figure 5-10).**

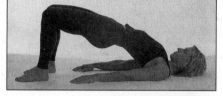

Figure 5-10:
The bridge.

Photograph by Raul Marroquin

7. **Do a spine toner for 5 breaths (see Figure 5-11).**

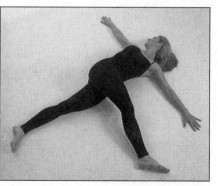

Figure 5-11:
The spine
toner.

Photograph by Raul Marroquin

Book IV

**Powering
Your Way
to Fitness:
Power
Yoga**

8. **Do one repetition of the missing link upward transition pose (see Figure 5-12).**

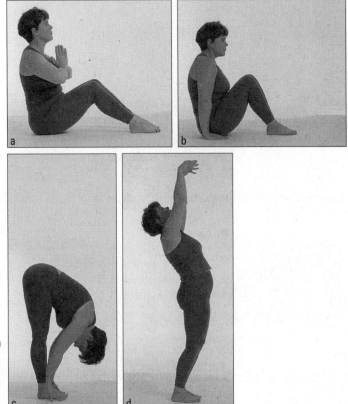

Photographs by Raul Marroquin

Figure 5-12:
The missing link upward.

9. **Move into an extended side angle and hold for 5 breaths (see Figure 5-13).**

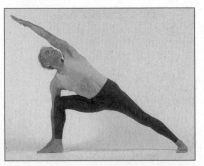

Figure 5-13:
The extended side angle.

Photograph by Raul Marroquin

10. Do one repetition of the missing link downward transition pose (see Figure 5-14).

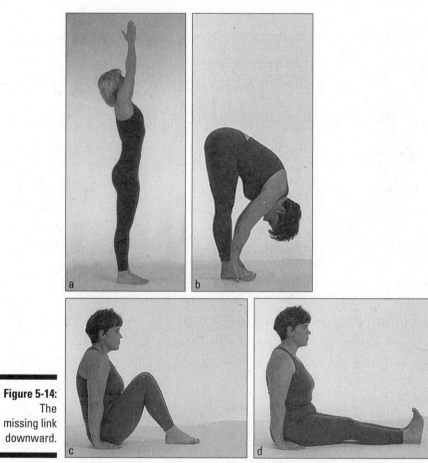

Figure 5-14: The missing link downward.

Photographs by Raul Marroquin

11. **Move into a shoulder stand and hold for 5 to 20 breaths (see Figure 5-15).**

    Choose whichever pose in Figure 5-15 is more comfortable.

Figure 5-15:
The
shoulder
stand.

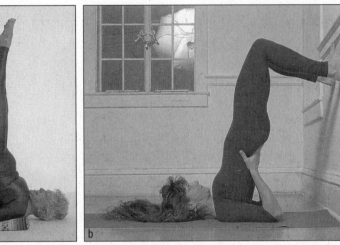

Photographs by Raul Marroquin

12. **Relax with yoga breathing for 5 breaths.**

    Refer to Book IV, Chapter 1 for instructions.

13. **Lie in the corpse posture for deep relaxation for 15 to 30 minutes (see Figure 5-16).**

Figure 5-16:
The corpse
posture.

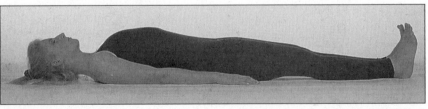

Photograph by Raul Marroquin

Book V

Yoga-ing Your Way to a Toned Body: Yoga with Weights

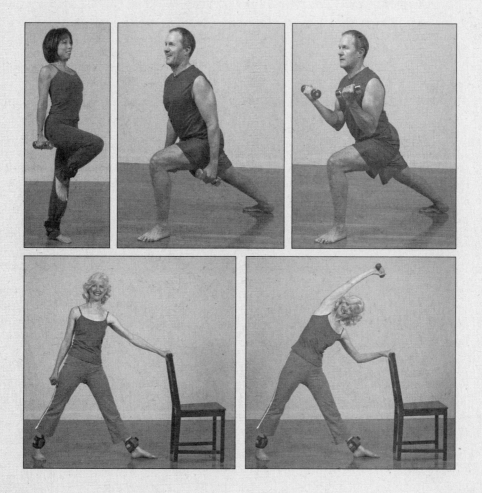

Contents at a Glance

Chapter 1

Introducing Yoga with Weights

*Y*oga with Weights is a hybrid of two powerful, time-tested exercise systems: yoga and bodybuilding. Working out with weights is one of the best ways to achieve overall physical fitness, and yoga is renowned as a system of personal development by which you can cultivate peak performance and achieve a higher quality of life. By combining these exercise systems, Yoga with Weights addresses the needs of your body, but it also goes beyond the physical dimension of your well-being.

Yoga with Weights calls for 1-, 3-, or 5-pound weights on your wrists and/or ankles. The weights stabilize your body and help you achieve a higher level of physical benefit and conditioning. Yoga with Weights is a system for the body, mind, and spirit. If you practice diligently, it can be a way of being and living through conscious exercise that leads you to discover your true self.

Everyone can benefit from Yoga with Weights exercises. No matter how flexible you are, how old or young you are, whether you're a paragon of good health or you're just starting down the road to a healthier, happier lifestyle, Yoga with Weights can help you.

Weighing the Benefits of Yoga with Weights

Adding weights to your yoga routine makes you feel the effect of the yoga training sooner. The weights train your muscles where to be and where to go more quickly than you would otherwise experience in a beginning yoga practice, where the same knowledge may take several months. The weights force you to engage the right muscles. The added weight also offers a deeper sense of physical grounding, and the weights challenge your balancing skills more intensely than traditional yoga. Yoga with Weights also offers many health benefits, outlined in this section.

Making you stronger

Adding weights gives an additional boost to the muscle strengthening and toning powers of yoga. When you stress a muscle with exercise or a repeated activity, the muscle increases in strength and diameter as the muscle fiber expands, becoming toned. The weight-bearing aspect of Yoga with Weights improves the oxygenation of muscles, which promotes the muscles' growth and repair. The stretching improves the flexibility and health of muscles and tendons. Yoga with Weights also reduces the risk of muscle tears and strains because weightlifting, when properly done, integrates the muscles closer to the bones.

Strengthening your core and toning your muscles

Your *core muscles* — the muscles of your trunk and torso that support your spine — are the major players in balancing and coordination. These muscles also support your shoulders and hips. And your abdominal muscles are very important for supporting your spine.

Your core muscles are responsible for good posture. They keep your back straight and your shoulders square, and they keep you from slouching. They support and protect your internal organs. Without strong core muscles, you're more susceptible to back problems.

Can yoga turn back time?

It's often said that yoga slows the aging process. What yoga really does is help maintain and improve your posture and general health through exercising and proper breathing. Yoga with Weights helps increase your vitality and overall well-being so you look and feel younger and more beautiful. It can give you self-confidence and poise, increase your self-awareness, and make the light inside you shine more brightly with each decade.

When most people think of getting stronger, they imagine being able to lift heavier weights or run faster. But before you can accomplish such feats, you need to develop the core muscles of your trunk and torso. In fact, unless your core muscles are strong, you can't develop the muscles of your arms and legs to their fullest potential, in much the same way that tree branches can't grow big unless the trunk of the tree is strong enough to support the branches. Remember, deep strength begins in these core muscles — your power source, the axis around which so many muscles move.

Yoga with Weights exercises are designed to work and tone all the muscles of your body. If you think your arms are too flabby, if you want to develop your abdominal muscles, or if you want to strengthen your legs, you can find many Yoga with Weights exercises that target those areas.

Addressing your flexibility and range of motion

Yoga is well known for making people more flexible, supple, lithe, and limber. Being flexible is necessary if you want to be comfortable in your body. Think of all the practical advantages of being flexible. You can reach higher, sit more comfortably on the floor, sit at your desk for longer periods of time with greater ease, or stand longer. You have the choice of bending at the waist or squatting when you want to pick up something from the floor.

Soreness, swelling, and pain relate to the loss of body tissue movement. To prevent injury and postural changes, it helps if your joints have a maximum range of motion.

You've probably seen photographs of human pretzels, contorting themselves into different yoga postures, and may, like many people, believe that being flexible enough to get into pretzel poses is the primary goal of yoga. The fact is, however, that you can be a good yoga practitioner without being

Indian club, anyone?

If you think Yoga with Weights is new under the sun, think again. As an exercise discipline, combining yogalike postures with weights is many centuries old, except that the ancient practitioners didn't lift weights as you know them. They lifted heavy wooden clubs called *gadas,* or *Indian clubs,* which are shaped like bowling pins, range in height from 2 to 2½ feet, and weigh between 1 and 7 pounds.

After the British colonized India, they recognized the value of exercising with Indian clubs, and swinging Indian clubs became an exercise activity in Britain and then in the United States in the late 19th and early 20th centuries. In some respects, Yoga with Weights is a return to an exercise program that was practiced in India for centuries and was well known to

American and British exercise enthusiasts 100 years ago.

Physical trainers liked the clubs because they permitted you to build muscle strength while maintaining the range of motion in your arms and shoulders. Exercising with Indian clubs was sometimes called *circular weight training.* In traditional weight training, sometimes called *linear weight training,* you isolate one muscle or one muscle group as you lift. This isolation can make you stiff or muscle-bound after you train for a while. But by swinging Indian clubs, you can build strength while retaining your grace of motion.

Yoga with Weights and circular weight training share some common traits. Both work your muscles, and both help your muscles retain their agility, flexibility, and range of motion.

especially flexible. Yoga with Weights combines basic master techniques from the yoga tradition with physical culture practices. The goal is to achieve the proper body alignment and breathe correctly in every move and exercise while cultivating an open mind and heart. You want to achieve a balanced and overall strengthening effect, not to be as flexible as a pretzel.

Improving your circulation

Whenever you exercise, you improve your blood circulation. After you stretch or contract a muscle in a Yoga with Weights exercise and the muscle relaxes, it becomes flooded with blood! "Flooded with blood" may sound like the title of a horror movie, but this blood inundation is good for you because it increases the flow of blood to your muscles, and blood delivers nutrients. Your muscles become stronger and healthier because they receive more nutrients. Stretching also helps renew muscles and muscle fiber.

Creating body awareness

Book V

Yoga-ing
Your Way
to a Toned
Body: Yoga
with
Weights

Yoga with Weights builds body awareness. You can think of Yoga with Weights as a dialogue between your mind and body. As you exercise, your brain sends a message to a part of your body telling it to move in a certain direction, and your body sends a signal back to your brain saying that the body part can make the desired motion or can't move any farther. When your brain receives its signal, it sends out another signal asking the part of the body to become more active or relax a little more. This ongoing dialogue amounts to a self-exploration of your body. In a very profound way, it makes you more aware of your body and enables you to extend the physical limits that you thought your body was incapable of reaching.

Focusing on your balance and coordination

Balancing is discovering how to work muscles in opposition to one another. When you balance on one leg, for example, you flex, or integrate, some muscles, and you relax others. If you flex or relax the wrong muscles, you lose your balance. Yoga with Weights helps you understand which muscles to contract or relax in an action, and in so doing it teaches balance and coordination.

Balancing improves your ability to direct your thoughts or stream of concentration. You develop skills of concentration in order to balance. Balancing fires the neurons of your brain. It helps clear the nerve highways and pathways so you can focus better. Recent studies in brain elasticity indicate that exercises that develop coordination and balance stimulate the brain to create new maps and communication pathways, keeping the brain healthy and vital.

Building bone density

Loosely speaking, "bone density" refers to how strong and dense your bones are. To be specific, *bone density* is a measure of how tightly packed the cells and molecules in a bone are. The more tightly packed the tissue is, the higher the bone density, and the healthier the bone. Low bone density increases your risk of fracturing or breaking a bone.

Weight-bearing exercises such as Yoga with Weights help bones retain density. When you lift a weight, your muscle pulls against your bones, which makes your bones experience stress. Detecting this stress, your body sends a signal to the cells in your bones that goes something like this: "Please get stronger and denser." Isn't it nice to know that some kinds of stress are actually good for your health?

As they age, most people lose bone density, partly because their bodies can't absorb the calcium and minerals they need for strong bones as readily as they once could. Bone density decreases gradually in men and women starting at age 30; in women, the decrease is more pronounced after menopause because estrogen, the ovarian hormone, plays a role in maintaining strong bones.

Promoting organ health

Squeeze-and-soak exercises are exercises that massage your internal organs — your liver, stomach, intestines, pancreas, and others. You'll find many squeeze-and-soak exercises in Book V because they help squeeze out the toxins in your internal organs and deliver more blood and oxygen to the organs.

When you bend forward or twist your spine, you squeeze and soak. When you return to a resting position, your organs open up and return to their normal shapes and sizes, and as they do so, they soak up oxygenated blood cells. This oxygenation restores and helps to maintain the organs' health and vitality.

Evaluating Your Readiness

"Can I really do this?" is a question many people ask themselves every day. Maybe you're new to yoga, new to weight training, or new to an exercise program, or maybe you've been lifting weights regularly for years. In each of these cases, you may wonder whether you can engage in Yoga with Weights. The discussion that follows is for people who can't quite decide whether Yoga with Weights is for them.

A few medical conditions may preclude you from doing Yoga with Weights. If you have a heart condition, you're obese, or you're pregnant, think twice before undertaking this form of exercise and proceed with caution. You may have to consult your doctor before doing the exercises.

You haven't studied yoga

Yoga with Weights is user-friendly, meaning it isn't intimidating, and you don't need a background in yoga. The door is always open. Anyone who's interested is welcome. Of course, if you've already studied yoga, studying Yoga with Weights is that much easier because the language and the concepts aren't completely new or unfamiliar. For example, you already understand the importance of breathing in exercise. If an exercise instructs you to breathe deep into your chest and lungs, you know what's what. And if a routine tells you to move into the downward-facing dog position, you know exactly what that is.

You haven't had weight training (or you lift weights regularly)

You don't need to have lifted weights before now to study Yoga with Weights. The weights you use are only 1 to 5 pounds and aren't difficult to get the hang of. If you've never picked up a weight before, rest reassured that holding a pair of hand weights or strapping on a pair of ankle weights doesn't take any expertise whatsoever. The weights help you feel more grounded but don't weigh you down.

One of the biggest attractions of Yoga with Weights is being able to lift weights and still maintain your flexibility. You get the same muscular tone you get from weight training and work on your flexibility as well. You won't get "bulked up" or muscle-bound, but your muscles will be toned, defined, and strengthened.

Yoga with Weights may also intimidate people who have lifted weights. Why? Because weightlifters aren't flexible. Here's some advice: Stepping out of your element and comfort zone is a challenge for everybody, bodybuilders included, but taking that first step is actually much easier than you may think. For people who lift weights regularly, engaging in Yoga with Weights allows them to reclaim full range of motion and flexibility while maintaining strength, which is just what they often need.

You're really out of shape

Even if you're very out of shape, you can still engage in Yoga with Weights. The key is to start slow. Go to Book V, Chapter 2 and start with gentle walking and breathing exercises. Try to observe a daily walking program of 20 to 45 minutes to get the ball rolling. When you build your confidence, go to Book V, Chapter 3 for the Balanced Workout. You may also want to check out Book V, Chapter 6, which offers low-impact exercises designed for seniors.

Are you a busy mom, CEO, or other dynamic person who struggles to find time to exercise? Then try this: Make a commitment in writing to show up. Enter your yoga class on your calendar and plan your time around yoga.

You're stiff as a board

Some people are by nature muscle-bound or tight, and they have a limited range of motion. They can hardly lean forward far enough to tie their shoes. People with tight muscles tend to be protective and guarded in their movements. They don't have the confidence to move freely. This lack of confidence hinders their movements and makes them even stiffer. Eventually, they may develop bad posture, which can lead to other health problems, including chronic back pain and chronic headaches. Bad posture can compress the internal organs, causing poor digestion, high blood pressure, and respiratory ailments.

If you're stiff by nature, Yoga with Weights can help you escape the cage that your body has become, spread your wings, and fly. Yoga breathing techniques (see Book II, Chapter 1) can improve the blood circulation in your body and bring new healthy cells to your muscles. Where flexibility is concerned, success breeds success. One muscle unknotting can cause the one beside it to loosen. Even people who are very stiff by nature can become limber if they stick with Yoga with Weights and practice it as little as twice a week. Eventually, your muscles will rest back against your bones and stretch out and elongate, and you'll be able to move more comfortably and freely.

You're loose as a goose

Some people are double-jointed. Their tendons and ligaments are more elastic. They can touch their noses to their knees without any distress or bend over backwards to touch the floor. People who are double-jointed, or *hyperflexible,* run the risk of hyperextending their knees, elbows, and other joints because their ligaments and tendons are too elastic. They're capable of flexing well beyond a joint's normal range. Unless they develop the muscular strength to support their supple joints, these people can injure their joints in the course of doing an exercise.

Yoga with Weights helps people who suffer from hyperflexibility strengthen supporting muscles. This extra muscle mass makes the joints more stable.

What You Need to Get Started

To get started with Yoga with Weights, you need a little willpower, an open mind, and a sense of adventure; at least, those are the only intangibles you need. Taking the first step in any new activity is usually the hardest part. As for the tangibles, you need some equipment to get going. At minimum, you need a quiet and comfortable place to exercise, hand weights, and ankle weights. A yoga mat, the right clothes, and good shoes (for warming up) are also beneficial. The good news for you? These items don't cost a bundle.

Read on for more information about the gear and equipment you need — some of it shown in Figure 1-1 — for a Yoga with Weights workout.

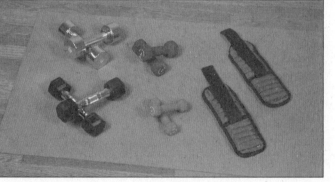

Figure 1-1: Some of the equipment you need for a Yoga with Weights workout.

Photograph by Bonnie Kamin (www.bonniekamin.com)

Choosing hand- and ankle-weights

You need two kinds of weights if you want to incorporate weight resistance into your yoga workouts: hand weights and ankle weights. Most sporting goods and athletic stores carry these weights. This section offers some guidelines.

Investing in weights of different sizes

Opt for three sizes of hand and ankle weights: a pair of 1-pound weights, a pair of 3-pound weights, and a pair of 5-pound weights.

Why not lift weights heavier than 5 pounds? Using 5-pound weights — in addition to the yoga poses — gives you a very solid workout. The 1-, 3-, or 5-pounders stretch your muscles, release tension in your muscles, and engage the muscles in the deep core of your body that you use for balance and stability. This added resistance from the weights forces your deep-core muscles to spring into action. Lifting weights heavier than 5 pounds may make you too top- or bottom-heavy and upset the balance and distribution of your body weight.

The exercise descriptions in this book don't tell you which of the three weights to use. The amount of resistance you want is up to you. Experiment with the different weights, and choose the size that gives you the best workout. Always start with the lightest hand or ankle weights and work your way up. Doing so allows you to start from your comfort zone and work your way into the weight that gives you the most fulfilling workout. If you start with the heaviest weight, you run the risk of straining yourself and pulling a muscle.

Knowing which size weight to use

How do you know which size weight (1-, 3-, or 5-pound) to use in a particular exercise? The size is ultimately up to you, but if you find yourself straining as you do an exercise, consider using a lighter weight. Some telltale signs that you should switch to a lighter weight include grunting, holding your breath, or experiencing shaking or cramping muscles.

Don't be afraid to experiment. Keep different sizes of weights at your side and test the different weights until you find the pair that engages you the best in an exercise. You may find yourself using different weights for different exercises. The surest way to know whether your choice of weights is the right one is to see how you feel after a workout. If your body feels weak and shaky, or you're too sore the next day, you need lighter weights. If you finish a workout with the feeling of "comfortable discomfort" — a feeling that you've met the challenge and given yourself a good workout — you know that your choice in weights was the right one.

Settling on the right yoga mat

You need a solid, supporting surface to exercise on, and for that reason, using a yoga mat is a good idea for your safety. Mats give you padding, comfort, and protection, especially for your knees and spine. However, it isn't necessary to have a yoga mat when you do Yoga with Weights exercises. You can exercise on a solid, non-slippery, close-weave type of carpet or clean, dry floor.

If you're taking a Yoga with Weights class in a gym, bring your own mat for hygiene purposes. Most gyms offer yoga mats, but they can get very sweaty. Rolling around in your own sweat is much more agreeable and hygienic than rolling around in a stranger's sweat.

When you shop for a yoga mat, look for one that stretches a little and gives you good support. Mats range from a fraction of an inch to an inch deep, but depth isn't the real issue — cushioning is. The idea is to get some relief from the hard floor, and although comfort is fine, a spongy mat can be a nuisance because it doesn't give you a solid base to work on. For your purposes, a quarter- to half-inch-thick mat is best because it offers comfort and stability; if you're uncomfortable sitting on the floor or on your knees, get a mat that's on the thick side. Also, the mat should be as long as you are tall plus about 6 inches; in other words, if you're 5-feet-6, find a 6-foot yoga mat.

Don't select a foam mat; they're too thick and too short for Yoga with Weights exercises. Foam mats are made for aerobic exercising.

Book V

Yoga-ing Your Way to a Toned Body: Yoga with Weights

Wearing clothing that preserves modesty and movement

Don't wear shirts and pants that restrict your movements in any way or drag on the floor, and never wear a belt; the waistband of your pants must be loose so your breathing isn't constricted or confined. For the sake of comfort, wear clothes with natural and breathable fibers. You can find these clothes in many sporting goods stores, outdoor outfitters, and yoga retail stores, as well as on the Internet.

Follow these guidelines when choosing your undergarments:

- **Women:** Women should wear an athletic or spandex bra that lifts their breasts and presses them into their bodies. For top-heavy women, this factor is important for balancing as well as for comfort.

- **Men:** Men should wear tightly fitting — but not too tightly fitting — underwear from which no, ahem, *items* may escape and see the light of day. Spandex running shorts are excellent for Yoga with Weights. They support your muscles and keep them warm, and they permit you to move without restriction.

Mastering Posture Alignment Techniques for Yoga with Weights

Posture alignment refers to how your muscles are integrated and your bones are aligned to support your body for optimal movement during exercise. The aim of good posture alignment is to establish a solid foundation with your body so you can support your limbs, back, and head while you exercise. You want your body to be safe, secure, and able to expand more fully and freely during each exercise.

To avoid injury and to get more out of Yoga with Weights exercises, it pays to practice proper posture alignment. The posture-alignment techniques presented here give you a greater sense of stability and balance not only when you exercise but also when you stand in lines or sit for long periods of time. The better your posture is, the fewer injuries you're prone to in exercise and in daily life. Here are the basic principles regarding posture alignment:

- ✔ **Engage your core muscles.** When you engage these muscles, it feels as though you're wearing a tight-fitting spandex suit on your body because you have a "hugged-in" feeling. You feel empowered when you move from your core muscles into all the exercises. Refer to the earlier section "Strengthening your core and toning your muscles" for more on the importance of core muscles.

- ✔ **Draw your belly in and up and your tailbone down.** As your tailbone drops toward the floor, your legs strengthen, and you press your leg muscles up against the bone where they can support your body. You should feel the muscles hugging the bones as the bones begin lengthening.

- ✔ **Press into all four corners of your feet.** You root downward through the soles of your feet to create depth and stability while you exercise. You should feel equal weight on the front and back of each foot as well as on the sides. Feel the corners of your heel and the ball or pad on the front of your foot — especially the area below your big toe and baby toes — pressing downward. You should also feel the arches of your feet gently lifting up as if energy from the front of your shins is pulling your arches up. The feeling continues through your knees as your thigh muscles gently lift your knees upward.

- ✔ **Stabilize and center your head between your shoulders.** You may read instructions that ask you to perform this action during standing exercises. When you do, gaze forward with your chin naturally down, not lifted or tilted. Draw your shoulders away from your ears and your shoulder blades down your back. Make sure your chest is comfortable, spread your collarbones wide, and give a slight lift to your breast bone or sternum, lifting naturally. Stand with your hips aligned over your knees and with your knees over your heels.

- ✔ **Spread your fingers wide.** When your hands are on the floor and you're supporting your body with your hands, spread your fingers wide so that each finger is active and pressing firmly on the floor to help support your body.

✔ **Place your shoulders over your wrists and hands and your hips over your knees.** You'll see this instruction when an exercise requires you to be on all fours. When you're in this position, make sure that you distribute your body weight evenly over your wrists, hands, and knees and that you fully engage the core muscles of your trunk.

When you're lifting a hand weight or an ankle weight, always make sure not to hurry. Lift the weight in a slow, controlled fashion. When you go slow, you make your body more stable and capable of supporting the weight, you isolate the muscle you want to work more effectively, and you don't cheat by relying on your momentum to lift the weight.

No matter what Yoga with Weights exercise you're doing, your entire body should be involved. In addition to keeping your core body engaged, before you do an exercise, direct your thoughts to the specific area that's most actively involved in that particular exercise. For example, if you're doing bicep curls, focus on your biceps. By directing your mind to the specific body action, you enhance your body-mind connection and create a more empowered workout. This technique is also excellent for mental conditioning.

Heeding the All-Important Safety Issues

Use common sense when practicing Yoga with Weights. If something doesn't feel right, don't do it. Work at your own level of ability and never push yourself too far. This section presents guidelines for making sure you practice Yoga with Weights safely. These guidelines can help you determine what's safe, but practically speaking, it's up to you to draw your own guidelines. As long as you stay in the moment and register the sensations in your body very carefully, your breathing, discomfort level, and pain level can tell you where the edge is and show you how to get the most from the exercises.

Listen to your breathing

Rapid breathing, short and shallow breathing, holding your breath, and gasping are signs of distress. If you can't take slow, deep, rhythmic breaths as you exercise, you're overexerting and subjecting yourself to injury. Ease away from what you're doing just enough to regain control over your breathing, and then continue with the exercise.

Be aware of your discomfort level

In Yoga with Weights, you make a distinction between comfortable discomfort and uncomfortable discomfort. Feeling comfortable discomfort, such as the uneasiness that accompanies breaking new ground in Yoga with Weights (or any other exercise technique), is fine. If you feel uncomfortable discomfort, however, you're straining yourself. Abandon the exercise you're doing and ask yourself whether you're doing the exercise correctly or pushing yourself too far.

Be aware of any pain you feel

As with other exercise techniques, you sometimes feel pain when you do Yoga with Weights exercises. Pay careful attention to any pain or discomfort you feel. Listen to it. Focus on the part of your body where the pain is located. Burning or stinging pain signals you to be careful, but not necessarily to back away from what you're doing. Sometimes you can control this kind of pain by breathing. Quivering or sharp pain means you've gone too far. You're pulling muscle off the bone and subjecting yourself to injury.

Practice at a slow but steady pace

When you're exercising, switching to automatic pilot and going through the motions is easy. When that happens, you increase your chances of injuring yourself, because you're not focusing on your body.

Listen to your body and focus on what you feel as you exercise. This, along with conscious breathing (refer to Book II, Chapter 1) and a steady exercise pace, helps prevent injuries. Timing and proper breathing are the keys to the depth and success of each workout and practice. Try not to speed up to get your workout over with quickly. At the same time, don't go so slowly that you lose your pacing and rhythm and make the workout boring.

Staying hydrated

All exercisers must pay attention to fluid intake, because as you lose water when you exercise, you run the risk of being dehydrated. Some yoga exercises squeeze and soak your kidneys, which releases toxins in your body. You need to drink water to help flush out those toxins. So make sure you have water on hand whenever you do Yoga with Weights exercises.

Many people make the mistake of drinking a lot of water right before they exercise. What they don't know is that the water they drink right before a workout or during a workout doesn't hydrate their bodies. The water you drink *three to four hours* before your workout quenches your body's thirst. Drinking slowly over the course of the day makes for better hydration and absorption of water by your body. Guzzling, on the other hand, doesn't give your body enough time to absorb the water. So get a 1.5-liter or 1-quart container of drinking water and sip from it throughout the day.

Book V

Yoga-ing Your Way to a Toned Body: Yoga with Weights

Chapter 2

Warming Up for Your Yoga with Weights Workout

. . . .

In This Chapter

▶ Looking at the benefits of warming up

▶ Walking as a prelude to working out

▶ Doing the Yoga with Weights warm-up exercises

. . . .

*W*arming up is recommended no matter what kind of exercise you intend to do. In Yoga with Weights, warming up is especially important because this style of yoga works your muscles and joints more than other exercise programs.

Warming up offers some real advantages. It helps prevent injuries by preparing your muscles, tendons, and ligaments and makes them more flexible and less susceptible to injury for the dynamic exercises that follow. It makes your body more supple and mobile so that your joints and muscles are better able to move through their full ranges of motion. And it helps stimulate the flow of blood — and of oxygen — to your muscles, thus making your body warmer and your muscles more pliable and giving you a better workout.

In this chapter, you discover several easy but effective warm-up exercises that get you ready for your Yoga with Weights workout.

Walking to Warm Up

Walking is the most natural of all exercises. It can also be one of the most — if not *the* most — enjoyable exercises. Walking doesn't require any particular expertise, either; it gives everyone the chance to be physically active.

If you have the time, make walking a prelude to every Yoga with Weights workout. You don't have to hike to the top of Mt. Everest; a short walk of 10 to 20 minutes will do. Getting in a walk daily or every other day has all kinds of benefits for your body and your mind. And if you combine walking with the other short warm-up exercises described in this chapter, you'll be well prepared for your Yoga with Weights workout. The combination of walking and Yoga with Weights as a daily and/or weekly workout program enhances the quality of your general health and mental well-being. It also helps keep your weight in check.

Try walking outside in nature, weather permitting. If you can't walk outside, a treadmill in your home or a gym works well.

Improving your mindfulness

Walking increases the oxygen to your brain and muscles, reduces stress, and slows bone mineral loss. The stimulus of seeing the world outside (if you decide to walk outside the confines of your house or office) calms your mind and body.

As you walk, be mindful of your breathing. Make your short walk a moving meditation by synchronizing your breathing with your steps. As you put one foot in front of the other, focus on the count of each breath. Take four counts to breathe in and four to breathe out. Being mindful of your breathing as you walk is good practice for being mindful of your breathing in your Yoga with Weights exercises and in everything you do. It also sharpens your awareness of breathing and increases your powers of concentration.

Shopping for shoes

Taking a short walk is a necessary warm-up exercise before working out, and assuming you want to walk outdoors, you need good shoes. Here's some advice for getting the right pair of walking shoes:

✔ Choose shoes with arch supports that are designed for exercising. And make sure you have enough room inside your shoes for socks and for swelling. Your feet swell when you exercise.

✔ Buy a new pair of shoes when your soles start to wear down. Walking and running in worn-out shoes can cause your feet and ankles to collapse, which can strain muscles and tendons in your feet and calves. Worn-out shoes can also cause problems in your lower back, upper back, and shoulders. If you walk and run daily, you probably need a new pair of shoes every six months.

Breathe through your nostrils, or take Complete Breaths (Book II, Chapter 1 explains what those are). You can also try saying the following sentence silently with each breath to get into the four-count rhythm: "Breathing in I calm body and mind; breathing out I cleanse and clear."

Preparing for a workout

For the first five minutes of your walk, stroll in an easy manner with your head held in whatever position feels most comfortable. Find your natural stride, feel your feet connecting with the ground, and gaze straight ahead. Gradually start to pick up speed, but never walk so fast that you're uncomfortable or have to strain to catch your breath. If you're walking with a companion, you should be able to carry on a conversation without having to stop to catch your breath.

As you walk, swing your arms gently alongside your body in a natural arc. Notice the movement of your arms, and develop an opposite-arm, opposite-leg movement — in other words, a coordinated stride. Walk with purpose and direction. Feel your chest lift up and open, and feel the energy flowing through your body.

Adding Warm-Up Exercises to Your Walk

Along with walking to warm up (the subject of the preceding section), you can do warm-up exercises. These warm-ups will keep your juices flowing after your walk and lead you comfortably into your Yoga with Weights workout. None of these exercises is difficult. None takes more than a minute to complete. Feel free to do as few or as many of these warm-up exercises as you want before your workout.

Choose exercises that warm up the parts of your body that feel tight or stiff. You can also choose exercises that make you feel better or relax you and prepare you physically and mentally for the workout to come.

Many of these warm-up exercises involve what yoga teachers call static holding. *Static holding* means you hold a position for three or more breaths. Simply stated, you push or contract a muscle against resistance and then hold that contraction for a few breaths. This technique requires a certain amount of concentration because you have to hold the pose and focus on your breathing throughout. Static holding gives you an opportunity to stretch out your muscles and develop your ability to balance. It also gives your muscles a chance to discover new ways of moving and holding as each exercise does its unique work for you. As you engage in static holding, listen carefully to your body, and feel your way to an understanding of which muscles you should contract and utilize fully and which muscles you should gently relax.

Chin-chest tuck

The purpose of the chin-chest tuck is to loosen up the back of your neck and upper spine area. Grab your hand weights and follow these steps:

1. **Stand looking straight ahead with your feet below your hips and your arms dangling at your sides, holding the weights with your palms facing inward.**

   This is the starting position. Make sure your feet are parallel to one another.

2. **Exhaling slowly, tuck your chin into your chest (see Figure 2-1).**

   If you can, touch your chin to your chest. Feel the back of your neck and upper spine stretching. Take two or three slow breaths while you're in this position.

3. **Inhaling slowly, return to the starting position (see Step 1).**

Repeat this exercise three to six times, pausing to rest between each repetition.

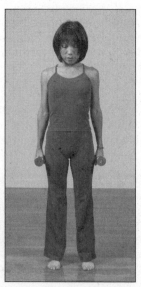

Figure 2-1:
The
chin-chest
tuck.

Photograph by Bonnie Kamin
(www.bonniekamin.com)

Head turner

Book V

Yoga-ing
Your Way
to a Toned
Body: Yoga
with
Weights

The head turner, as you may expect, increases the mobility of your neck, which is important for many of the Yoga with Weights exercises that require you to look in different directions. Use the hand weights as you follow these steps:

1. **Stand looking straight ahead with your feet below your hips and your arms dangling at your sides, holding the weights with your palms facing inward.**

   This is the starting position. Make sure your feet are parallel.

2. **Exhaling slowly and being careful not to drop your chin, turn your head and look over your right shoulder (see Figure 2-2).**

   Feel the muscles of your neck contracting and stretching. Hold this pose for two or three slow breaths.

3. **Inhaling slowly, return to the starting position (see Step 1).**

Alternating shoulders after each repetition, repeat this exercise three to six times for each shoulder.

Try the head turner after you've been sitting at your desk for a long time to give your neck a little exercise.

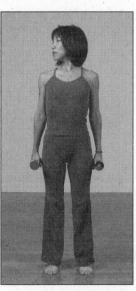

Figure 2-2:
The head
turner.

Photograph by Bonnie Kamin
(www.bonniekamin.com)

Lateral neck release

Like the two previous warm-up exercises, the lateral neck release also loosens up your neck. Grab your hand weights and follow these steps:

1. **Stand looking straight ahead with your feet below your hips and your arms dangling at your sides, holding the weights with your palms facing inward.**

   This is the starting position. Make sure your feet are parallel.

2. **Exhaling slowly, lower your right ear toward your right shoulder (see Figure 2-3).**

   Concentrate on the left side of your neck stretching and your left ear lifting up. Don't allow your chin to droop toward your chest.

   Hold this pose for two to three slow breaths, and concentrate on your breath opening and relaxing your neck and shoulders.

   Don't stay in this position for more than three breaths; it's easy to overstretch your neck in this position.

3. **Inhaling slowly, return your head to the starting position (see Step 1).**

Alternating sides after each repetition, repeat this exercise three to six times with each side of your neck.

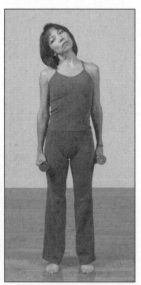

Figure 2-3:
The lateral neck release.

Photograph by Bonnie Kamin
(www.bonniekamin.com)

Book V

Yoga-ing
Your Way
to a Toned
Body: Yoga
with
Weights

Backward shoulder roll

The backward shoulder roll loosens and relaxes the back of your shoulders and the upper back region. Pick up your hand weights and follow these steps:

1. **Stand looking straight ahead with your feet below your hips and your arms dangling at your sides, holding the weights with your palms facing inward; inhale to a count of four.**

   This is the starting position. Make sure your feet are parallel.

2. **Exhaling slowly, roll your shoulders up, back, and then down (see Figure 2-4).**

   Allow the hand weights to draw your shoulders down when you lower your shoulders; the weights allow for a deeper stretch.

3. **Continue the rolling motion — moving your shoulders up, back, and then down — until they're loose as a goose.**

   Don't roll your shoulders forward; in other words, don't slouch.

Repeat this exercise three to six times.

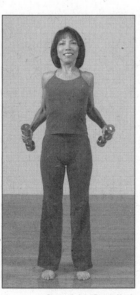

Figure 2-4:
The
backward
shoulder
roll.

Photograph by Bonnie Kamin
(www.bonniekamin.com)

Forward shoulder roll

The forward shoulder roll, like the backward shoulder roll (see the preceding exercise), loosens up and helps relax the muscles of the front of your shoulders, your upper chest, and your back. The forward shoulder roll and the backward shoulder roll go hand in hand, creating a balanced workout for this area of your body.

Grab your hand weights and follow these steps (be sure to engage your abdominal muscles throughout this exercise to support your back):

1. **Stand looking straight ahead with your feet below your hips and your arms dangling at your sides, holding the weights with your palms facing inward; inhale to a count of four.**

    This is the starting position. Make sure your feet are parallel.

2. **Exhaling slowly, roll your shoulders up, forward, and then down (see Figure 2-5).**

    As you roll your shoulders forward and down, allow the weights to pull your shoulders in the proper direction. Concentrate on your shoulder blades widening.

3. **Continue this motion — going up, forward, and then down — until your shoulders feel loose.**

Repeat this exercise three to six times.

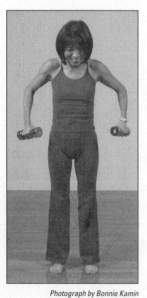

Figure 2-5:
The forward
shoulder
roll.

Photograph by Bonnie Kamin
(www.bonniekamin.com)

Side bender

The side bender concentrates on loosening the trunk of your body, from your hips to your shoulders. Pick up your hand weights for this exercise and follow these steps:

1. **Stand looking straight ahead with your feet below your hips and your arms dangling at your sides, holding the weights with your palms facing inward.**

   This is the starting position. Make sure your feet are parallel.

2. **Exhaling slowly, turn your head to the right as you lean gently to your right (see Figure 2-6).**

   Allow the weight to stretch the left side of your body. You should feel your waistline stretching. Be careful not to lean forward or backward; lean straight to your side. Pretend you're between two walls, one in front of you and one behind.

   Take two or three slow breaths in this position.

3. **Inhaling slowly, lift your body back to the starting position (see Step 1), turning your head as you lift.**

Alternating sides after each repetition, repeat this exercise two to four times with each side of your body.

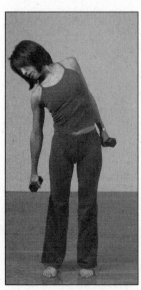

Figure 2-6:
The side bender.

Photograph by Bonnie Kamin
(www.bonniekamin.com)

Body twister

The object of the body twister is to loosen your hips and improve the flexibility of your trunk as a whole. Pick up your weights and follow these steps:

1. **Stand looking straight ahead with your feet below your hips and the weights held at hip level, palms facing inward.**

   This is the starting position. Make sure your feet are parallel.

2. **Pressing down on your left foot, twist your trunk, neck, head, and shoulders to the right (see Figure 2-7).**

3. **Hold this pose for two or three relaxed breaths, and then return your upper half to the starting position (see Step 1) and take the pressure off your left foot.**

Alternating from side to side, repeat this exercise six to eight times on each side of your body.

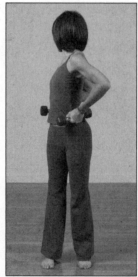

Figure 2-7:
The body
twister.

Photograph by Bonnie Kamin
(www.bonniekamin.com)

Wrist rotator

The wrist rotator loosens and relaxes your wrists, a must for the times when you have to maneuver hand weights or support your body with your hands. Pick up your hand weights and follow these steps:

1. **Stand looking straight ahead with your feet below your hips and your arms dangling at your sides, holding the weights with your palms facing backward.**

   This is the starting position. Make sure your feet are parallel.

2. **Breathing slowly and steadily, rotate your wrists in a counter-clockwise fashion (see Figure 2-8).**

   Rotate until the backs of your hands are facing each other. Enjoy feeling the muscles of your wrists loosen.

3. **Continuing to breathe slowly and steadily, rotate your wrists in the clockwise direction.**

   Rotate until your palms are facing forward.

Repeat this exercise three to six times in each direction.

If you have carpal tunnel syndrome or another wrist condition, use light hand weights to prevent injury or no hand weights at all.

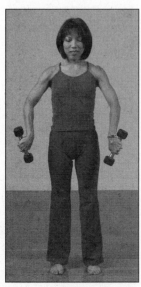

Figure 2-8:
The wrist rotator.

Photograph by Bonnie Kamin
(www.bonniekamin.com)

Big shoulder release

The big shoulder release is designed to eliminate the tension in your shoulders, shoulder joints, and upper back. Grab your hand weights and follow these steps:

1. **Stand looking straight ahead with your shoulders squared, your feet directly below your hips, and your arms hanging to your sides, holding the weights with your palms facing backward.**

   This is the starting position. Press down onto all four corners of your feet, and draw your belly in and up to support your back. Make sure your feet are parallel.

2. **Inhaling to a count of four, raise your arms forward and up, following the weights with your eyes as you lift (see Figure 2-9).**

   Lift, don't throw, your arms so they're straight over your shoulders, and hold them there for a moment.

   Don't jerk your arms, overextend the weights, or slouch. Performing these actions with weights in your hands can cause muscle or joint injury.

3. **Exhaling to a count of four, lower your arms and head to the starting position (see Step 1).**

Repeat this exercise three or four times.

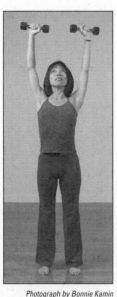

Figure 2-9:
The big
shoulder
release.

Photograph by Bonnie Kamin
(www.bonniekamin.com)

Y shoulder release

The Y shoulder release is designed to strengthen and improve the flexibility of your shoulders and upper back. Pick up your hand weights and follow these steps:

1. **With your shoulders squared and feet below your hips, stand looking straight ahead with your arms hanging to your sides, holding the weights with your palms facing inward.**

   This is the starting position. Press onto all four corners of your feet, and draw your belly in and up to support your back.

2. **Inhaling to a count of four, raise your arms away from your sides until they form a *Y* with your body, looking toward the ceiling as you lift (see Figure 2-10).**

   Be careful not to jerk your arms, which can cause muscle or joint injury.

   If you can't lift your arms above your shoulders, lift them as high as you comfortably can.

3. **Exhaling to a count of four, lower your arms and gaze to the starting position (see Step 1).**

Repeat this exercise three or four times.

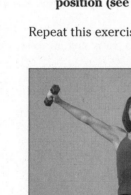

Figure 2-10:
The Y shoulder release.

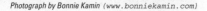
Photograph by Bonnie Kamin (www.bonniekamin.com)

Quad stretcher

The quad stretcher warms up your quads (or quadriceps), the large muscles on the front of your legs above your knees, by stretching them and strengthening them with the help of ankle weights.

To perform this exercise, you need ankle weights and a chair for balance. When you're ready, follow these steps:

1. **Stand directly behind the back of the chair with your feet directly below your hips and your arms at your sides.**

   This is the starting position.

2. **Bend your right knee, reach back with your right hand to hold your foot, and hold the chair with your left hand for balance (see Figure 2-11).**

   Make sure your shoulders are over your hips and your knees are close to one another. Feel your quad muscle stretching.

   If you can't reach your foot, grab a pant leg. You can also put a towel around your ankle and hold the towel.

3. **Hold this position for three or four deep, full breaths, and then return to the starting position (see Step 1).**

Alternating legs after each repetition, repeat this exercise four to six times with each leg.

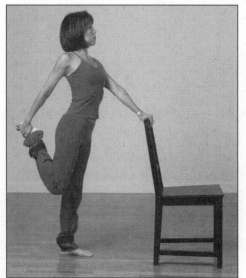

Figure 2-11:
The quad
stretcher.

Photograph by Bonnie Kamin (www.bonniekamin.com)

Back and hamstring stretcher

The back and hamstring stretcher works your hamstrings and, in the process, stretches and strengthens your back. Your *hamstring* is the long muscle on the back of your leg that runs from your knee to your buttock.

Grab a chair, strap on your ankle weights, and follow these steps:

1. **Stand directly behind the back of a chair with your feet directly below your hips and your arms at your sides.**

2. **Grab the back of the chair with both hands and step backward by one arm's length, making sure your arms and the trunk of your body are parallel with the floor.**

   This is the starting position. Fix your gaze on the floor.

3. **Step forward with your right leg, and flex your right foot.**

   Draw your belly in and up and your tailbone down for support.

4. **Lean back onto both of your heels (see Figure 2-12).**

   Concentrate on your hamstrings and back stretching.

5. **Hold this position for three or four slow breaths, and then return to the starting position (see Step 2).**

Alternating legs after each repetition, repeat this exercise four to six times with each leg.

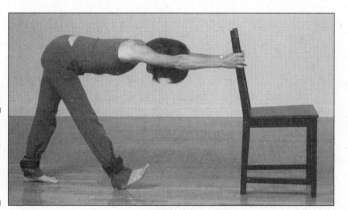

Figure 2-12: The back and hamstring stretcher.

Photograph by Bonnie Kamin (www.bonniekamin.com)

All-out hamstring stretcher

The all-out hamstring stretcher stretches your hamstrings — an important task because these muscles help you move comfortably in many of the exercises where you need to step, stand, or bend over.

Put on your ankle weights, find a chair, and follow these steps:

1. **Face the front of the chair with your feet below your hips and your hands on your thighs.**

   This is the starting position.

2. **Put your right heel on the chair's seat.**

   Keep your foot flexed and your toes pointing toward the ceiling. Pull your belly in and up and draw your tailbone down to anchor your legs.

3. **Bend forward as far as you can to stretch your hamstring, keeping both legs as straight as possible (see Figure 2-13).**

   If you can, put both of your hands on the chair. You should also feel your back stretching.

4. **Hold this pose for three or four slow breaths, and then return to the starting position (see Step 1) by slowly raising your body and taking your right heel off the chair.**

Alternating legs after each repetition, repeat this exercise four to six times with each leg.

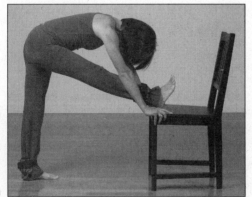

Figure 2-13:
The all-out hamstring stretcher.

Photograph by Bonnie Kamin (www.bonniekamin.com)

The big stretcher

Book V

**Yoga-ing
Your Way
to a Toned
Body: Yoga
with
Weights**

The big stretcher warms up your shoulders, back, and spine. The pose may seem difficult at first if you aren't limber, but the discomfort is worth it because the exercise stretches many different muscles that help you in Yoga with Weights workouts.

Strap on your ankle weights and follow these steps:

1. **Stand with your shoulders squared, your feet below your hips, and your arms hanging to your sides.**

2. **Interlace your fingers behind your back, with your palms facing each other.**

   This is the starting position. You may have to raise your shoulders — in other words, shrug them — to do this.

   If you can't interlace your fingers, grab a hand towel behind your back with both hands.

3. **As you slowly exhale, bend your knees and move the trunk of your body forward as far as you can (see Figure 2-14).**

   If you can go forward until you're looking at your feet like the model in Figure 2-14, great. If not, don't worry; go as far as you can. Your arms should remain together and be pointing toward the ceiling. Press into all four corners of each foot.

4. **Hold this pose for three or four breaths, and then slowly inhale as you return to the starting position (see Step 2).**

Repeat this exercise six to eight times.

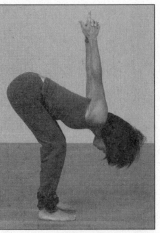

Figure 2-14:
The big
stretcher.

Photograph by Bonnie Kamin
(www.bonniekamin.com)

Marching legs

The marching legs exercise warms up your hips and *glutes* (the muscles on your buttocks).

You need ankle weights and hand weights for this exercise. When you're ready, follow these steps:

1. **Stand looking straight ahead with your feet below your hips and your arms hanging to your sides, holding the hand weights with your palms facing inward.**

   This is the starting position. Make sure your feet are parallel and that your shoulders are squared.

2. **As you slowly inhale to a count of four, lift your right knee (see Figure 2-15).**

   Pull your belly in for support, and keep your shoulders squared.

3. **As you slowly exhale to a count of four, lower your right leg to the starting position (see Step 1).**

Alternating legs after each repetition, repeat this exercise six to eight times with each leg.

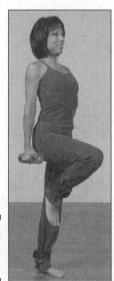

Figure 2-15: Marching legs.

Photograph by Bonnie Kamin
(www.bonniekamin.com)

If you want to go for a jog or do some other aerobic activity in place of Yoga with Weights, marching legs is an excellent warm-up for running activities.

Hip opener

The hip opener is an excellent stretch for your buttocks and hamstrings. It provides freedom and a greater range of motion in those areas, which in turn supports the well-being and healthy movement of your hips.

You need ankle weights for this exercise. When you're ready, follow these steps (keep your belly muscles engaged at all times during this exercise):

1. **Lay on the floor with your knees bent and your feet flat on the floor.**
2. **Place your right ankle on the top of your left knee (see Figure 2-16a).**

    This is the starting position.

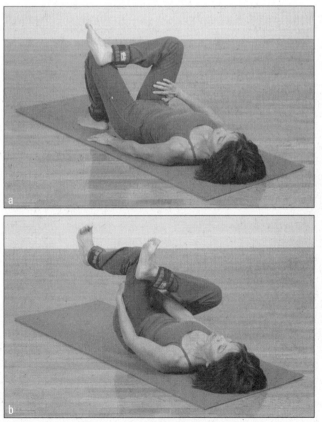

Figure 2-16: The hip opener.

Photographs by Bonnie Kamin (www.bonniekamin.com)

3. **Draw your left knee toward your chest (see Figure 2-16b).**

   Hold the underside of your left thigh with both hands to help bring your thigh closer to your chest. Pull your belly in for support.

4. **Hold this pose for two or three long, slow breaths, and then slowly lower your left foot back to the floor and put your right leg back in the starting position (see Figure 2-16a).**

Alternating legs after each repetition, repeat this exercise six to eight times with each leg.

Lower back release

The object of the lower back release is to gently stretch your lower back, hips, and pelvis and to relieve tension in these areas.

You need ankle weights for this exercise. When you're ready, follow these steps:

1. **Lay on your back with your knees bent and your heels a few inches away from your buttocks (see Figure 2-17a).**

   This is the starting position.

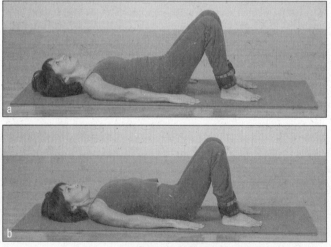

Figure 2-17:
Your lower back supports you during many Yoga with Weights exercises.

Photographs by Bonnie Kamin (www.bonniekamin.com)

2. **Slowly inhaling to a count of four, lift the lumbar curve of your back toward the ceiling (see Figure 2-17b).**

   The *lumbar curve* of your back is the part of your back between your waist and the base of your spine. Let your back rise to the rhythm of your breathing. Pull your belly in and up for support, and tilt your tailbone and pubic bone toward your navel.

3. **Slowly exhaling to a count of four, lower your back to the starting position (see Figure 2-17a).**

   Let your back fall to the rhythm of your breathing.

Repeat this exercise six to eight times.

For a better stretch, keep your buttocks on the floor throughout this exercise.

Chapter 3

From Head to Toe: The Balanced Workout

The Balanced Workout exercises and tones your entire body in one workout session. In this workout, you exercise all the major muscle groups of your body, from head to toe. If you do these exercises on a regular basis, you'll take a giant step toward the goal of getting in shape and cultivating a calm mind and beautiful body.

This workout takes 20 to 30 minutes. Ideally, you should practice it every other day.

As you engage in the Balanced Workout, follow these recommendations:

✔ **Breathe correctly.** In the Balanced Workout, you use the Complete Breath, which fills your body from your chest to your belly (head to Book II, Chapter 1 for information on what the Complete Breath is). Breathing Complete Breaths is a mindful practice that harmonizes body, mind, and spirit; improves your circulation; and de-stresses your mind.

✔ **Engage in a moment or two of silent meditation at the end of your workout.** Head to Book VII for more on meditation.

The Mountain

The mountain is a warm-up exercise that loosens and relaxes your spine, shoulders, and neck. Because it opens up your chest, back, and spine for vitality, it's good for your posture, as well as establishing a foundation that enables you to focus on concentration and develop balance and coordination.

Grab your hand weights and follow these steps:

1. **Stand with your legs as far apart as your hips and your toes pointing straight ahead, and let the hand weights dangle at your sides with your palms facing backward (see Figure 3-1a).**

   This is the starting position. Look straight ahead with your chin neither lifted nor lowered.

2. **As you inhale to a count of four, step forward with your right leg and lift the weights above your shoulders (see Figure 3-1b).**

   Keep your arms straight and raise them directly above your shoulders. Draw your belly in and up and your tailbone down for support. Focus on how you distribute your body weight as you step forward.

   If you feel any pinching in your shoulders or neck, you can lift the weights halfway up, perpendicular to your body.

   As you lift, the heel of your back foot may leave the floor, but keep the ball of your foot planted (see Figure 3-1b). Concentrate on your breathing and alignment during the lift. Make sure your breathing is steady and even. Don't shrug your shoulders.

3. **As you exhale to a count of four, lower your arms and step back into the starting position (see Figure 3-1a).**

   Lower the weight in time to your breathing. Don't look up or look down; gaze straight ahead.

Alternating legs, repeat this exercise six to eight times with each leg. Pause to rest, and then do six to eight more repetitions with each leg.

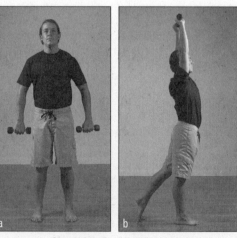

Figure 3-1:
The mountain is a head-to-toe exercise that loosens your body.

Photographs by Bonnie Kamin (www.bonniekamin.com)

Heaven and Earth

This exercise is called heaven and earth because you reach to the sky and root to the earth at the same time. It stretches the side of your body and brings oxygen to your back and spine; it helps you warm up and focus on your breathing; and it gets the energy flowing through your body.

Grab your hand weights and follow these steps:

1. **Stand with your legs as far apart as your hips and your toes pointing straight ahead, and let the hand weights dangle at your sides with your palms facing inward (see Figure 3-2a).**

   This is the starting position.

2. **Inhaling to a count to four, extend the weight in your right hand forward and then above your right shoulder, following the weight with your eyes (see Figure 3-2b).**

   Stretch out your arm and shoulder as much as possible without lifting your heels off the ground, and press your right foot into the ground as you look to the sky. You should finish inhaling as the weight reaches its peak. Feel your hip and the side of your body stretch as you lift the weight.

   If your neck feels too tight, look toward your elbow; in other words, look as high as you comfortably can. If your shoulders are tight, practice this exercise without a weight or raise the weight halfway.

3. **Exhaling to a count of four, lower the weight back to your side and return to the starting position (see Figure 3-2a).**

Keep your feet squarely on the floor throughout this exercise. Don't throw the weight; gently lift it. Focus on your breathing so that you have smooth transitions as you inhale (when you lift the weight) and exhale (when you lower the weight). Try to time your breathing so that you never hold your breath. Your breathing helps you relax and do the stretching portion of this exercise.

Repeat this exercise six to eight times with each arm, pause to rest, and then do six to eight more repetitions with each arm.

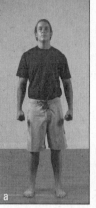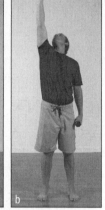

Figure 3-2:
The heaven
and earth
exercise
invigorates
your body
and helps
you breathe.

a   b

Photographs by Bonnie Kamin
(www.bonniekamin.com)

The Rag Doll

The rag doll releases tension in your neck and spine. It helps you relax and also works your abdominal muscles and the core muscles of your torso for a total upper-body workout.

Pick up your hand weights and follow these steps:

1. **Standing with your feet directly below your hips and your toes pointing forward, let your hand weights dangle at your sides with your palms facing inward (see Figure 3-3a).**

   This is the starting position. Don't let your belly collapse in this exercise; sculpt your belly in and up. Let your abdominal muscles support your spine. You should feel an "energetic girdle" around your abdomen.

   Throughout this exercise, keep your feet parallel to one another, both pointing straight ahead. Don't turn them out.

2. **Inhaling to a count of four, slowly roll your shoulders up and forward (see Figure 3-3b).**

   Pause your breath momentarily when you reach the top of the shoulder roll.

3. **Exhaling to a count of four, bend your knees and roll your torso forward with your shoulders leading the way (see Figure 3-3c).**

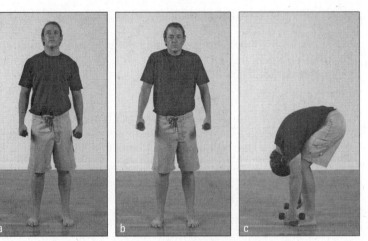

Figure 3-3:
The rag doll releases tension in your neck and spine and improves your flexibility and mobility.

Photographs by Bonnie Kamin (www.bonniekamin.com)

Now you're in the rag doll position, with your neck, head, and shoulders feeling loose and relaxed. Don't shrug your shoulders — roll them forward, using the weights to help extend your body forward and lengthen your spine.

You should feel your spine stretching as the weights hang. Keep your knees slightly bent and move your hips back.

4. **Inhaling to a count of four and pressing through your legs, roll your shoulders up, back, and down as you return to the starting position (see Figure 3-3a).**

   Feel the breath filling your lungs during this part of the exercise.

5. **Exhale to a count of four as you rest in the starting position.**

Do this exercise six to eight times, pause to rest, and then repeat the exercise another six to eight times.

The Airplane

The airplane stimulates feel-good chemistry in your brain and works your biceps, triceps, and upper torso.

You need the hand weights for this exercise; ankle weights are optional. Use the ankle weights if you want additional tone and strength.

Follow these steps to fly the airplane:

1. **Stand with your feet together and directly below your hips, and hold the weights in front of your chest with the knuckles of each hand touching (see Figure 3-4a).**

   This is the starting position.

2. **Slowly inhaling to a count of four, bend your left knee, extend your right leg behind you as you lean forward, and open your arms to a C position (see Figure 3-4b).**

   While you're extending your leg, look slightly upward toward your forehead and brow. To achieve the C position, imagine you're crunching a soda can with your shoulder blades.

   To help with balancing, press your standing foot into the floor, draw your belly in and up, and draw your tailbone down. If you feel pinched in your neck and shoulders or you otherwise experience distress as you maneuver the hand weights, use lighter weights or no weights at all.

3. **Slowly exhaling to a count of four, return the hand weights to your chest as you lower your leg to the floor and assume the starting position (see Figure 3-4a).**

Repeat this exercise six to eight times with each leg, pause to rest, and then do the exercise six to eight more times with each leg.

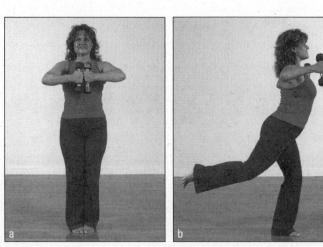

Figure 3-4: In the airplane, you work your balancing muscles and strengthen your upper body.

a

b

Photographs by Bonnie Kamin (www.bonniekamin.com)

Book V

**Yoga-ing
Your Way
to a Toned
Body: Yoga
with
Weights**

The Triangle

The triangle is an extended side angle pose that beginners can enjoy. The exercise works many muscles in your body, but it concentrates on the core muscles of your trunk, your shoulders, and your legs. As you balance, the triangle also helps you trace and explore the physical feeling and sensation of your body.

You need hand weights for this exercise, so grab them and follow these steps:

1. **With your feet parallel to each other, stand with your legs as wide apart as you comfortably can, and hold the weights at your waist with your palms facing inward.**

2. **Turn both feet to the right and bend at the right knee until you align your knee over your ankle (see Figure 3-5a).**

3. **Rotate your torso to the right and rest your right forearm on your right thigh or knee; let the weight in your left hand hang to the ground with your arm straight and your palm facing inward (see Figure 3-5b).**

   This is the starting position.

   Draw your belly in and up and your tailbone down to stabilize your legs, trunk, and spine. If you feel a burning sensation along the top of your supporting leg, your leg is doing too much support work. Focus on the core muscles of your torso and trunk so that they do more of the lifting and balancing work.

4. **Exhaling to a count of four, lift the weight in your left hand to your torso, bending your elbow toward the ceiling and drawing your shoulder slightly back, over, and downward as you lift (see Figure 3-5c).**

   Look toward the ceiling and imagine that you're pulling back an arrow on a bow. You should feel a solid pulling action that goes up, over, and back with each lift.

5. **Inhaling to a count of four, bring your head and torso back down as you turn to the right and lower the weight to the starting position (see Figure 3-5b).**

   Follow the weight with your eyes. Don't drop the weight; lower it slowly to the floor.

REMEMBER

To anchor yourself, press down onto all four corners of your right foot and onto the balls of your left foot as you do this exercise. Don't let your supporting knee wobble from side to side or extend over your toes. If you're flexible enough, straighten both legs as you do this exercise. If you feel a strain in your neck, use lighter weights.

Do this exercise six to eight times on each leg, pause to rest, and then do the exercise six to eight more times on each leg.

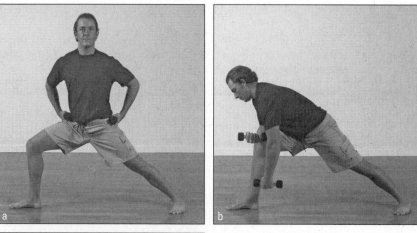

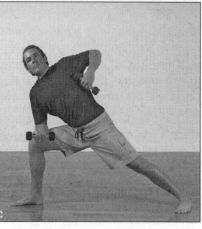

Figure 3-5: The triangle is a yoga master pose (with a few variations) that beginners can master.

Photographs by Bonnie Kamin (www.bonniekamin.com)

The Exalted Warrior

Book V

Yoga-ing
Your Way
to a Toned
Body: Yoga
with
Weights

The exalted warrior makes use of a classic yoga pose: the victorious warrior (for a video showing how to prepare for and move into this posture, visit www.dummies.com/go/yogaaiofd. This Yoga with Weights variation sends a surge of power through your entire body. It strengthens and tones your upper torso, opens your collarbone, teaches you to work the core muscles of your trunk for balance, and strengthens your legs.

Pick up your hand weights for this exercise and follow these steps:

1. **Stand with your feet together and your toes pointing forward, and allow the hand weights to dangle at your sides with your palms facing backward.**

2. **Gently step back with your right foot, keeping your legs straight.**

   Turn your back foot slightly out for balance and stability. Align your shoulders with your hips.

   Make sure your legs are strong and engaged. Let your back and your front leg support you.

3. **Raise your arms forward until they're directly above your shoulders (see Figure 3-6a).**

   This is the starting position. Draw your belly in and up and point your tailbone down throughout the rest of the exercise.

4. **As you exhale to a count of four, pull your arms down, bending your elbows and holding the weights at ear level (see Figure 3-6b).**

   This movement is what weightlifters call a *back-lat pull-down.* Pull down with your *lats* — the muscles on your back around your shoulder blades — as well as with your shoulders. Don't let your wrists flop or cock back as you do this exercise; keep them aligned with your forearms.

5. **As you inhale to a count of four, press the weights back up to the starting position (see Figure 3-6a).**

Do this exercise six to eight times on each leg, pause to rest, and then do the exercise six to eight more times on each leg.

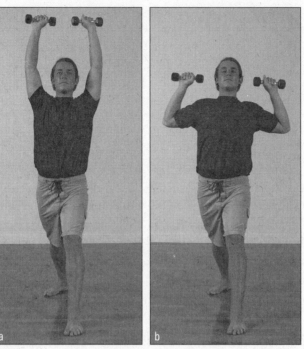

Figure 3-6:
Feel the
strength and
courage of
the exalted
warrior
surging
through
your whole
body.

Photographs by Bonnie Kamin (www.bonniekamin.com)

The Warrior II

The warrior II is a variation of the exalted warrior, the preceding exercise in this workout. This version works your biceps, legs, and the core muscles of your trunk and torso. It looks easy, but if you do it right, the exercise works your entire body and teaches you the power of concentration.

Pick up your hand weights for this exercise and follow these steps:

1. **Stand with your legs as far apart as you comfortably can and your feet pointing forward, and hold the weights at your waist with your palms facing forward.**

2. **Turn both of your feet to the right and bend your right knee until you align it vertically with your ankle.**

   Your back foot should be pointing at a 45-degree angle, and your right foot should be pointing straight ahead to your right. Keep your torso centered equally between your heels and your hips rotated wide open. You're in a lunge position.

Book V

Yoga-ing
Your Way
to a Toned
Body: Yoga
with
Weights

3. **Raise your arms to shoulder height with your palms facing upward and your arms extended away from your body (see Figure 3-7a).**

   This is the starting position. Concentrate on your legs to keep them strong and stable as you move your arms.

4. **Exhaling to a count of four, draw your hands to your shoulders with a bicep curl (see Figure 3-7b).**

   Draw your belly in and up and your tailbone down to support yourself and maintain your balance. The warrior II is a total body exercise, not just a biceps exercise. Don't let your front knee wobble or move forward over your toes.

5. **Inhaling to a count of four, return to the starting position (see Figure 3-7a).**

Do this exercise six to eight times on each leg, pause to rest, and then do six to eight more repetitions on each leg.

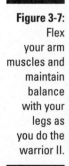

Figure 3-7:
Flex
your arm
muscles and
maintain
balance
with your
legs as
you do the
warrior II.

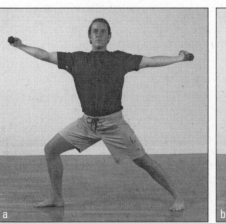 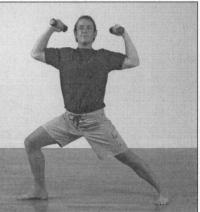

Photographs by Bonnie Kamin (www.bonniekamin.com)

The Camel

The camel is a simple exercise that has real benefits. It stretches out your spine; tones your thighs and backside; opens up your chest, armpits, and back; and improves circulation to your lungs and heart region. In most daily activities, you lean forward, but this exercise gives you an opportunity to stretch the other direction.

If you have sensitive knees, don't sit on your heels during this exercise. Try straddling a rolled-up yoga mat, a stack of books, or a briefcase.

Grab your hand weights for this exercise and follow these steps:

1. **Sit on your knees with your buttocks resting on your heels and your legs flat on the floor, and hold the weights at your sides with your palms facing backward (see Figure 3-8a).**

   This is the starting position. Look straight ahead, and keep your spine erect.

2. **As you inhale to a count of four, rise to your knees — using the power and strength of your thigh muscles — and lift the weights straight above your shoulders (see Figure 3-8b).**

   Let your breath establish a rhythm as you rise and lift.

3. **As you exhale to a count of four, sit down on your legs, and lower the weights to the starting position (see Figure 3-8a).**

   Don't swing the weights. Carefully control the release as you kneel and sit back down.

Do this exercise six to eight times, pause to rest, and then do it six to eight more times.

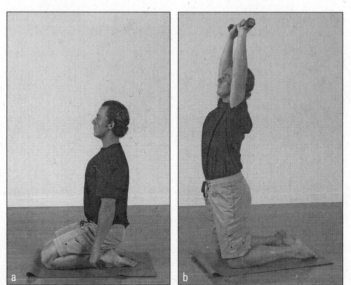

Figure 3-8:
Focus on your breathing as you lift your body off the ground for the camel.

Photographs by Bonnie Kamin (www.bonniekamin.com)

The Table

The table works and tones your buttocks, hips, and thighs; it exercises your back and spine to develop core-strength conditioning; and it helps you develop the muscles that support your trunk.

Time to grab your ankle weights. After you're strapped in, follow these steps:

1. **Get on all fours with your hands directly below your shoulders and your knees directly under your hips.**

   Lift your waistline so that your back feels flat. Spread your fingers wide so they support your weight.

2. **Lift your right leg up to the height of your hip, keeping the plane of your body flat (see Figure 3-9a).**

   This is the starting position.

3. **Inhaling to a count of four, bend your knee backward and push your leg up (see Figure 3-9b).**

   Press your foot up so it's higher than your hip, without rolling your hip to the side. Keep your leg directly behind you and your hips squared. Flex your foot as if you're standing on the floor.

   If you feel discomfort in your lower back, don't raise your leg as high. Use a lighter weight if you have trouble lifting your leg.

4. **Exhaling to a count of four, unbend your knee and bring your leg back to the starting position (see Figure 3-9a).**

Let your breathing guide you. Slowly move your foot upward as you inhale; move it back down slowly as you exhale. Count to four as you complete each inhale and exhale.

Don't push with your arms or bend your elbows. Use them only for stability and maintaining your balance. Don't sag as you do this exercise.

Do this exercise six to eight times with each leg, pause to rest, and then do it six to eight more times with each leg.

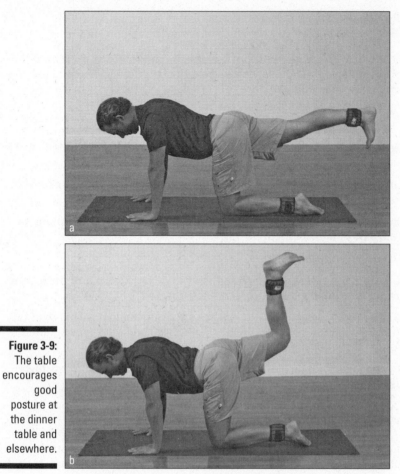

Figure 3-9:
The table
encourages
good
posture at
the dinner
table and
elsewhere.

Photographs by Bonnie Kamin (www.bonniekamin.com)

The Cat

The cat stretches out your spine, back, neck, and shoulders. This exercise works the same muscles as the table (see the preceding exercise in this workout), but you also stretch your spine and belly.

Strap on your ankle weights for this exercise and follow these steps:

1. **Get on all fours with your knees directly under your hips and your hands directly below your shoulders.**

   Make sure your fingers are spread wide for support.

Book V

Yoga-ing
Your Way
to a Toned
Body: Yoga
with
Weights

2. **Extend your right leg behind you, and look forward and up (see Figure 3-10a).**

   This is the starting position. Draw your belly in and up and your tailbone down for support.

   Don't rotate your leg (what a dog does next to a fire hydrant). Make sure it's in line with the rest of your body.

3. **Exhaling to a count of four, draw your right leg deep into your chest as you arch your back and look toward your navel (see Figure 3-10b).**

   Point your nose at your pelvis as you move toward your bent knee. Don't swing your leg; move it slowly in rhythm with your breathing.

4. **Breathe four counts in and four counts out while in the tucked position.**

5. **Inhaling to a count of four, lift your head, flatten your back, and extend your right leg back to the starting position (see Figure 3-10a).**

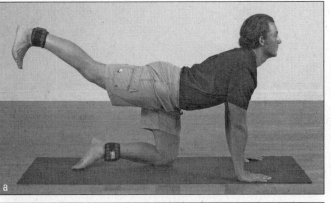

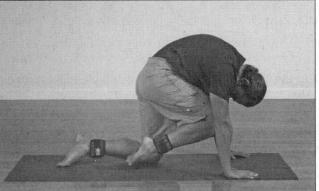

Figure 3-10: Stretch your back like a cat in this exercise.

Photographs by Bonnie Kamin (www.bonniekamin.com)

Keep your arms straight to stabilize and balance your body throughout this exercise. Make sure they stay directly below your shoulders.

Do this exercise six to eight times with each leg, pause to rest, and then do it six to eight more times with each leg.

The Dog

The dog introduces ankle weights to a classic yoga master pose — the downward-facing dog. The dog strengthens, stretches, and tones all parts of your body, but especially your *rhomboids* (the muscles behind your thighs) and *hamstrings* (the muscles on the back of your legs above the knees). The exercise also improves circulation to your head and chest, which helps you feel strong and mentally awake.

Grab your ankle weights and follow these steps:

1. **Get on all fours with your knees directly under your hips and your hands directly below your shoulders.**

   Make sure your fingers are spread wide for support.

2. **Pressing through your palms and the balls of your feet, lift your hips, push your thighs backward, press your sitting bones up to the sky, and move your belly in and up until you're in an upside-down *V* position (see Figure 3-11a).**

   This is the starting position. Your ears should now be between your arms.

   Stand on the balls of your feet if you can't stretch your hamstrings far enough to keep your feet flat. If your hamstrings and Achilles tendons are tight, feel free to spread your legs a little farther apart.

3. **Inhaling to a count of four, lift your right leg directly behind you toward the ceiling without rotating your hips (see Figure 3-11b).**

   Try to keep your leg straight, and square your hips. Press your hands into the floor and keep your elbows straight. If you're collapsing in your arms, lift up your armpits as if you're shrugging your shoulders.

4. **Exhaling to a count of four, slowly lower your leg to the starting position (see Figure 3-11a).**

If you feel like your arms are working too hard, bend your knees more, pull your belly in, press into your hands, and move your thighs back.

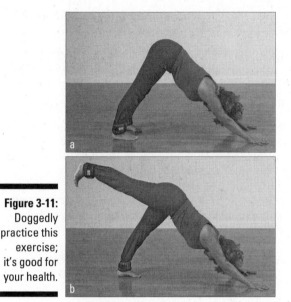

Figure 3-11: Doggedly practice this exercise; it's good for your health.

Photographs by Bonnie Kamin (www.bonniekamin.com)

Breathe fully — four counts inhaling and four counts exhaling — as you do this exercise. Alternating legs, perform six to eight repetitions with each leg, pause to rest, and then do six to eight more reps with both legs.

The Bridge

The bridge is designed to stretch your spine to make it more elastic. The exercise also stretches your rib cage and chest and strengthens your upper back, torso, hamstrings, and calves.

If you have a lower back problem, do this exercise tentatively at first, and engage your buttocks muscles as you engage your abdominals; this helps stabilize your lower back.

You need your hand weights to cross this bridge; ankle weights are optional. After you've prepared, follow these steps:

1. **Lie on your back with your knees bent, your feet planted flat on the floor, and your palms facing downward while holding the weights on the floor (see Figure 3-12a).**

   This is the starting position. Make sure your lower back is flat against the floor. Look straight up at the ceiling.

2. **Inhaling to a count of four, raise your hips and buttocks to knee height and lift both arms above your head (see Figure 3-12b).**

   Your hands should move 180 degrees to the floor behind you. Press down into your feet as you lift your hips and buttocks, and rely on your shoulders to bear most of the burden.

   If you feel any discomfort in your shoulders, neck, or arms, lift your arms halfway.

3. **Exhaling to a count of four, lower your back to the floor one vertebra at a time and bring your arms forward and back down to the starting position (see Figure 3-12a).**

Keep your tailbone down and your abdominal core strong to take the strain off your lower back during this exercise. And keep your knees stable and in their starting position; they shouldn't wobble.

Do this exercise six to eight times, pause to rest, and then do it six to eight more times.

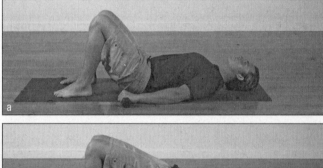

Figure 3-12: The bridge aims to make your spine more elastic.

Photographs by Bonnie Kamin (www.bonniekamin.com)

The Frog

This particular exercise, aptly named the frog, opens up, stretches, and relaxes your groin, hips, and pelvis. It also lengthens your spine. You'll feel your blood coursing through your body as you do the frog.

Strap on your ankle weights for this exercise and follow these steps:

1. **Lie on your back and, with your knees bent and spread wide, lift your legs to your chest so you can hold your feet, ankles, or calves (see Figure 3-13a).**

   This is the starting position. Draw your belly in and up for support. The bottom of your spine should feel elongated.

   If your knees or inner groin muscles feel tight, extend your legs halfway. You can also hold your inner thighs rather than your feet, ankles, or calves.

2. **Exhaling slowly to a count of four, straighten your right leg as far as you comfortably can while still holding your toes, calves, or ankles (see Figure 3-13b).**

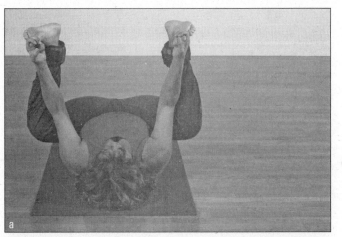

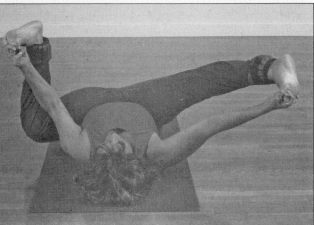

Figure 3-13: The frog is a hoppin' good exercise for your torso.

Photographs by Bonnie Kamin (www.bonniekamin.com)

Pull your belly in; this exercise works your belly muscles, which you need to support your legs and keep them from getting overextended.

Don't lift your back off the floor or rock your body from side to side.

3. **Inhaling slowly to a count of four, return your right leg to the starting position (see Figure 3-13a).**

Do this exercise six to eight times with each leg, pause to rest, and then do another six to eight repetitions with each leg.

The Zen

Your Balanced Workout is over; time to relax and enjoy how great your workout has made you feel. As you do this last cool-down exercise, feel the gentle rise and fall of your breath. In yoga, transitions are always important. During this exercise, see if you can make a smooth transition from exercising to whatever activity you want to do next.

You need ankle weights for this exercise, but don't put them on. Follow these steps:

1. **Lie on your back with your ankle weights resting on your diaphragm (see Figure 3-14).**

The weight is to make you aware of your breathing.

2. **Take in eight to ten Balancing Breaths.**

Taking Balancing Breaths is a great way to relax (for more detail, see Book II, Chapter 1).

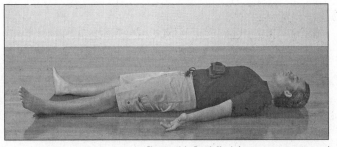

Figure 3-14:
Time to
relax with
the Zen.

Photograph by Bonnie Kamin (www.bonniekamin.com)

Chapter 4

Waking Up Your Mind and Body: The Energy Workout

In This Chapter

▶ Reenergizing your mind and body

▶ Releasing tension in your body through breathing

*W*hen you start to feel listless in the afternoon or early evening, forgo the cup of coffee or the sugar-filled snack and do the body shaping, mentally awakening exercises in this chapter instead. The Energy Workout takes 20 to 30 minutes and can be a mini-break that makes a positive difference in how you feel because the exercises take only a few minutes of your day. They benefit your circulation and nervous system, allow you to let go of your anxieties, and help you de-stress. The deep breathing brings calm and quiet to help you deal with stress, which gives you more energy and sharpens your senses. After you do this energy-boosting workout a few times, you'll feel more fit and energized, and your spiritual batteries will be recharged. You'll discover a keener awareness of the world around you. You'll feel refreshed and renewed.

Practice the exercises in the Energy Workout with thoughtfulness and care. Heed this advice:

✔ Don't push yourself too far; take the time to feel your muscles at work, and understand where your exercise limits are.

✔ Breathing is an essential element in all the workouts in Book V, but especially in this one because of the demand you place on your body. In this workout, you use the Ocean Breath, which you can read about in Book II, Chapter 1. This kind of breathing maximizes the potential of your upper chest for breathing and exercising.

✔ Be sure to engage in a moment or two of silent meditation at the end of your workout. Head to Book VII for more on meditation.

The Chair

The chair is a total-body strengthening exercise that particularly benefits your shoulders, arms, and legs. It also exercises your buttocks, abs, and hamstrings. As you do the chair, press into the ground on all four corners of your feet as you raise and lower the weights.

You need hand weights for this exercise. Follow these steps:

1. **Stand with your feet below your hips, your toes pointing forward, and the weights held at your sides with your palms facing inward (see Figure 4-1a).**

   This is the starting position. Draw your belly in and up and your tailbone down for support.

2. **As you inhale to a count of four, sit on an imaginary seat, and slowly raise your arms above your shoulders until they align with your ears (see Figure 4-1b).**

   Raise your arms in front of your body, keeping your palms inward. Imagine that a chair is behind you and you're touching it with your buttocks.

   If your knees bother you, don't crouch as far; take your tailbone down and pull your belly in more. You can also raise your arms only to shoulder height if you have trouble lifting the weights.

3. **As you exhale to a count of four, stand up and slowly lower the weights back to the starting position (see Figure 4-1a).**

Be patient as you do this exercise; let the rhythm of your breathing lift you up and lower you down. As long as you focus on your breathing, you won't throw the weights upward. Inflate your body as you breathe in, letting the intake of air raise your arms as if someone were blowing you up like a balloon.

Repeat this exercise six to eight times, pause to rest, and then do another six to eight repetitions.

Book V

Yoga-ing
Your Way
to a Toned
Body: Yoga
with
Weights

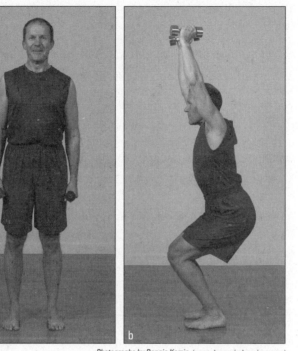

Figure 4-1:
Use the
chair to
work your
entire body
from the
(imaginary)
seat of your
pants.

Photographs by Bonnie Kamin (www.bonniekamin.com)

The Skater

The skater is an aerobic exercise that works the muscles of your buttocks. The skater is similar to the chair (see the preceding exercise in this workout), but here you lift a leg behind you. The balancing aspect of this exercise fires and stimulates your brain's nerve connections.

Focus on inhaling and exhaling so you don't do this exercise too fast and throw the weights. Keep your chest open as you inhale and exhale throughout this exercise.

Strap on your ankle weights and grab your hand weights. Then follow these steps:

1. **Stand with your feet below your hips, your toes pointing forward, and the hand weights at your sides with your palms facing backward (see Figure 4-2a).**

This is the starting position. Spread your toes wide, pressing hard into the ground through all four corners of both feet — your heels and your toes. You should actively engage both feet. Also, for support, draw your belly in and up and point your tailbone down.

2. **As you inhale to a count of four, lift the weights above your head while you bend your left leg for support and lift your right leg behind you as high as you can without losing balance (see Figure 4-2b).**

   Lift your arms in front of your body until they reach the height of your ears. As you lift, sit back a little bit with your buttocks behind your heel. Feel your buttocks squeezing as your hips are parallel to the floor.

   Keep your leg behind you (don't lift it to your side as a dog does beside a fire hydrant).

3. **As you exhale to a count of four, return to the starting position (see Figure 4-2a).**

   Keep your chest open as you exhale.

If you have trouble balancing, try using lighter weights, or do the exercise without the hand weights and rest your hands on your hips. You can also do this exercise without the ankle weights.

Alternating legs with each repetition, repeat this exercise six to eight times with each leg, pause to rest, and then do another six to eight repetitions with each leg. You're imitating the gliding motion of an ice skater.

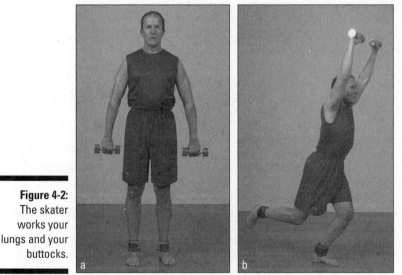

Figure 4-2:
The skater works your lungs and your buttocks.

Photographs by Bonnie Kamin (www.bonniekamin.com)

The Crow

The crow is a weighted version of a classic yoga posture that works your buttocks, your upper shoulders, your belly, and your legs. It stretches and conditions your hamstrings and calves and also works your spine. The exercise may seem difficult to do at first, but you can master it with a little practice.

With your ankle weights strapped in place, follow these steps:

1. **Stand with your feet touching or as close to touching as possible, and let your arms fall to your sides.**

2. **Crouch down with your knees parted, put your elbows inside your knees, and rest your hands at shoulder width on the floor (see Figure 4-3a).**

   This is the starting position. You should be squatting deep into your heels. Do your best to keep your heels down while you're in the squatting position.

   If your knees bother you or you have trouble squatting, try squatting halfway. You can also try this exercise without ankle weights if they cause too much trouble for you.

3. **As you inhale to a count of four, straighten your left leg and raise your right leg behind you (see Figure 4-3b).**

   Push through your right foot like a swimmer pushing off the side of the pool. Don't rotate your hips; keep them square. Be careful not to kick out your back leg.

   Support yourself with your hands and shoulders as well as your left leg, and sculpt your belly in and up for stability. Keep your supporting leg and your hands flat on the floor. If you can't keep your supporting leg straight and maintain your flat hand position, bend your knee a little.

4. **As you exhale to a count of four, lower your extended leg and return to the starting position (see Figure 4-3a).**

Alternating legs, do this exercise six to eight times with each leg, pause to rest, and then do another six to eight reps with each leg.

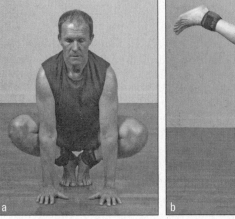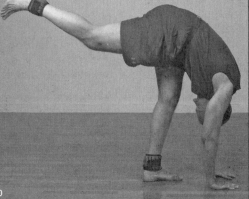

Figure 4-3:
The crow is a full-body exercise that improves your balance and co-ordination.

a b

Photographs by Bonnie Kamin (www.bonniekamin.com)

The Runner

This exercise is called the runner because the starting position makes you look like a sprinter in the starting blocks and because you get the feeling of freedom and exhilaration that comes from running in an open field. The exercise strengthens your arm and belly muscles and develops your timing, rhythm, and coordination. The runner also stretches out your hamstrings, works your legs, and won't upset your allergies like the field.

Strap on your ankle weights and follow these steps:

1. **Start on all fours with your shoulders directly over your wrists and your hips directly over your knees.**

   Spread your fingers wide for support.

   Make sure the inside creases of your elbows face each other. In other words, don't turn your elbows out. If you're limber, you run the risk of tearing a ligament if you turn your elbows out.

2. **Lean back, bringing your heels toward the ground as you draw your knees toward your belly and your buttocks toward your heels (see Figure 4-4a).**

   This is the starting position. Your knees should be deeply bent. Draw your belly in and up and your tailbone down for support.

3. **Exhaling to a count of four, straighten your left leg as you lift your right leg toward the ceiling (see Figure 4-4b).**

   As best you can, keep both legs straight. Focus your eyes on your left knee and shin. Feel your spine stretching.

Remove the ankle weights or wear lighter weights if lifting your leg up high proves too difficult.

4. **Inhaling to a count of four, lower your right leg and return to the starting position (see Figure 4-4a).**

   Look forward as you squat.

Alternating legs, do this exercise six to eight times with each leg, pause to rest, and then do another six to eight reps with each leg.

Figure 4-4:
Feel the exhilaration of a race as you do the runner.

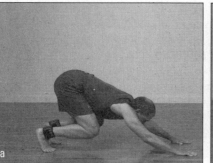
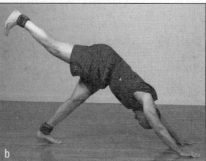

Photographs by Bonnie Kamin (www.bonniekamin.com)

The Eye of the Needle

The eye of the needle massages your organs (see Book V, Chapter 1 for more on squeeze-and-soak exercises), loosens your spine, opens up your chest and shoulders, and strengthens and conditions your whole upper torso and shoulder-rotation mechanism.

Don't hold your breath in this exercise (be conscious of breathing in and out). Keep your hips over your knees at all times, and remember that your supporting arm should be active the entire time as you look through the eye of the needle; don't let this arm go limp.

Grab one hand weight, and strap on your ankle weights. Then follow these steps:

1. **Start on all fours with your hips directly over your knees and your hands on the floor directly below your shoulders; hold a weight in your right hand (see Figure 4-5a).**

   In this position, you should draw your belly below your navel in and up for abdominal stability. Your toes should be pointing straight back.

2. **Inhaling to a count of four, press your left palm down as you slowly raise your right arm up (along with the weight), keeping it straight, and roll your right shoulder back (see Figure 4-5b).**

   This is the starting position. Rotate your shoulder and open your chest to the right side as you look toward the ceiling.

3. **Exhaling to a count of four, slowly bring your right hand under and past your body as you stretch out your back and roll onto the backside of your right shoulder (see Figure 4-5c).**

   Your head and the weight should move onto the floor. Feel your back and shoulder stretching as you move the weight onto the floor.

   Watch the weight with your eyes as you roll down. This way, your head flows with the movement of your shoulder and arm. Tuck your chin in slightly to loosen your neck.

   If your shoulders are too tight to roll all the way down, you may want to rest your head on a rolled-up blanket or towel so your neck isn't straining and then gently rotate as far as you can. You can also move your supporting hand forward and out from your body to make the needle loop bigger.

4. **Inhaling to a count of four, return to the starting position (see Figure 4-5b).**

   Pull the weight back through the loop in rhythm with your breathing.

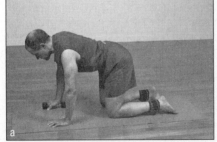
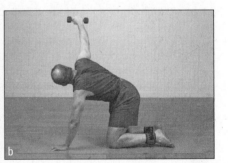
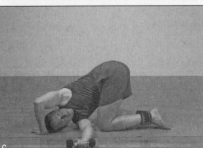

Figure 4-5:
You massage your internal organs as you thread the eye of the needle.

Photographs by Bonnie Kamin (www.bonniekamin.com)

Do this exercise six to eight times with each arm, pause to rest, and then do the exercise six to eight more times with each arm.

The Dog to Plank

The dog to plank is a powerful upper-body strengthener. It sculpts and tones the entire trunk of your body and also works your buttocks. Along with the strength benefits, the dog to plank gives you an endurance exercise with aerobic benefits, and it develops your ability to concentrate.

Strap on your ankle weights and follow these steps:

1. **Begin on all fours with your hands directly below your shoulders, your knees directly underneath your hips, and your toes planted on the ground (see Figure 4-6a).**

   Spread your fingers wide for support.

2. **Move into the downward-facing dog position by lifting your hips and buttocks as you straighten your legs, bring your thighs back, and move your heels toward the floor.**

   Your ears should be between your arms. Draw your belly in and up and your tailbone down for support.

3. **As you inhale to a count of four, lift your right leg up as high as you can without twisting your hip open (see Figure 4-6b).**

   This is the starting position. Push your leg straight back, and flex your foot to keep it fully engaged; it shouldn't be limp.

4. **As you exhale to a count of four, bring the trunk of your body forward so that your shoulders are over your wrists (see Figure 4-6c).**

   You're in the plank position. Keep your lifted leg parallel to the floor if you're strong enough; otherwise, tap your toe on the floor. You should feel your abdominal and arm muscles working.

   Don't bend your elbows; support your weight through your shoulders and across your back without using your chest muscles.

5. **As you inhale to a count of four, return to the starting position (see Figure 4-6b).**

   Don't lunge backward. Be patient, and move in rhythm with your breathing.

You can do this exercise without ankle weights if you have too much trouble.

Do this exercise six to eight times with each leg, pause to rest, and then do another six to eight repetitions with each leg.

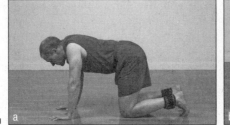

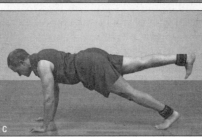

Figure 4-6:
The dog to plank is a powerful exercise for your upper and lower body.

Photographs by Bonnie Kamin (www.bonniekamin.com)

The Twisted Triangle

The twisted triangle is a squeeze-and-soak exercise, which means that it massages your internal organs. Along with warming your insides, it lengthens, tones, stretches, and conditions your legs, back, and spine. Talk about an all-around body conditioner!

If you discover that you're not ready for this exercise, don't rush. Take it slowly. You can injure your lower back if you do the twisting motion in this exercise incorrectly.

You use one hand weight in this exercise. Follow these steps:

1. **Stand with your feet as far apart as you comfortably can, with your arms extended straight away from your body forming a straight line with your shoulders (see Figure 4-7a).**

   Make sure you have the weight resting in front of your right foot.

2. **Turn the trunk of your body to face your right leg and, as you bend your right knee, gently lean forward.**

3. **Rest your left hand on the outside of your right foot, and grasp the weight with your right hand (see Figure 4-7b).**

   This is the starting position. Draw your belly in and up and your tailbone down for stability and balance.

If you can, square your hips, with your right hip back and your left hip forward. Not everyone can square his or her hips in this position, however, and if you can't, do your best and don't worry about it.

4. **Exhaling to a count of four, bend your right elbow and lift the weight as you rotate your shoulder and trunk (see Figure 4-7c).**

   Imagine you're an archer pulling back the string of a bow. Twist your trunk, starting at the bottom of your spine and working your way up, one vertebra at a time. Lift your head to the right with the weight as you twist.

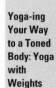

Book V

Yoga-ing
Your Way
to a Toned
Body: Yoga
with
Weights

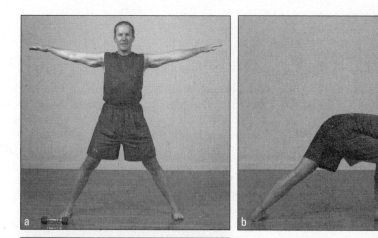

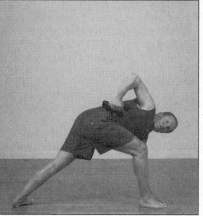

Figure 4-7:
The twisted
triangle
conditions
your entire
body.

Photographs by Bonnie Kamin (www.bonniekamin.com)

Your left hand should remain by your right foot as you lift. Press down into the balls of your feet for balance and stability.

5. **Inhaling to a count of four, unwind and lower the weight to the starting position (see Figure 4-7b).**

Be patient as you return to the starting position. Focusing on your breathing helps you return to the starting position in rhythm. Your left hand should remain by your right foot as you lower.

Try straightening your front leg to stretch your hamstring. If you can't rotate your trunk, lift the weight to exercise your triceps without rotating your shoulder and chest.

Do this exercise six to eight times on each leg, pause to rest, and then do the exercise six to eight more times on each leg.

The Warrior I

The warrior I, a relatively simple exercise, is a weighted variation of the classic warrior yoga pose. As you do this exercise, you tap the energy of your heart and feel the strength, honor, and courage of a warrior. On a more practical note, the warrior I works your biceps and legs. (For tips on preparing for and moving into the classic warrior pose, go to www.dummies.com/go/yogaaoifd.)

If you can, keep your hips squared throughout this exercise; neither hipbone should be forward of the other. If squaring your hips is too hard, however, forget it and do your best.

Grab your hand weights and follow these steps:

1. **Standing with your feet below your hips, your toes pointing forward, and the hand weights hanging at your sides with your palms facing inward, step back with your right foot and bend your left leg for support (see Figure 4-8a).**

   This is the lunge position — and the starting position. Turn out your back foot slightly and keep looking forward.

   Your bent knee shouldn't be forward of your ankle. Also, press in with all four corners of your foot.

2. **As you exhale to a count of four, bend your elbows and work your biceps as you lift the weights to shoulder level (see Figure 4-8b).**

   Draw your belly in and up and your tailbone down for support. Keep your elbows locked in; rocking isn't allowed.

3. **As you inhale to a count of four, lower the weights to the starting position (see Figure 4-8a).**

   Don't let your back sag; keep it straight.

Do this exercise six to eight times, pause to rest, and then do six to eight more repetitions.

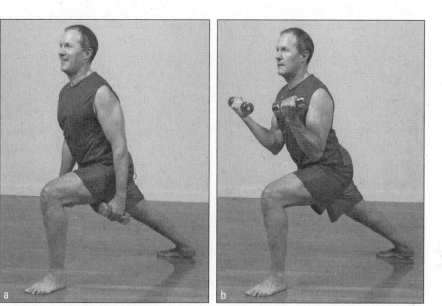

Figure 4-8: Feel the courage and strength of a warrior while you work your biceps.

a   b

Photographs by Bonnie Kamin (www.bonniekamin.com)

The Rise and Shine

The rise and shine is a transitional exercise that helps you relax after your strenuous workout. The exercise massages your internal organs and helps you unwind. Imagine you're greeting the morning sun as you do this exercise, feeling its warm rays relaxing your body.

Do a yogic Balancing Breath as you do this exercise (Book II, Chapter 1 explains the yoga breaths). Don't rush; take your time and relax.

You need both hand weights for this exercise. When you're ready, follow these steps:

1. **Crouch with your feet about 6 inches apart, your buttocks behind your heels, your elbows outside of your knees, and the weights in your hands with your palms turned inward (see Figure 4-9a).**

   This is the starting position. You should be looking slightly downward. Keep your toes pointing straight ahead throughout this exercise.

2. **As you inhale, pull your belly in and press down through your feet as you rise to a standing position and extend your arms away from your body to the *T* position (see Figure 4-9b).**

   Your palms should be facing downward at this point.

3. **Continue to inhale as you turn your palms upward and bring your arms together above your head, looking up as you do so (Figure 4-9c).**

   Steps 2 and 3 should be one continuous motion.

4. **As you exhale, slowly lower your arms, turn your palms downward again, and return to the starting position (see Figure 4-9a).**

   Feel your body deflating as you exhale; slowly lower yourself to the ground in rhythm with your breathing.

Repeat this exercise six to eight times.

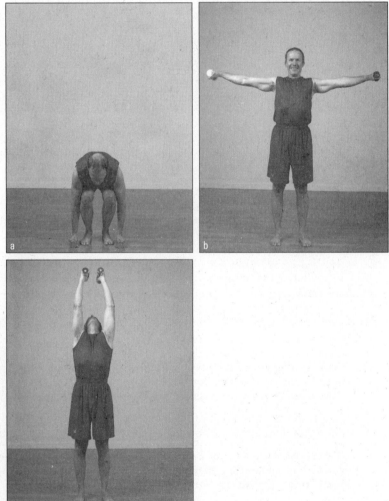

Figure 4-9:
Greet the morning sun and say goodbye to your high-energy workout as you do the rise and shine.

Photographs by Bonnie Kamin (www.bonniekamin.com)

Chapter 5

Exercises for Seniors

In This Chapter

▶ Improving blood circulation throughout your body

▶ Strengthening your spine and improving your range of motion

▶ Concentrating on your coordination and focus

*N*o matter your age, Yoga with Weights exercises can help you stay strong and supple. Therefore, the exercises in this chapter are designed specifically for seniors. Here, you find a workout that emphasizes the importance of stretching, relaxing, and strengthening for promoting the general health and well-being of seniors. Still not convinced? Okay, the exercises also slow down and prevent premature aging!

Reaping the Rewards of the Senior Workout

An old saying in the yoga tradition says that you're as youthful as your spine is supple and flexible. The exercises in this workout increase the strength and suppleness of your spine. It feels great to have a limber spine that's free to move in all directions, but a spine that moves with ease is important for safety reasons, too. For example, you'll be able to sit on the floor and get up without assistance, and you'll feel more youthful so you can do the physical activities that you really love.

The exercises in this workout also increase bone density. An excessive loss of bone density in the process of aging leaves your bones weakened and susceptible to fracturing and breaking. However, there is good news: Because bone is living tissue, it's in a constant state of regeneration. In a Yoga with Weights workout, your muscles have to work against the weights you carry, which puts stress on your bones and therefore increases bone density. You increase blood circulation to your muscles as well, which also builds bone density and muscle strength.

Along with building up your bone and muscle, the exercises in this chapter improve your coordination. Maintaining good coordination reduces your risk of falling and allows you to be more confident and sure of yourself. How's that for a feel-good prescription?

To ensure that you get the maximum benefit from the exercises in this chapter, keep these points and suggestions in mind:

- ✔ **Try to do these exercises every other day.** When you begin to practice the exercises, you'll notice a greater level of mobility and strength. And the exercises help you maintain the strength and mobility that you already have, giving you healthy support for years to come.

- ✔ **Use a sturdy chair for these exercises.** The chair should be short enough so you can sit on it without leaving your feet dangling (if you're short, you may need to place a footstool under your feet) and have a strong back. (You'll grasp the back of the chair in some exercises.)

- ✔ **Maintain a concentrated focus on the alignment of your spine.** Imagine or visualize your spine lengthening and realigning as you gently breathe in each exercise.

- ✔ **Use the gentle, empowering Complete Breaths as you do this workout (go to Book II, Chapter 1 for details).** Remember, breathing is a barometer of how you're doing. If you're breathing too rapidly or holding your breath, you're probably working too hard, but if your breathing is steady and calm, you're probably working just right.

- ✔ **Use light weights to start.** As you get stronger, gradually increase the size of the weights. Always work at your own level of ability and take into account the energy you have that day.

- ✔ **Engage in a moment or two of silent meditation at the end of your workout.** Head to Book VII for more on meditation.

- ✔ **Never force yourself or push too hard as you do this workout.** Use your experience to recognize when you should rest or press forward. The goal is to challenge yourself to do the exercises with a little more intensity and concentration each time you do them.

Candle Blowing

Candle blowing warms you up for all the exercises in the senior Yoga with Weights workout. In this exercise, you focus on your breathing. Throughout the exercise, you breathe in and out with pursed lips as if you're blowing out the candles on a birthday cake. As you concentrate on your breathing and warming up your body, you work your bicep muscles and increase your blood circulation.

You need hand weights for this exercise. Follow these steps:

1. **Sit in a chair with your elbows bent and the weights held at your thighs, palms facing upward (see Figure 5-1a).**

   This is the starting position. Sit upright with your shoulders squared, but don't allow your shoulders to creep up to your neck. Purse your lips for the proper breathing technique.

2. **Exhaling to a count of four, curl the weights to the level of your shoulders (see Figure 5-1b).**

   In weightlifting, this action is called a *bicep curl*. Pull your belly in, and use your belly as well as your arms to support the weights. Feel the air leave your lungs as you exhale.

3. **Inhaling to a count of four, lower the weights to the starting position (see Figure 5-1a).**

   Inhale slowly and deeply into your abdomen as you slowly lower the weights in rhythm with your breathing.

Repeat this exercise four to six times, pause to rest, and then do four to six more repetitions.

Book V

Yoga-ing Your Way to a Toned Body: Yoga with Weights

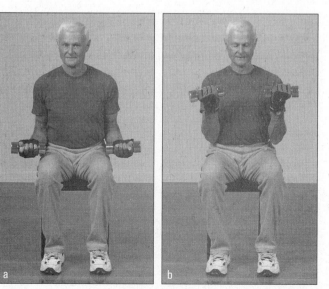

Figure 5-1: Focus on your breathing as you do bicep curls.

Photographs by Bonnie Kamin (www.bonniekamin.com)

The Mirror

The mirror opens your chest and lungs, as well as the sides of your body, aiding in free breathing and improved flexibility. It also creates better range of motion in your neck and shoulders, making the exercise excellent for people who suffer from stiff necks and "frozen shoulders." Having more room to breathe deeply makes it easier to relax.

You need hand weights for this exercise. Follow these steps:

1. **Sit in a chair with your elbows bent and the weights held at your thighs, palms facing upward, and fix your gaze on your right hand (see Figure 5-2a).**

   This is the starting position.

2. **Inhaling to a count of four, lift your right arm in a half-arc position until your hand is above your right shoulder, watching your right hand along the way (see Figure 5-2b).**

   Draw your belly in and up as you lift the weight, and reach only to a comfortable height. If you can, raise your hand straight up, as the model does in Figure 5-2. The goal is to reach as high as you can without forcing or straining.

   Always keep your eyes on the weight you're lifting. This keeps you focused on what you're doing.

3. **Exhaling to a count of four, lower your right arm and turn your head forward to return to the starting position (see Figure 5-2a).**

   Don't slump your shoulders; keep them wide open so it feels as if your chest is smiling.

Repeat this exercise four to six times with each arm, pause to rest, and then do four to six more repetitions with each arm.

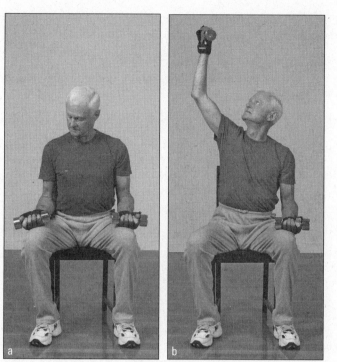

Figure 5-2: The mirror improves motion, breathing, and flexibility.

a   b

Photographs by Bonnie Kamin (www.bonniekamin.com)

The Ticking Clock

Smooth, rhythmic movements are known to massage away stiffness in the body and aid in your ability to balance. The ticking clock gets its name because you move your body similarly to a clock pendulum. This exercise is about timed movement and the timeless quality of "being." It warms up the sides of your body and helps your neck and spine feel more flexible. It also stretches your shoulders and tones the muscles of your torso.

Grab your hand weights for this exercise and follow these steps:

1. **Sit in a chair with your arms hanging at your sides, the weights in your hands, and your palms facing inward (see Figure 5-3a).**

   This is the starting position. Look straight ahead.

2. **Turn your head to look over your right shoulder.**

   As you turn, keep your shoulders squared.

3. **As you exhale to a count of four, gently arc your torso to your right side (see Figure 5-3b).**

   Look down at the weight in your right hand, and feel your spine stretching.

4. **As you inhale to a count of four, return to the upright starting position (see Figure 5-3a).**

   Turn your head and look forward as you return to the starting position.

Alternating sides with each repetition, repeat this exercise four to six times on each side of your body, pause to rest, and then do four to six more repetitions on each side of your body.

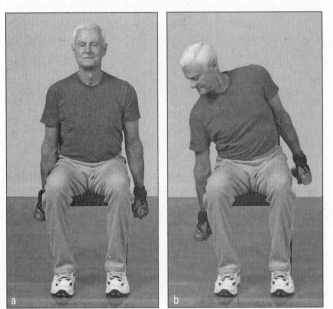

Figure 5-3:
The ticking clock uses smooth, rhythmic movements.

Photographs by Bonnie Kamin (www.bonniekamin.com)

The Wave

The wave stretches your back and spine and releases tension from your head, neck, and shoulders. The rhythmic motion of the exercise also teaches you balance, coordination, and stability. For muscle benefit, the wave strengthens and tones your abdominal muscles.

You need hand weights to do the yoga wave. Follow these steps:

1. **Sit in a chair with your back separated from the back of the chair and your arms hanging down at your sides, holding the weights with your palms facing inward (see Figure 5-4a).**

   This is the starting position. Look straight ahead. If your back is touching the back of the chair, you may be tempted to rely on the chair for support, which would defeat the purpose of this exercise.

2. **Exhaling to a count of four, roll your shoulders up and over as you slowly lower the trunk of your body onto your thighs; let the weights hang beside your body as you lean forward (see Figure 5-4b).**

   Allow the weights to slowly pull you down. As you exhale, slowly push the air from your lungs so that by the time your body touches your thighs, you're pushing out the last bit of air.

   Anchor your buttocks to the chair to keep from slipping forward.

   Your head can hang down in this position. If you can't hang your head all the way, hang it as far as is comfortable, or lift your head slightly as you bend forward.

3. **Inhaling to a count of four, sit up and roll your shoulders up and back down again to return to the starting position (see Figure 5-4a).**

   Move your feet forward or backward if it helps you maintain your balance.

Figure 5-4:
Move to the
rhythm of a
wave, not a
tsunami.

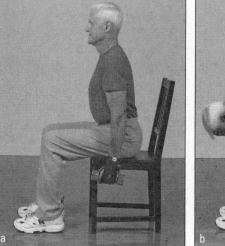 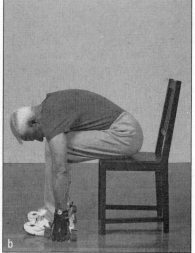

Photographs by Bonnie Kamin (www.bonniekamin.com)

Repeat this exercise four to six times, pause to rest, and then do four to six more repetitions.

The Egyptian

If your declining range of motion is starting to make everyday tasks — like grabbing objects out of the cupboard — difficult to manage, you can fight back with exercises like the Egyptian. This exercise tones and strengthens your back, arms, chest, and shoulders. It also expands your chest and gives your shoulders a wider range of movement.

Draw your belly in and up throughout this exercise. Engaged belly muscles help you lift the weights and maintain stability.

Use your hand weights for this exercise and follow these steps:

1. **Sit in a chair with your arms hanging down to your sides, the weights in your hands, and your palms facing inward (see Figure 5-5a).**

   This is the starting position. Look straight ahead. Don't shrug your shoulders, lean against the back of the chair, or lean forward during this exercise.

2. **Inhaling to a count of four, lift your arms out to the sides until you join your hands above your head (see Figure 5-5b).**

   Rotate your hands so that your palms are facing up by the time your arms are halfway lifted. Look up so that you're gazing at your hands above your head.

   If you can't reach above your head, lift your arms as high as you comfortably can.

3. **Exhaling to a count of four, slowly lower your arms to the starting position (see Figure 5-5a).**

   Rotate your hands again as you lower your arms so they end up facing inward at the starting position. Lower your gaze so that you're looking straight ahead as you lower your arms.

Repeat this exercise four to six times, pause to rest, and then do four to six more repetitions.

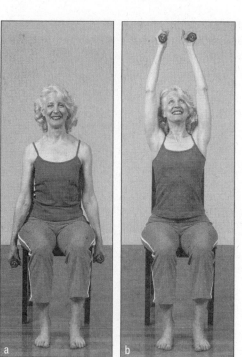

Figure 5-5: The Egyptian improves your posture and your range of motion.

Photographs by Bonnie Kamin (www.bonniekamin.com)

The Pigeon

The Yoga with Weights pigeon increases the range of motion in your hips; if you're tight in this area, the pigeon opens you up. The exercise also increases blood circulation to your hips and pelvic girdle, which helps you when you're climbing stairs or walking your dog.

Don't attempt this exercise without the permission of your primary caregiver if you've recently had a hip replacement.

Pick up both your hand weights and grab one ankle weight for this exercise. When you're ready, follow these steps:

1. **Sitting in a chair, place your right ankle over your left knee, and place the ankle weight on your right thigh.**

   The ankle weight helps anchor your thigh in place. By placing one leg over the other, you open and stretch out your hip and groin.

   If you can't lift your ankle onto your knee, cross your ankles instead or put your foot on a footstool.

2. **Grab your hand weights, separate your arms as far apart as you can, and lift them to shoulder height with your elbows bent and palms facing forward (see Figure 5-6a).**

   This is the scarecrow position, and also your starting position. Make sure your spine is erect and that you're relaxed.

3. **Inhaling to a count of four, lift your arms overhead (see Figure 5-6b).**

   Lift to a place that's comfortable for you. In weightlifting terminology, this action is called an *overhead press* or *military press*.

4. **Exhaling to a count of four, lower the weights to the starting position (see Figure 5-6a).**

   Lower the weights slowly so you can feel your muscles working. Keep your belly muscles engaged for stability and balance.

Repeat this exercise four to six times with each leg, pause to rest, and then do four to six more repetitions with each leg.

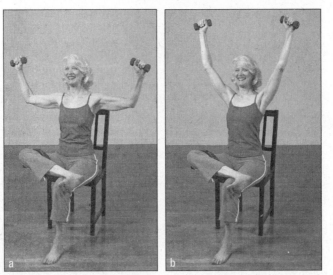

Figure 5-6:
Look straight ahead as you press your way to better mobility and circulation.

Photographs by Bonnie Kamin (www.bonniekamin.com)

The Heart Lift

The heart lift is a great exercise for people of all ages, but it's especially helpful for seniors because it brings a balance of oxygen and blood to your heart. The exercise opens and expands your chest and helps you to breathe more deeply. It also strengthens your spine, abdominal muscles, and quads.

You need ankle weights for this exercise. Follow these steps:

1. **Sit on the edge of a chair, and reach backward to grasp the back of the chair with your hands.**

   If you can't hold the back of the chair, hold the sides of the chair seat.

2. **Roll your shoulders up, back, and down; lift your chest; and raise your chin (see Figure 5-7a).**

   This is the starting position. Sink your buttocks deeply into the chair so you can lean forward slightly. Feel the front of your body stretching, and enjoy breathing in this position as your heart opens up.

3. **Exhaling to a count of four, lift your right knee a few inches and then straighten your right leg (see Figure 5-7b).**

   Press forward through your heel, and continue to hold on to the chair for balance.

4. **Inhaling to a count of four, lower your right leg to the starting position (see Figure 5-7a).**

   Lower your leg slowly to the rhythm of your breathing; don't drop it.

Alternating legs with each repetition, do this exercise four to six times with each leg, pause to rest, and then do four to six more repetitions with each leg.

Book V

Yoga-ing Your Way to a Toned Body: Yoga with Weights

Figure 5-7:
Feel your heart open up as the oxygen enters and leaves your body.

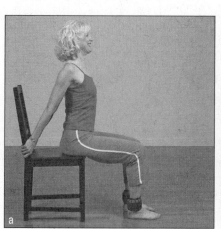
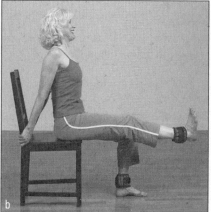

Photographs by Bonnie Kamin (www.bonniekamin.com)

The Hacker

The hacker is a simple exercise that builds strength and flexibility in your lower body. The exercise works your quad and hamstring muscles while toning your belly and increasing the range of movement in your hips. The hacker helps build the necessary strength for climbing up and down stairs and ladders.

Strap on your ankle weights for this exercise. Adding hand weights is an option for people who feel strong enough (the model in Figure 5-8 explores this option). When you're ready, follow these steps:

1. **Sit on a chair with your back separated from the back of the chair, your feet flat on the floor, and your arms hanging at your sides (see Figure 5-8a).**

   This is the starting position. Make sure your spine is erect and your shoulders are squared. If you want to use hand weights, hold them with your palms facing inward.

2. **Exhaling to a count of four, lift your right knee toward your chest (see Figure 5-8b).**

   Engage your belly muscles; you should feel these muscles working as you lift. Keep your foot flexed to engage your leg muscles.

3. **Inhaling to a count of four, lower your leg to the starting position (see Figure 5-8a).**

   Lower your leg slowly; keep your leg muscles fully engaged all the way down.

Be careful not to lean forward as you do this exercise. Breathe deeply into your lower back.

Alternating legs with each repetition, do this exercise four to six times with each leg, pause to rest, and then do four to six more repetitions with each leg.

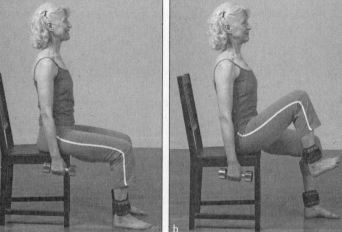

Figure 5-8:
Work your belly muscles and legs as you keep your trunk straight.

Photographs by Bonnie Kamin (www.bonniekamin.com)

The Champion

The Yoga with Weights champion strengthens, conditions, and tones the trunk of your body, your shoulders, and your arms; refines the integrity of your muscles; contributes to the structure of your bones; and brings more blood to your pelvic girdle, which helps with movement.

You need hand weights and ankle weights for this exercise. Follow these steps:

1. **Straddle the right corner of a chair seat with your bent right knee in front of you over the chair, your left leg bent and at your side, and the toes of your left foot curled under for support.**

   Your left knee should be a couple of inches from the floor in this position. Make sure you have the hand weights in your hands at this point.

2. **Twist the trunk of your body slightly to the left, and lift and extend both of your arms to shoulder height, palms facing upward (see Figure 5-9a).**

   This is the starting position. Your shoulders should be directly above your hips. Look ahead toward the arm in front of you — your right arm in this case.

3. **Exhaling to a count of four, bend your elbows and lift the weights toward your shoulders (see Figure 5-9b).**

   In weightlifting terminology, this action is called a *bicep curl*.

4. **Inhaling to a count of four, extend your arms and return to the starting position (see Figure 5-9a).**

Repeat this exercise four to six times, pause to rest, and turn your body to the opposite side of the chair to do four to six more repetitions for the other side of your body.

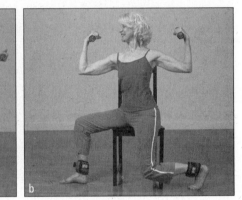

Figure 5-9:
Flex your arms like a champion for better health.

Photographs by Bonnie Kamin (www.bonniekamin.com)

The Body Builder

The body builder exercises your buttocks and tones your legs, back, and thighs. This part of the workout builds the bone density in your back, spine, and legs, which allows you to feel free to be active without worrying about injury.

Wear ankle weights for this exercise. Follow these steps:

1. **Standing behind a chair, hold the top of the chair with both hands and, bending at your waist, step backward far enough so that your trunk and arms are parallel to the floor (see Figure 5-10a).**

   This is the starting position.

   Put the chair against a wall so that it doesn't slide when you do this exercise, which could cause you to slip and fall. (The model in Figure 5-10 didn't take this advice, but she's a daredevil.)

2. **Inhaling to a count of four, lift your right leg behind your body as high as you can without straining or causing too much discomfort (see Figure 5-10b).**

   Ideally, your leg should be parallel to the floor, but if you can't lift it that high, don't worry about it. You can bend your knee if you need to.

3. **Exhaling to a count of four, lower your leg to the starting position (see Figure 5-10a).**

   Lower your leg slowly and gently; don't drop it down.

Alternating legs with each repetition, do this exercise four to six times with each leg, pause to rest, and then do four to six more repetitions with each leg.

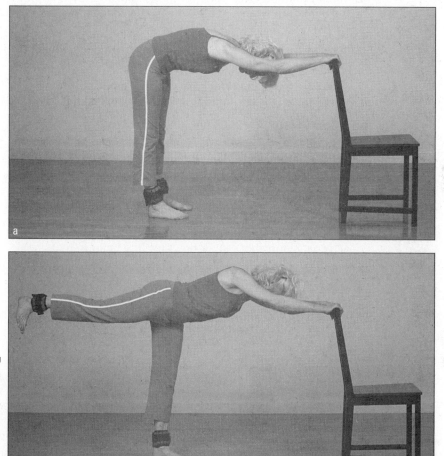

Figure 5-10: Who says body builders can't be graceful doing yoga?

Photographs by Bonnie Kamin (www.bonniekamin.com)

The Triangle

The triangle gives you the chance to really challenge your muscles and build strength. The exercise stretches the sides of your body and creates strength and stability in your arms, legs, and trunk.

You need both ankle weights and one hand weight for this exercise. Follow these steps:

1. **Stand behind a chair with your legs apart, your right foot pointing to the chair, and your left foot at a 45-degree angle with respect to the chair.**

   Your body should be facing left when positioned behind the chair in this position. Your feet should be a little wider than your hips.

2. **Grasp the top of the chair with your left hand; with your right hand, hold the hand weight at your side, palm facing your body (see Figure 5-11a).**

   This is the starting position.

3. **Exhaling to a count of four, stretch the right side of your body by lifting the hand weight over and around your head. As you lift, turn your head to the left and bend your left elbow (see Figure 5-11b).**

   Press into your legs as you lift the hand weight, and try to arc the weight over the back of the chair.

   If you can't lift the weight over your body or over the chair, lift it as high as you comfortably can, or don't use the hand weight.

4. **Inhaling to a count of four, slowly return to the starting position (see Figure 5-11a).**

Repeat this exercise four to six times, pause to rest, and turn around to do four to six repetitions with the other side of your body.

Figure 5-11:
Don't be
a square;
being a
triangle
strengthens
your body.

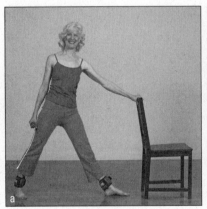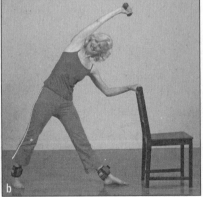

Photographs by Bonnie Kamin (www.bonniekamin.com)

The Lift

The lift is a full-body exercise that lengthens the quad muscles in your legs and opens your groin. The exercise also tones and strengthens your spine and chest. As it tones your lower-body muscles, the lift also exercises your arms — specifically your triceps.

You need both ankle weights and one hand weight for this exercise. Follow these steps:

1. **Straddle the right corner of a chair seat with your bent right knee in front of you over the chair, your left leg bent and at your side, and the toes of your left foot curled under for support.**

   Your left knee should be close to the floor in this position. Make sure you're seated firmly in the chair with your right leg.

2. **Holding the hand weight with both hands, lift your hands above your head and bend your elbows so the weight goes behind your head (see Figure 5-12a).**

   This is the starting position. Your elbows should be near your ears; don't drop your head.

   If you can't reach your arms back far enough, reach them as far as you feel comfortable. You can also do this exercise without the hand weight.

3. **Inhaling to a count of four, straighten your arms and raise the weight over your head (see Figure 5-12b).**

4. **Exhaling to a count of four, lower the weight to the starting position (see Figure 5-12a).**

   Be careful not to hit yourself in the head on the way down.

Repeat this exercise four to six times, pause to rest, and then do four to six more repetitions.

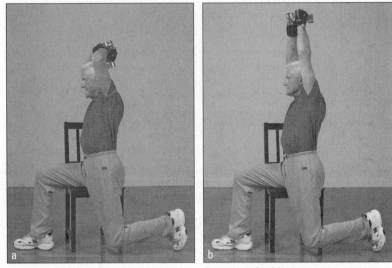

Figure 5-12:
Enjoy the
uplifted
feeling you
get from
working
your whole
body.

Photographs by Bonnie Kamin (www.bonniekamin.com)

The Seated Twist

The seated twist aims to wring your body out like a wet rag to make you feel more relaxed. The exercise loosens your neck and spine and releases tension from your shoulders and neck. It also increases the circulation in your legs, because when you cross and uncross your legs, you stimulate blood flow. Twisting and releasing your torso does the same.

Strap on your ankle weights and follow these steps:

1. **Sitting toward the front of a chair, cross your right leg over your left leg.**

   The weights on your ankles help anchor you into the chair.

2. **Place your left hand on the outside of your right knee, and reach your right hand behind you so you can hold the back of the chair at a location and level that's comfortable for you (see Figure 5-13a).**

   This is the starting position. Draw your belly in and up for support, and make sure that your spine is erect and your chin is slightly lifted.

3. **Exhaling to a count of four, turn your back, neck, and head one vertebra at a time to look over your right shoulder (see Figure 5-13b).**

Start your twist in the area behind your navel, and move upward in a spiraling direction. Imagine that your spine is twisting like a spiral staircase, with your mind climbing the stairs one step at a time. Twisting with an engaged abdomen protects your lower back and neck.

You can use your left hand, holding your crossed leg back, as leverage, which lengthens your spine and engages your core muscles even more.

4. **Inhaling to a count of four, rotate your back, neck, and head to the starting position (see Figure 5-13a).**

   Slowly unwind as you return to the starting position; don't jerk.

Repeat the exercise four to six times with this side of your body, pause to rest, and turn your body to the opposite side of the chair to do four to six more repetitions with the other side of your body.

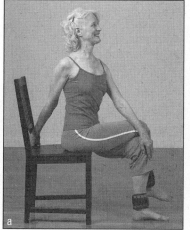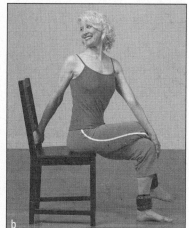

Figure 5-13: Wring the tension from your body with the seated twist.

Photographs by Bonnie Kamin (www.bonniekamin.com)

Book VI
Ancient Practices in the Modern World: Hot Trends in Yoga

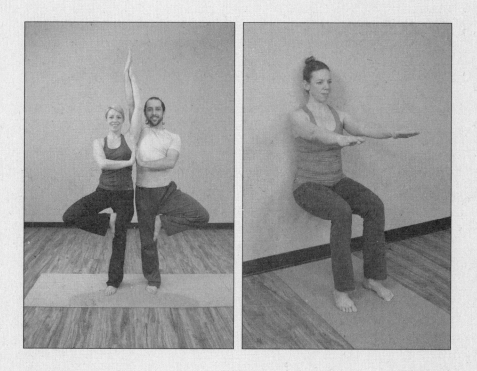

Contents at a Glance

Chapter 1

Partnering Up for Yoga

*Y*oga need not be a solitary practice. *Yoga* means "union," and partner yoga fosters unity. *Partner yoga* is a modern American development of the late 20th century, although some people trace its roots back to ancient yoga lineages. Its modern expression may even have developed independently with different practitioner-teachers, but clearly, it's an idea whose time has come. As with other varieties of yoga postures, partner yoga is suitable for all levels of complexity and challenge. This chapter presents the many benefits and joys of practicing partner yoga and illustrates several safe postures you and a partner can try.

Defining Partner Yoga

Partner yoga is a joyful practice that brings two people together to create a new posture. Unlike what's referred to as assisted yoga, in partner yoga each person gives support and receives benefits as the two create a posture together. When you and your partner try this approach, you discover and enjoy one of the requirements and lessons of partner yoga: dialogue and clear communication.

Consider the benefits of partner yoga:

✔ **It can be good for your health.** By its very nature, partner yoga is a playful practice and can even evoke laughter. Laughter can be a very healing experience, as Norman Cousins has taught the world.

✔ **It fosters your ability to trust and feel secure with another person.** It gives you the opportunity to surrender to another individual and feel supported. That experience of trust on the mat can spill over to your life *off* the mat.

✔ **It can add an element of delight when practiced by romantic couples.** How comfortable are you with being touched? Partner yoga isn't sexual, but it involves touching. Because of differences in personality, personal experience, upbringing, and culture, the idea of touching another person during your yoga routine may be more or less comfortable than the practice of going solo. Although partner yoga can help you address issues with intimacy, only you know your limits and what's right for you. As with all other aspects of your yoga practice, listen to and respect your inner voice.

Partner yoga as a metaphor for how we live in the world

According to Cain Carroll and Lori Kimata, authors of *Partner Yoga,* the first axiom of partner yoga is "All things are interdependent." Partner yoga gives you immediate feedback on how you interact with your partner and, by extension, with others in your life. If one person pushes too far, both will fall over. How's that for immediate feedback?

Consider the opportunities for feedback that partner yoga offers:

✔ Do you communicate your needs?

✔ Do you listen when your partner communicates his or her needs?

✔ Are you sensitive to the subtle adjustments and movements of your partner?

✔ Do you give support when needed?

✔ Are you flexible enough to allow your partner to move with ease yet maintain your own integrity?

✔ Can you find that healthy medium between rigidity and flexibility?

Exploring 12 Ways to Pose with a Partner

This section illustrates and describes 12 safe and fun yoga postures that you can practice with a partner. Feel free to mix and match, and sprinkle them within a more traditional practice session in which you each practice on your own.

Partner yoga is best practiced with someone your same size, but differences in height and weight can stimulate creativity to make the postures work.

Partner suspension bridge

The partner suspension bridge decompresses the entire spine, provides traction, and stretches the hamstrings. It also builds strength in the arms and shoulders. You can see it illustrated in Figure 1-1 and watch trust and leverage in action at www.dummies.com/go/yogaaiofd.

1. **Face your partner standing, and hold on to one another's wrists with corresponding right and left hands (known as the *fireman's grip*).**

2. **Begin to bend forward, and walk backward until you're both parallel to the floor.**

3. **Lean back with your hips, and communicate with your partner to arrive at a stretch that's a comfortable maximum for you both.**

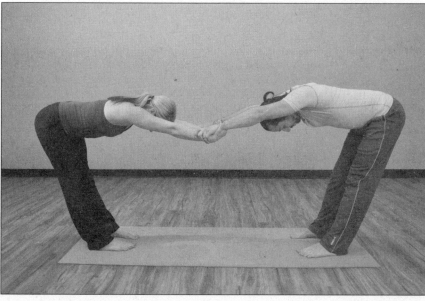

Figure 1-1: The partner suspension bridge gives both partners a delicious stretch.

4. **Stay for 6 to 8 breaths.**

5. **To come out of the pose, walk back toward one another and release one another's wrists.**

When you're comfortable in the partner suspension bridge, try wiggling your hips a few times to stretch your hips and lower back.

Avoid the partner suspension bridge if you have back or shoulder problems, or if you feel pain in your lower back or shoulders when executing the posture.

Partner teeter-totter

The partner teeter-totter decompresses the lower back and builds strength in the arms and shoulders. Take a peek at Figure 1-2 to see what it looks like: You start as in the suspension bridge in the preceding section and add a flourish.

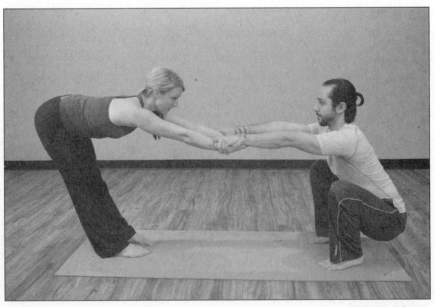

Figure 1-2: The partner teeter-totter is nearly everyone's favorite on the yoga mat (as well as in the playground).

© John Wiley & Sons, Inc.

1. **Face your partner standing, and hold on to one another's wrists with corresponding right and left hands.**

2. **Begin to bend forward, and walk backward until you're both parallel to the floor.**

3. **Lean back with your hips, and communicate with your partner to arrive at a stretch that's a comfortable maximum for you both.**

4. **Now one partner bends at the knees and goes down into a half or full squat.**

   Communicate to decide who goes first. Squat only as far as you feel comfortable. Stay focused on your partner for the best communication.

5. **When you're ready to come out of the pose, let your partner know; when you're both standing, step forward and release each other's wrists.**

6. **After 6 to 8 breaths, switch and have the other partner move into a squat for another 6 to 8 breaths.**

Book VI

Ancient Practices in the Modern World: Hot Trends in Yoga

It's perfectly fine if only one partner wants to squat.

Avoid the partner teeter-totter if you have back or knee problems, or if you feel pain in your lower back, knees, or shoulders.

Hugasana

Hugs teach us how to give and receive. And if that's not enough, research suggests that touch (and what is a hug, if not touch?) can contribute to healing sickness, disease, loneliness, depression, anxiety, and stress.

1. **Stand and face your partner; move close to one another.**

2. **Open your arms wide and wrap them around each other in a nice embrace, as in Figure 1-3.**

3. **Stay for 4 to 5 breaths.**

Smiling and laughter are also good for your health, so let loose and go with the flow as you perform the hugasana with your partner.

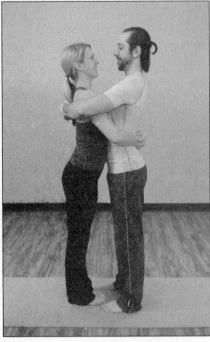

Figure 1-3:
A hug is a simple and delightful partner posture.

Partner warrior II

Warrior II as a partner pose blends the many benefits of this powerful posture — especially improvements in strength, stamina, and balance — with the interpersonal benefits of partner yoga. You can see its final expression in Figure 1-4.

1. **Stand sideways with your partner, facing the same forward direction.**

2. **Touch your inside feet together.**

3. **Reach with your inside hand and place it on your partner's upper arm.**

4. **Turn your outside foot out and away from your partner about 90 degrees, and raise your outside arm so it's parallel to the floor.**

5. **Inhale deeply and, as you exhale, bend your outside leg to a right angle as your back hand slides along your partner's arm toward his wrist.**

6. **Stay in the final posture, firmly gripping your partner's wrist, for 6 to 8 breaths.**

7. **When you're finished, straighten your legs, release your hands, switch places, and repeat on the other side.**

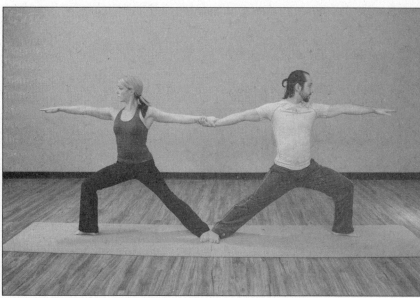

© John Wiley & Sons, Inc.

Figure 1-4:
What's mightier than a warrior? Two warriors!

TIP

When you're holding the posture in Step 6, try tucking your tail to allow your hips to open. Also think of lengthening through the top of your head and widening with your arms.

Partner table pose

The partner table pose stretches the upper back and shoulders, relieving neck tension. It also stretches the hamstrings. It differs from the partner suspension bridge (see Figure 1-1) in that it doesn't decompress and provide traction to the lower back. You can see it illustrated in Figure 1-5.

1. **Standing, face your partner; move toward one another and place your hands on your partner's shoulders.**

2. **Bend forward from the hips until you're both parallel to the floor; soften your knees if necessary and let your neck and head relax downward to a comfortable position.**

3. **Stay for 6 to 8 breaths.**

4. **When you're ready to come out of the pose, let your partner know and step forward as you release your hands from one another's shoulders.**

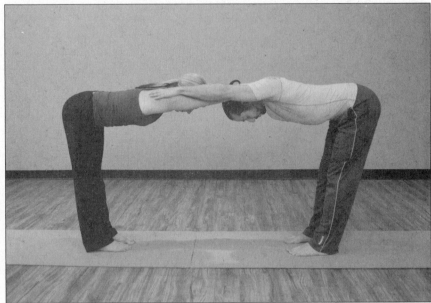

Figure 1-5:
You form a table with a friend in the aptly named partner table pose.

© John Wiley & Sons, Inc.

Double triangle

The double triangle provides an excellent side stretch to the body and the spine. It strengthens the legs, helps the digestive system, and improves stability and balance. You can see it illustrated in Figure 1-6.

1. **Turn back to back with your partner as both of you spread your legs to a comfortable distance, about 3 to 5 feet apart; open one foot on the same side, and turn in the back foot about 45 degrees or less.**

2. **Place your bottom hand on your forward thigh, bring your top arm up, and entwine your arm with your partner's top arm and hand.**

3. **Lean back gently, and slide your bottom hand down your forward leg as far as you feel comfortable.**

4. **Stay for about 6 to 8 breaths, and then repeat on the other side.**

Avoid this pose if you're suffering from a back condition, migraines, high blood pressure, or neck injuries.

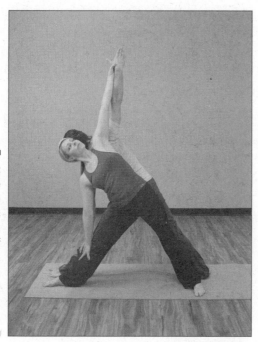

Book VI

Ancient Practices in the Modern World: Hot Trends in Yoga

Figure 1-6:
The double triangle delivers all the benefits of the triangle, plus the fun of practicing with a partner.

© John Wiley & Sons, Inc.

Partner tree pose

This simple-looking posture brings a bounty of benefits. It creates stability and balance, improves concentration, opens the hips, and strengthens the ankles. You can see it illustrated in Figure 1-7.

1. **Stand side to side with your partner, facing the same way, about 1 to 2 feet from each other.**

2. **Bring your inside arms straight up, with your hands extended, and touch your partner's palms (or anywhere on the inside of the arms, depending on your size matchup).**

3. **Bend your outside leg and bring your outside heel into your groin, or to a comfortable spot between your groin and your knee.**

   If you can't reach that high, place your heel between your ankle and your knee — just not on the knee joint, which can cause injury.

4. **Bring your outside arms to the middle, and touch palms in the prayer, or namaste, position.**

   If you're feeling unstable, entwine your inside extended arms.

5. **Focus on a spot on the floor about 6 to 8 feet in front of you to help your balance.**

6. **Stay for 6 to 8 breaths and then get out of the pose by taking down the outside bent leg and placing that foot on the floor, releasing the inside palms that are touching, and finally releasing the outside arms and hands that are touching or entwined.**

7. **Switch places, and repeat on the other side.**

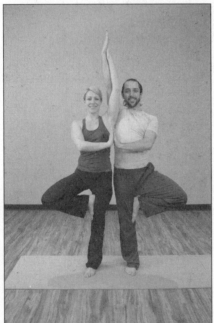

Figure 1-7: The elegant partner tree pose creates stability and builds strength.

© John Wiley & Sons, Inc.

TIP

The partner tree pose makes a great photograph of you and your partner for your next holiday card!

Yoga miracle pose

This pose gives a deep stretch to the hamstring muscles, which helps you with the rest of your practice. After all, the hamstrings are the most influential muscle group for all yoga postures. You can see this pose in Figure 1-8.

1. **Start with one partner lying face up, with one leg bent and the other leg straight up.**

2. **The other partner stands in a lunge position, with the forward leg bent and close to the extended leg of the partner on the floor.**

3. **The lunging partner places a hand at the back of the extended leg and provides resistance; the lying partner pushes steadily and comfortably for 10 seconds.**

   Just a steady medium push of your heel against your partner's hand is fine. This pose isn't competitive!

4. **At the end of 10 seconds, the lying partner releases the push and allows the lunging partner to push the extended leg to a new flexibility point; do both legs.**

5. **Switch positions, and repeat Steps 1 through 4.**

Book VI

Ancient Practices in the Modern World: Hot Trends in Yoga

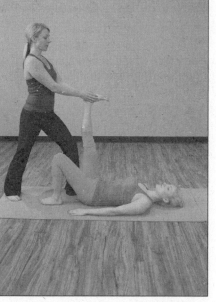

Figure 1-8: The hamstring stretch you get in the yoga miracle pose benefits the rest of your practice.

© John Wiley & Sons, Inc.

Seated straddle pose

This pose improves hip and hamstring flexibility and stretches the entire back as well as the arms and shoulders. You and your partner first rotate together to warm up, and then you alternate leaning forward and back. You can see it illustrated in Figure 1-9.

Figure 1-9: The seated straddle pose benefits the hips, hamstrings, and upper body.

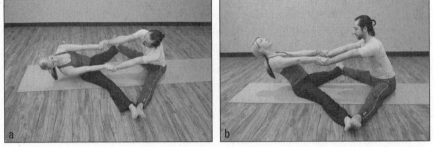

© John Wiley & Sons, Inc.

1. **Sit on the floor, facing your partner, with your legs wide and your feet touching your partner's feet or ankles.**

2. **Reach forward with both hands and hold your partner's corresponding wrists.**

3. **Slowly circle your torsos together, taking turns leaning forward and backward as you rotate in your comfort zone; circle three times in each direction (see Figure 1-9a).**

4. **After the rotation, sit up straight while one partner slowly leans back, gently pulling the other partner forward for 4 or 5 breaths (see Figure 1-9b); then repeat in the other direction.**

Communication is the key here: Convey to your partner how you're doing with something along the lines of "Stop, that's enough" or "More, more."

Avoid this pose if it causes back pain.

The partner diamond

The partner diamond opens the hips, hamstrings, and inner thighs. Figure 1-10 shows this posture.

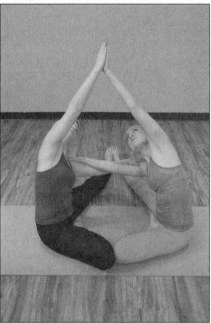

Figure 1-10: The partner diamond is good for opening and stretching.

© John Wiley & Sons, Inc.

1. **Sit on the floor and face your partner with your legs open wide.**

2. **On the same side as your partner, bend one leg and bring that foot into your groin; let the inside of your foot touch the inner part of your extended leg.**

3. **Bring the hand closest to your extended leg up to your partner's shoulder on the side that's closest to your partner's extended leg.**

4. **Raise your outside arms straight up and touch hands.**

5. **As you exhale, lean together sideways toward your extended legs; inhale back up, and repeat this step three times before staying in the folded sideways position for 4 to 5 breaths.**

When you're in the final step and are leaning together toward your extended legs, think of twisting gently away from your partner.

6. **Repeat Steps 1 through 5 on the other side.**

Avoid this pose if it causes back pain.

Partner seated twist

The partner seated twist rejuvenates the spine and stimulates the abdominal organs and digestion. Figure 1-11 shows you how it looks.

1. **Sit on the floor in a comfortable position, back to back with your partner (see Book II, Chapter 2 for more on sitting).**

2. **Raise your right hand and put it on your own left knee, palm down.**

3. **Move your left arm out to the left as far possible, and then place that arm palm down on your partner's right knee.**

4. **Take a deep breath together and, as you exhale, twist to your left as far as you comfortably can.**

5. **Stay for 4 to 5 breaths, and then repeat Steps 1 through 4 on the other side.**

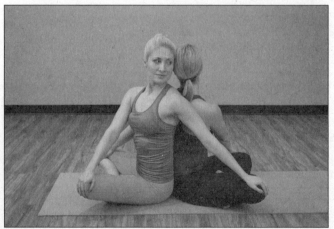

Figure 1-11:
A seated twist with a partner doubles the fun.

© John Wiley & Sons, Inc.

TIP

As you perform the partner seated twist pose, think of lengthening through the top of your head and then rotating your spine and shoulders.

WARNING!

Avoid this pose if it causes back pain.

Easy partner camel

The easy partner camel extends the back and stretches the abdomen, chest, and throat. It also stimulates the organs in the abdomen and neck. You can see it in Figure 1-12.

Figure 1-12:
The easy camel gives you a stretch while it stimulates your internal organs.

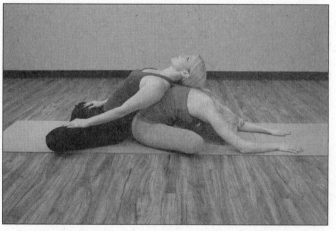

© John Wiley & Sons, Inc.

1. **Sit on the floor in a comfortable posture, back to back with your partner (see Book II, Chapter 2 for more on sitting).**

2. **One partner places her hands on the floor in front of her, while the other partner places her hands on her own knees.**

3. **The partner with her hands on her knees simply leans backward while the other partner bends forward, sliding her hands forward on the floor.**

   4. **Communicate about how far you each want to bend, and then stay in the final posture for 4 to 5 breaths.**

   5. **Repeat Steps 1 through 4, switching direction and hand positions.**

Avoid this pose if it causes back or neck pain.

You can make this pose more challenging by hooking bent elbows with your partner.

Chapter 2

Yoga against the Wall

I n the 1940s, Indra Devi (the first foreign woman taught by Professor Sri T. Krishnamacharya, the father of modern yoga) opened a studio in Hollywood, where she offered yoga adapted to the needs of Westerners. Among her students were Gloria Swanson and Marilyn Monroe. One posture she used was the headstand in the corner, to give the practitioner the support of two walls. Since then, the wall has become an integral, no-cost prop in the yoga tool kit. In this chapter, you discover the ways in which using the wall as a prop can support your yoga practice and give you new pose possibilities. You also find a variety of safe postures you can easily do at the wall.

The World Is Your Yoga Studio

In Wall Yoga, the wall is your friend — one you can always turn to when you need a little extra support or a confidence boost — and one that doesn't shy away from giving you some honest and direct feedback. The wall can give you some welcome benefits:

✔ Provides safety and stability

✔ Supports your balance

✔ Gives you feedback on your alignment

✔ Adds variety to reinvigorate your practice

When you embrace the wall as a prop, you open up a world of possibilities for practice. For starters, a wall allows you to practice when you're not dressed for yoga. Some postures you can easily do in business dress in an office setting. Imagine the benefits of taking a few minutes to stretch and breathe before attending a high-powered business meeting or delivering an important presentation.

Wall Yoga is a great option when the floor surface isn't inviting. Attention all backpacking travelers: How great does a few minutes of Wall Yoga sound when you're staying in a super-budget hotel that's seen better days? Don't have a wall? Don't worry; if the walls in your home or hotel room are flush with furniture and framed artwork, you can always use a door. In addition, a tree or the side of a building can stand in for a wall.

You can do many categories of postures, and the wall helps in each instance.

✔ **Standing postures:** The wall provides feedback on your alignment and orientation in space.

✔ **Safe inversions:** The wall provides safety and allows you to experience the benefits of inversions (refer to Book II, Chapter 6) without doing traditional inversions that can be risky for many people.

✔ **Forward bends and hamstring stretches in hanging postures:** The wall provides safety, precision, and guidance for your alignment.

A Wall-Supported Yoga Workout

You can do these postures in sequence for a full and varied yoga session, sprinkle them into your floor-based practice, or use them as desired.

Most people spend way too much time leaning forward. Maybe you spend hours in front of a computer entering data, writing, or simply gaming or surfing. Or perhaps you're a health professional who leans in toward patients a good part of the day. Chances are your posture is suffering because of it, and you're feeling those effects. The first two yoga postures illustrated — the wall mountain pose and the mountain posture flow — in this section are a perfect way to check your posture and remind yourself which way is up.

Wall mountain pose

Doing the mountain pose against the wall gives you feedback on your body's alignment, improves posture and balance, and facilitates yoga breathing. You can see it illustrated in Figure 2-1.

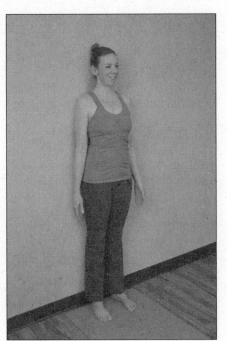

Figure 2-1: In wall mountain posture, you get valuable feedback on your posture and alignment.

© John Wiley & Sons, Inc.

1. **Stand tall with your back up to the wall but relaxed and with your feet hip distance apart; hang your arms at your sides, with your palms turned toward your legs.**

2. **Touch the wall with your hips and shoulders; visualize a string lifting the tip of your head and keeping your feet reaching down to the earth.**

3. **Choose a yoga breathing technique from Book II, Chapter 1 to use throughout the routine.**

4. **Stay in this posture for 6 to 8 breaths.**

Mountain posture flow

This posture is great for everyone with a desk job. Try it two or three times a day, and you'll notice a dramatic improvement in your posture.

In addition to aligning the body and improving posture, mountain posture flow relieves stress and tension in the neck and shoulders. You can see it illustrated in Figure 2-2.

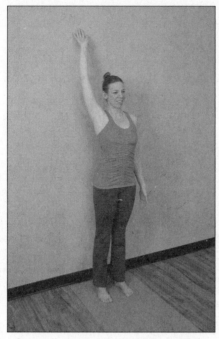

Figure 2-2:
Mountain posture flow helps relieve tension in the neck and shoulders.

© John Wiley & Sons, Inc.

1. **Stand in the mountain pose, with your feet and body about 6 inches away from the wall.**

2. **As you inhale, raise your right arm and touch the wall behind you with the back of your hand.**

   Adjust your distance from the wall as needed so that you can touch the wall with your extended hand.

3. **As you exhale, bring your hand back down to your side; repeat with your left arm, and then raise both arms and touch the wall.**

4. **Repeat the sequence of one arm, then the other arm, and then both arms two or three times.**

Try turning your head away from your arm as you raise your right arm and then your left to add in a nice neck stretch.

Wall warrior flow

Wall warrior flow is a simple series of movements that warm you up before athletic activities, indoors or out, as well as within your longer yoga session. It strengthens and stretches the legs, back, shoulders, and arms; it also improves flexibility in the hamstrings, calves, and Achilles. You can see it illustrated in Figure 2-3.

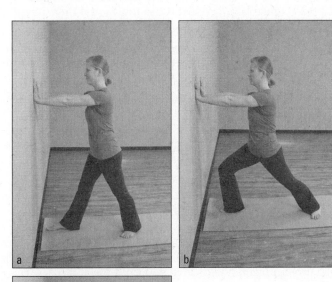

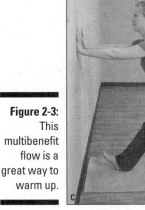

Figure 2-3: This multibenefit flow is a great way to warm up.

1. **Stand facing a wall about 3 feet away; place the toes of your right foot close to the wall, and place the palms of both hands on the wall, with your arms parallel at shoulder height.**

2. **Turn your left foot out about 45 degrees (see Figure 2-3a).**

    Both legs should be straight, and you should be looking straight ahead.

3. **Take a deep breath and, as you exhale, bend your right (front) leg to a 90-degree angle while keeping the outside edge of your back foot down (see Figure 2-3b); repeat three times, and then stay in the warrior posture, looking straight ahead, for 6 to 8 breaths.**

4. **Slowly straighten your right leg and raise the front half of your right foot off the floor as you bend your back leg and drop your left hip (see Figure 2-3c).**

5. **Stay in this posture for 6 to 8 breaths, and then repeat Steps 1 through 5 on the left side.**

Try this sequence on a wall or a tree outside to prepare for golf, tennis, or a hike.

Standing side bend at the wall

The standing side bend at the wall, also called the willow pose, stretches and tones the muscles along the sides of the abdomen, rib cage, and spine. It facilitates breathing and helps give you a supple spine. See Figure 2-4 for an illustration.

1. **Stand tall sideways next to a wall, with your feet hip distance apart and your inside arm extended until you touch the wall with your hand.**

    Keep your palm and fingers pointing up at shoulder height.

2. **As you inhale, bring your outside arm up toward the ceiling; as you exhale, bring it toward the wall in alignment with your ear.**

    If you need to, you can bend your inside arm (at the wall) and your legs.

3. **Repeat Step 2 three times, and then stay with your top arm toward the wall for 6 to 8 breaths.**

4. **Turn in the opposite direction and repeat Steps 1 through 3.**

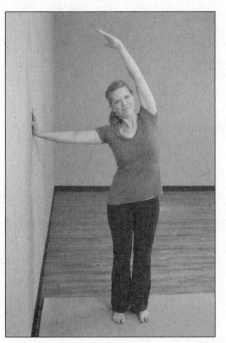

Figure 2-4:
The standing side bend at the wall tones you on the inside.

© John Wiley & Sons, Inc.

As you get more limber, straighten your inside arm at the wall more while holding the posture.

Avoid this posture if it causes back pain.

Half chair at the wall

The half chair at the wall helps improve your overall stamina and strengthens your back, legs, shoulders, and arms. See Figure 2-5 for an illustration.

1. **Start with your back to the wall and your feet hip distance apart.**

2. **As you inhale, extend both arms forward and parallel to the floor. As you exhale, slide down the wall to a half squat position.**

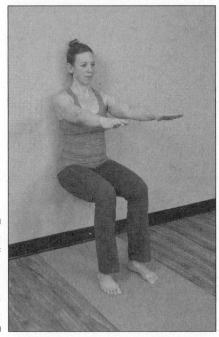

Figure 2-5:
The half
chair at the
wall posture
builds
stamina.

© John Wiley & Sons, Inc.

If you can't see your toes when you're at 90 degrees, move your feet farther from the wall. This posture also is great to use when you need to clean the walls.

3. **Repeat Steps 1 and 2 three times, and then stay in the half squat position for 6 to 8 breaths.**

Avoid this posture if it causes knee or hip pain.

Wall warrior III

Wall warrior III is a perfect illustration of how the wall can prepare you to eventually practice a highly beneficial posture away from the wall, without the extra support. With or without the wall, it's a good posture for overall stability and balance, and it strengthens the legs and arms. You can see it illustrated in Figure 2-6.

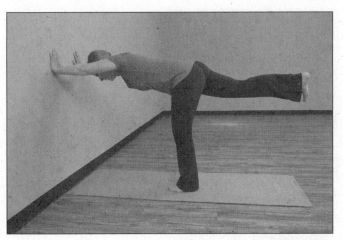

Figure 2-6:
Wall warrior III is a go-to posture for improving stability and balance.

1. Stand in the mountain posture (see Figure 2-1) and face the wall, about 3 to 4 feet away.

2. As you exhale, bend forward from your hips and extend your arms forward until your palms are flat against the wall.

   Alternatively, you may be comfortable with only your fingertips touching the wall for support. Your folded upper torso makes a 90-degree angle with your legs and hips.

3. As you inhale, raise your right leg back until it's parallel to the floor, as in Figure 2-6.

4. Stay in Step 3 for 6 to 8 breaths, and then repeat Steps 1 through 4 with the opposite leg.

Wall hang

The wall hang lengthens the entire spine and stretches the hamstrings, shoulders, neck, and arms. Because the head is below the heart in this pose, it also offers the benefits of inversion (refer to Book II, Chapter 6 for more on inversion). You can see the wall hang illustrated in Figure 2-7.

1. Stand with your back to the wall about 6 to 12 inches feet away, with your feet hip distance apart or slightly wider.

2. Keep your feet planted, and move your hips backward until they rest on the wall.

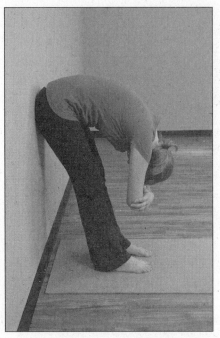

Figure 2-7:
This total body stretch offers benefits of inversion, too.

© John Wiley & Sons, Inc.

3. **Bend forward from the hips, bend your arms, and hold your opposite elbows as you hang.**

4. **Soften your knees and breathe slowly; stay for 8 to 10 breaths.**

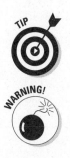

For a shorter, simpler stretch, just hang your chest, head, and arms downward and stay a few breaths.

Avoid this posture if it causes back pain.

Yogi wall sit-ups

The yogi wall sit-ups strengthen the abdomen (especially the upper abdomen) and the neck and shoulders. Check out Figure 2-8 for an illustration.

1. **Lie on your back about 3 feet away from the wall; place your feet on the wall, and adjust your floor position so you can bend your knees at a 90-degree angle.**

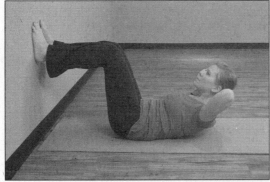

Figure 2-8:
The stability of the wall enhances this variation of the sit-up.

© John Wiley & Sons, Inc.

2. **Interlace your hands behind your head lightly. Inhale deeply and, as you exhale, sit up slowly, keeping your elbows wide so you don't throw your head forward; draw in your belly as you sit up.**

3. **Repeat six to ten times.**

To make this posture more challenging, stay folded at the top for an extra breath, and then return to the floor on the next exhalation.

To strengthen the oblique muscles of the abdomen, try twisting with one elbow as you come up.

Avoid this posture if it hurts your back.

Wall splits

This simple supported posture does a body much good! Wall splits stretch the hips, hamstrings, calves, and inner thighs (called *adductors*). You can see it illustrated in Figure 2-9.

1. **Sit sideways, close to the wall, with your legs straight; when you're ready, swing both legs up on the wall, turn your upper body away from the wall, and lie flat on your back, with your palms down.**

2. **Scoot your hips as close to the wall as you comfortably can; as you inhale slowly, open your legs into a split until you reach your comfortable maximum.**

3. **Upon exhalation, slowly bring your legs straight up again.**

4. **Repeat Steps 2 and 3 three times, and then stay in the open position for 6 to 8 breaths.**

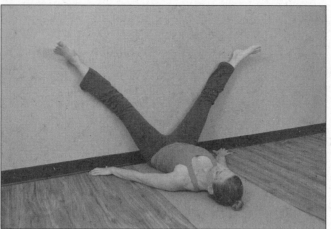

Figure 2-9: With the support of the wall, the benefits of the splits are widely accessible.

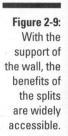

Don't force this posture. Take it nice and easy, allowing for gradual movement when you're opening your legs.

If your hamstrings are tight, you can move farther away from the wall and soften your knees in the splits.

Inverted hamstring pose at the wall

This wall inversion enables you to stretch your hamstrings, hips, calves, and ankles. See Figure 2-10.

1. **Lie flat on your back, with your hips about 3 feet away from the wall.**

2. **Place the soles of your feet up on the wall, with your knees bent at a right angle and your thighs parallel to one another.**

3. **As you exhale, straighten your right leg, bring it back toward you, and reach with both arms to hold your leg evenly.**

   Be sure to keep your hips on the ground and your shoulders dropped as you hold your right leg.

4. **Stay for 6 to 8 breaths, and repeat Steps 1 through 3 with the other leg.**

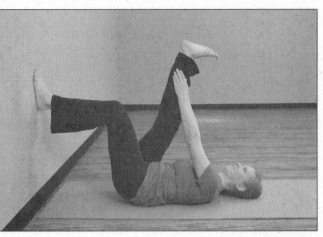

Figure 2-10:
The inverted hamstring pose does just what the name implies — and more.

If you have difficulty reaching your extended leg, try using a strap behind the heel of your foot.

Legs up against the wall

The legs up against the wall posture calms the nervous system and improves circulation to the legs, hips, and lower back. Imagine the possibilities if everyone, especially world leaders, spent 5 minutes each day breathing with his or her feet up the wall; the world would be a more peaceful place. Figure 2-11 illustrates this posture.

1. **Sit sideways as close as possible to the wall, with both legs extended forward; swing both legs up on the wall, and lie flat on your back.**

2. **Turn your palms up, soften your knees as necessary, and close your eyes.**

3. **Stay in this posture for 2 to 10 minutes.**

Try adding an eye pillow while you're relaxing in the pose. Eye pillows block out the light, and the gentle pressure they provide promotes relaxation. See how to move into this position, using a bolster or a few blankets for support, at www.dummies.com/go/yogaaiofd.

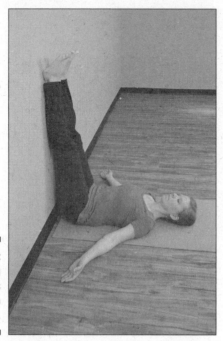

Figure 2-11:
This relaxing
pose has
circulation
benefits.

Avoid this pose if you have high blood pressure; have problems with your eyes, such as retinopathy or other conditions sensitive to pressure; or are more than 3 months pregnant.

Chapter 3

Yoga off the Mat, in the Heat, and outside the Box

* * *

* * *

*Y*oga in its newest incarnations isn't your parents' yoga. Worlds away from classically practiced yoga are the emerging trends of yoga practiced in a hammock slung from the rafters, yoga practiced atop the water on a moving board, and the renewed attention to Hot Yoga.

If you're a person who climbs the mountain to see what's on the other side and you have the requisite strength, stamina, and moxie, you just may find yourself in your element with these fun variations. However, just as the mountain climber adheres to safety guidelines, so should you when exploring these outer reaches of yoga.

Swinging through Yoga without Gravity

Anti-gravity, or *Aerial, Yoga* is a way of stretching, extending, folding, twisting, and inverting with the support of a 10-foot-wide silk hammock suspended from the ceiling. Strikingly new and New World, it was conceived in 1991 by gymnast and dancer Christopher Harrison, who later launched it in 2007. It combines yoga with dance and gymnastics, resulting in a novel hybrid that engages the mind and the body in challenging and delightful ways.

Think of the hammock as a multipurpose prop. It's sometimes a barre, as when supporting leg extensions; sometimes a spotter, as when providing safety with inversions; and sometimes an opposable surface that enables expansive stretches. Sometimes it's a swing — just for fun.

Although a gymnast developed Anti-gravity Yoga, it's practiced by people of all ages and body types.

Getting the unique experience of yoga in a hammock

Anti-gravity Yoga could just as well be called Yoga in a Cocoon. In certain positions, you find yourself safely nestled within the soft confines of the silk hammock. According to Kimberley Simonetti, Los Angeles-based Aerial Yoga teacher and yoga therapist, the physical sensation of being enveloped and contained within the hammock makes this form of practice comforting and even therapeutic for children with autism and adults with post-traumatic stress disorder (PTSD).

You find some notable differences when experiencing familiar postures with the hammock. For instance, in traditional yoga practice, warrior poses tend to be grounding. When you do them leaning into the bunched-up cloth of the hammock, extension becomes more dominant, and balance is challenged in surprising ways. The often-heard instruction in a mat-based yoga class — to feel each foot supported by all four corners — takes on new relevance when practicing with the hammock. Without the strong pull of gravity, you need a greater awareness to stand firmly.

Laying out the benefits of yoga in the hammock

Many reasons draw people to practice Aerial Yoga. Here are just a couple:

✔ **The "yum" factor:** Practicing yoga in a hammock has an element of deliciousness. With the support of the soft, smooth cloth, the body can stretch more deeply and enjoy greater release with both extension and flexion (folding). Some may find that the gentle give of the fabric makes a seated forward bend a more accessible and rewarding experience than the classic version, which is a challenging posture for many.

✔ **The fear factor:** Aerial Yoga is also a way to develop trust, first in the hammock and then in yourself. If you're a person who saunters to the end of the diving board and goes head first into the pool without hesitation, feel free to skip this paragraph. But if you're someone who walks gingerly to the end of the board and then thinks twice or even three times before diving (or heading back down the ladder), practicing Anti-gravity Yoga with a teacher you trust may be a liberating experience for you.

Knowing intellectually that the hammock can hold up to 1,000 pounds isn't enough for everyone to automatically feel free to flip and invert using the hammock for support and leverage. These acts may look effortless, and with practice, they may become so. But many people can take up to 10 or 12 classes to develop the confidence to figuratively let go and flip. (***Warning:*** *Figuratively* is the key word here; *do not* let go of the cloth.)

Selecting an Aerial Yoga teacher and your class gear

Decide what kind of experience you want in the practice and choose your teacher accordingly. Because Aerial Yoga is a hybrid style of practice, teachers may come to it through backgrounds in Pilates, pole and other aerial forms of practice, or traditional yoga.

Unlike conventional yoga practiced on a mat with the teacher in clear view, you can't always see what's beyond the cloth when you're in the hammock, which means the instructor, other students, and your own reflection (if you're in a mirrored room) are out of view for some of the positions. Thus, the teacher's ability to clearly articulate precise instructions is particularly important for the students' safety. Your ability to listen and follow directions is equally important. Listening carefully and following the instructions given — where to grasp the fabric, how tautly to pull it, how many handfuls of fabric to grab, and so on — is what keeps you safe.

Although you may equate hammocks with naptime, don't zone out during practice. Inattention and lack of focus may lead you to tumble out of the hammock. That's not a huge problem, because beginners' hammocks are close to the floor, but it's still one you want to avoid.

Be comfortable in setting your own limits. If you're an adventurous sort, go for it. But if you tend to be more cautious, take your time and allow your sense of trust to grow. Regardless of the form of practice, any good teacher will respect your limits while encouraging you to find your own individual edge.

One way to make your practice a little more comfortable is to put some forethought into your workout clothes. The last thing you want to worry about is inadvertently giving the class an eyeful while you're twisting and turning. Here are a few tips:

- Close-fitting tops are important for modesty because you're upside-down at some points.

- Cotton or cotton blends are preferable to synthetics because synthetics may be slippery and make staying in position difficult.

✔ Sticky gloves help your grip.

✔ Leave the valuable jewelry at home; you'll be asked to remove your jewelry before getting into the hammock to avoid damaging the fabric, so don't bring anything you don't want to let out of your sight.

What's SUP? Floating through Yoga on a Stand Up Paddleboard

SUP is short for stand up paddleboarding. Not surprisingly, it began in Hawaii as an offshoot of surfing. Initially used as a way to get farther out into the ocean to catch the waves, it's now practiced on bodies of water of all sorts, including lakes, rivers, and canals, and in the ocean, parallel to the shore on the other side of the breakers. *SUP Yoga,* then, is the global phenomenon of yoga practice on a board atop the water.

Before you can even think about practicing yoga on a paddleboard, you have to have the necessary swimming skills and confidence in the water so you don't panic if you fall in at a distance from the shore. Have a life jacket or equivalent safety device within reach, if not already on you. You can also get waistbands with safety features that can be activated should the need arise.

Understanding the physical requirements of SUP Yoga

Not unlike many beautiful and graceful things in life, stand up paddleboarding is more challenging than it looks. Those with skill make it look simple, but it actually requires a fair amount of core, thigh, and upper body strength. Strong thighs help you move from kneeling to standing quickly without losing your balance. Your core helps you balance after you're standing, and your upper body strength helps you hoist yourself back up onto the board after you fall off.

Even if you don't fall off, safety concerns require that all boarders know how to get back on safely. But expect to fall. Enjoy the fall. It's freeing and fun!

As with yoga postures on the mat, your forward steady gaze helps you maintain balance as you bring yourself to standing and navigate the waters.

Starting out with SUP Yoga

Begin in still water, such as in a swimming pool, until you can negotiate the board. Starting with stillness helps you notice where you're already strong and where you want to develop further before taking your SUP Yoga practice onto moving water. When you add the elements of underwater currents and wind, it's a whole other game.

You can also get accustomed to the board by doing your yoga practice on the board while it's on the sand. It's a different sensation from practicing on the mat.

Sweating with Hot Yoga

One of the beautiful things about yoga is its great variety in ways to practice. Hot Yoga, though definitely on the mat, is an out-of-the-box variation that is many practitioners swear by. It's not everyone's cup of tea, but it's the variety some folks want to brew every time.

Despite its popular image, Hot Yoga practitioners come in all sizes and ages. If it strikes your fancy, don't hesitate just because you don't think you're magazine cover material.

Getting at the how and why of Hot Yoga

Besides being trendy, Hot Yoga is literally hot. The thermostat is set to maintain a temperature range of 104 to 109 degrees Fahrenheit, and a set level of humidity is piped in. Feel free to contact the studio where you intend to practice Hot Yoga to find out the temperature used at that location.

Why the heat? Various explanations detail why heat is an essential element in this style of yoga.

- **Standardizing body heat:** The heat in the room substitutes for the heat that the body itself would eventually generate though rigorous practice. This internally heated state may be more available to some practitioners than others, especially those who are less fit and more reserved in their practice. Hence, the hot practice environment.

- **Recreating a traditional environment:** The heated practice space mimics the heated physical environment of southern India, replicating as much as possible what some consider to be the ideal practice environment.

✔ **Making the body malleable:** In anatomical terms, the heat allows the superficial soft tissue structures to warm up quickly, allowing greater flexibility and a greater range of motion.

Bikram Choudhury, the originator of Hot Yoga as a distinct style, offers this explanation: "Yoga changes the construction of the body from the inside out, from bones to skin and from fingertips to toes. So before you change it, you have to heat it up to soften it, because a warm body is a flexible body. Then you can reshape your body any way you want."

Theories abound as to why Hot Yoga is beneficial to health. Among them are that the heat is thought to

✔ Lubricate the tendons and ligaments, allowing greater range of motion and flexibility and making you less prone to injury

✔ Improve muscle tone and strength

✔ Exercise the heart as a muscle by increasing blood circulation

✔ Speed up metabolic processes of vital organs and glands and help the body eliminate toxins

✔ Facilitate fat loss by activating fat stores

✔ Boost the immune system

Hot Yoga: Not necessarily a weight-loss cure-all

A July 2014 *Time* magazine article described the science behind the health claims by Bikram and other forms of Hot Yoga as surprisingly scant. Reporting on a study conducted by Dr. Brian L Tracy, an exercise scientist at Colorado State University, the article indicates that results were positive but weaker than expected. A group of sedentary individuals took 24 Bikram sessions over a period of eight weeks. At the end of the eight-week study period, subjects had much-improved balance and modest improvements in strength and muscle control, but only a slight drop in body weight. One possible explanation for the disappointing results in weight loss is that the intensity of the heat and complexity of the postures make practitioners think the exercise is more intense than it really is.

Comparing Bikram and other Hot Yoga classes

Bikram Yoga, developed and trademarked by Bikram Choudhury, is the first and most commonly known variety of Hot Yoga. Its trademarked sequence of 26 postures draws from a much broader range of classical Hatha Yoga postures. In each class, Bikram-trained and certified instructors follow the same script without any variation. It's a routine you can count on being the same each time, regardless of where you take a class.

If variety is the spice of your life, Bikram Yoga and other Hot Yoga varieties that offer unvarying routines may not be appealing. However, for some, having all outside factors held constant is a way to observe and mark progress over time.

In order to offer Bikram classes, a studio must be franchised and follow the Bikram formula to the last detail, including what teachers say and what kind of carpet is on the floor. The legal issues surrounding Bikram Choudhury's trademarking of his sequence has raised concerns about the legitimacy of claiming ownership of a piece of India's cultural heritage. Other studios offering Hot Yoga take the essence of practicing in a heated room and offer what they feel are improvements to the practice and environment.

Book VI

Ancient Practices in the Modern World: Hot Trends in Yoga

These classes use a different selection of postures. Other differences you may find include the following:

- ✔ Freedom from the exact Bikram teacher's script.

- ✔ A different type of flooring. Bikram specifies that a certain kind of carpet be used for slip resistance, which is important when you're dripping with perspiration. Other Hot Yoga classes deal with the need to create traction in other ways.

- ✔ Different types of air circulation systems.

The postures in Bikram and other Hot Yoga classes that draw on a set sequence are taught in their full expression of the pose. In other words, the emphasis in this style is on getting into and holding relatively advanced postures rather than approaching a posture in a step-wise fashion with modifications and even different forms for practitioners at different levels of skill, flexibility, and strength. This emphasis represents a fundamental philosophical difference from the style and approach more generally advocated in yoga classes today and from that presented in *Yoga For Dummies* by Larry Payne and Georg Feuerstein (Wiley). Instead of being an inward experience, the classes pay a lot of attention to what the pose looks like.

Preparing for a Hot Yoga class

A bit of forethought is helpful when practicing in the superheated environment. Here are some things to put on your to-do list prior to your Hot Yoga practice:

- ✔ Bring a large towel, a washcloth or two, and ample water in addition to your yoga mat.

- ✔ Dress lightly — lighter than you think. In some areas, people even wear swimsuits. You won't be sorry. (If you're unsure about what to wear, check with the studio to see what attire is recommended.)

- ✔ Prepare your digestive system by not eating for one to three hours before class and eating only lightly at the meal prior to that period.

- ✔ Keep yourself well hydrated, both before and during class. Don't arrive at the class in a dehydrated state. When you're sweating profusely and expelling body toxins, you run the risk of upsetting your electrolyte balance. Dehydration and loss of electrolytes can result in feelings of nausea, dizziness, headache, and muscle cramping.

At Bikram classes, you are allowed to drink water and rest only at specified times. However, you're in charge of your body, what you choose to do, and when you choose to rest. So pace yourself and take a break when you need to. If you go to a Bikram class, or any yoga class for that matter, and get dizzy, nauseated, or otherwise hurt, take care of yourself, regardless of what the instructor says. You always have the choice to leave and not return for another class if the teacher objects. As with any extreme sport, you can gain a lot with an attitude of good sense and a modicum of caution.

Book VII
Meditation, Mindfulness, and Letting Go of Stress

Five Characteristics of a Mindful Exercise Program

A mindful exercise should incorporate at least one — and preferably several — of the following components:

- **Mindfulness:** The mind is part of the routine in a noncompetitive and nonjudgmental way that is introspective and not goal-oriented, called *mentative*.

- **Body awareness:** Participants focus on sensing what the body and its muscles are doing in all of the movements, called *proprioceptive awareness*.

- **Breath focus:** The sounds and feeling of full and conscious breathwork as a centering activity, called *breath centering*.

- **Method-appropriate form:** Self-discipline allows the body to be aligned to conform to a method's particular pattern of movement, called *anatomic alignment*.

- **Energy flow:** A movement of your own personal inner energy helps achieve the centering, calm, and focus common to mind-body fitness, called *energy centric or bliss*. In addition, research indicates that the best mind-body awareness isn't accomplished during vigorous exercise, but rather needs a low to moderate intensity to be successful. That means if you rate your intensity on a scale of 0 to 10 (with 10 being very hard), it should not feel any harder than about a 6.

Discover ways you can maintain a meditative mindset in everything you do — and reap the benefits — at www.dummies.com/extras/yogaaio.

Contents at a Glance

Chapter 1

How Your Mind Stresses You Out and What You Can Do about It

. . . .

In This Chapter

▶ Scuba-diving through your thoughts and feelings
▶ Checking out the many ways your mind causes stress
▶ Using mediation to ease your stress and suffering

. . . .

For thousands of years, pundits and sages in both the East and West have been saying that problems originate in the mind, that your mind by itself "can make a heaven of hell and a hell of heaven" (as English poet John Milton put it). But how, you may be wondering, can this cute little truism help you when you don't know what to do about it? "Sure, my mind's the problem," you may say, "but I can't exactly have it surgically removed."

You can begin by becoming familiar with how your mind works. As you may have noticed, it's a rather complex assortment of thoughts, ideas, stories, impulses, preferences, and emotions. Without a diagram, it can be as difficult to negotiate as the jumble of wires and hoses under the hood of your car.

When you have a working knowledge of how your mind is structured, you can begin to notice how those thoughts and feelings distort your experience and keep you from achieving the happiness, relaxation, effectiveness, or healing you seek. Then you can discover how meditation can teach you to change all that by focusing and calming your mind, and ultimately by delving more deeply and unraveling the habitual stories and patterns that keep causing you suffering and stress. Who knows? You may not need a lobotomy after all!

Taking a Tour of Your Inner Terrain

Natural metaphors actually lend themselves quite nicely to describing meditation. Practicing meditation can be compared to climbing a mountain, for example or journeying to the bottom of a lake. In either case, the lake or the mountain being referred to is *you* — you're journeying to the heights or depths of your own *being*.

Sifting through the layers of inner experience

When you meditate, in addition to developing your concentration and calming your mind, you may find yourself delving deeper into your inner experience and uncovering layers you didn't even know existed. What do you suppose lies at the bottom? The great meditative traditions have different names for it: essence, pure being, true nature, spirit, soul, the pearl of great price, and the source of all wisdom and love. The Zen folks call it your original face before your parents were born. You may like to picture it as a spring that gushes forth the pure, refreshing, deeply satisfying water of *being* without reservation.

This wellspring of *being* is who you really are in your heart of hearts before you became conditioned to believe that you're somehow deficient or inadequate, as so many folks do. It's your wholeness and completeness before you

Is it higher or deeper?

Spiritual teachers and personal growth advocates have a dizzying fondness for up and down metaphors. Some talk about digging down into your inner experience like a miner, or having profound insights, or feeling or knowing things deeply. Others talk about higher consciousness or transcending the mundane or having a mind like the sky.

To some degree, the difference lies in the personal preferences of the particular writer or teacher. But it can also refer to an attitude toward inner experience: If you believe that the wellspring of *being* lies deep inside you, beneath the personal, then you talk about *down*. If you believe that it exists in the upper echelons of your being or comes down like grace or spirit from above, then you talk about *up*.

In the end, if you dive deep enough, you find yourself at the top of the mountain. And if you rise high enough, you find yourself at the bottom of the sea. In the end, it's the same place anyway. Ultimately, pure *being* has no location — it's everywhere in everyone all the time.

began to feel separate or lonely or fragmented. It's the deep intuition of being inextricably connected with something larger than yourself and with every other being and thing. And it's ultimately the source of all peace, happiness, joy, and other positive, life-affirming feelings (even though you may think they're caused by outside circumstances). Of course, people experience this source differently, which explains why there are so many words to describe it.

Connecting in some way with this source or spring of pure being is actually the point of meditation, whether you're aspiring to become enlightened or just trying to reduce stress, enhance your performance, or improve your life. And meditation definitely takes you to this source, as explained later in this chapter. But when you meditate, you also begin to encounter material that seems to come between you and the experience of being, just as you may encounter layers of sediment, algae, fish, and debris on your way to the bottom of a lake. These layers don't pose a problem unless the inner water is turbulent, in which case they can make it difficult to see clearly. (In this context, *turbulence* refers to a busy, agitated mind or a troubled, frightened, defended heart.)

In more or less the order in which you may encounter them in meditation, the following sections cover these layers.

Mind chatter

When you turn your attention inward, the first thing you're likely to encounter is the ceaseless chattering of your mind. The Buddhists like to compare the mind to a noisy monkey that swings uncontrollably from thought-branch to thought-branch without ever settling down.

Most of the time, you may be so caught up in this chatter that you're not even aware it's happening. It may take the form of reliving the past or rehearsing for the future or trying to solve some problem in the present. Whatever the content, your mind is constantly talking to itself, often spinning a story with you as the hero or the victim. (Research indicates that a very small percentage of people experience no inner dialogue at all, but have only images or feelings instead.)

Intense or recurring emotions

Just as an action film or a romantic comedy takes you on a rollercoaster ride of emotions, so the *dramas* your mind keeps spinning out evoke their own play of feelings. If you're trying to figure out how to make a killing in the stock market, for example, or how to ask out that attractive man or woman you just met at work, you may feel fear or anxiety, or possibly excitement or lust. If you're obsessing about the injustices or unkindnesses you suffered recently, you may experience sadness, grief, outrage, or resentment. Together with these emotions, of course, go a range of bodily sensations, including tension, arousal, contraction in the heart, or waves of energy in the belly or the back of the head.

Book VII

Meditation, Mindfulness, and Letting Go of Stress

Some of these feelings may be pleasurable; others are unpleasant or even painful. But emotions in themselves don't pose a problem. It's just that as long as you keep reacting to the dramas inside your head, you may be cutting yourself off from others and from deeper, more satisfying dimensions of your being. You may miss what's really going on around you as well. (For more on working with emotions in meditation, see Book VII, Chapter 5.)

Many people have trouble distinguishing between thoughts and feelings. For example, if someone asks you, "What are you feeling?" you may reply, "I feel like I shouldn't be so open with my partner anymore." Even though this insight begins with the right word, it's actually a judgment rather than a feeling.

Here are a few pointers for telling the difference:

✔ **Feelings occur as a set of recognizable sensations in your body.** When you're angry, for example, you may feel tension in your shoulders and jaw and experience a rush of energy in the back of your head. When you're sad, by contrast, you may feel a heaviness in your chest and heart and a congested feeling in your sinuses and throat. Through meditation, you can discover how to experience your feelings directly as sensations, separate from the thoughts and stories that perpetuate them. (For more on meditating with thoughts and feelings, see Book VII, Chapter 5.)

✔ **Thoughts are the images, memories, beliefs, judgments, and reflections that float through your mind and often give rise to your feelings.** If you follow the word *feel* with the word *like*, you're probably voicing a thought or a belief rather than a feeling. You can practice breaking strong feelings down into their component parts by asking these questions: What are the thoughts and images in my mind that keep me feeling the way I do? And what am I actually experiencing in my body right now, aside from my thoughts?

Thoughts not only generate feelings but they also often masquerade as feelings (so you won't actually feel the ones you have), attempt to talk you out of your feelings, judge your feelings, or suppress them entirely. The more you can disentangle your thoughts and feelings, the more clearly and consciously you can relate with (and express) your inner experience.

Grasping and pushing away

At a somewhat subtler level of experience than thoughts and emotions lurks a perpetual play of like and dislike, attachment and aversion. The Buddhists teach that the key to happiness and contentment lies in wanting what you have and not wanting what you don't have. But often, we're somehow dissatisfied with what we have. We yearn for what we don't have and we struggle to get it. Or we may become deeply attached to what we have and then suffer when time and circumstances change it or take it away. Because change is unavoidable, this tendency to either hold on tight to experience or push it away can cause constant suffering.

Negative beliefs and life scripts

Imagine that your thoughts and emotions and even the dramas that keep running through your brain form the leaves and branches of some inner, subterranean bush or tree. (Think wild and uncontrollable here, like black-berries or bamboo.) What do you suppose constitutes the root from which the leaves and branches relentlessly spring?

Well, you may be surprised to discover that the root is a cluster of beliefs and stories, many of them negative, that have formed as the result of what people — especially people who are significant in your life, like loved ones and friends — have done to you and told you over the years. These beliefs and stories have intertwined over your lifetime into a kind of life script that defines who you think you are and how you view the people and circumstances around you.

The point is this: Your tendency to identify with your life script actually limits your range of possibilities and causes you suffering by acting as a *filter* through which you interpret your life in negative ways. To return to the bush metaphor, you can keep pruning back the branches, but you'll keep living out the same old story until you pull it up by the roots.

The sense of separation

Even deeper than your stories — some would say the soil in which the stories grow — lies a feeling of being cut off or separate from life or being itself. Although the meditative traditions teach that separation is actually an illusion and that everyone is inextricably connected to one another, the sense of being separate runs deep. Often it dates back to early childhood experiences, such as when you were forced by circumstances to separate prematurely from your mother or some other nurturing figure. Sometimes it can be traced to the birth trauma itself, such as when you had to exchange your placental paradise for a colder, harsher reality. Or maybe, as some traditions contend, it comes packaged with the embryonic hardware.

Whatever its origins, this feeling of separation may give rise to a kind of primordial fear: If I'm separate, then I must end at my skin, and everything out there must be *other*. Because these others are often bigger than I am, and I have only the most limited control over their actions, my survival must be at stake, so I need to protect myself at all costs.

Life scripts, which are discussed in the preceding section, evolve as strategies for surviving in a world of apparent separation, in which others are perceived as potentially unfriendly, withholding, demanding, or rejecting.

Becoming aware of your inner dialogue

Begin this meditation by paying attention to your thoughts. After several minutes, notice what the voices inside your head are telling you. (If you're not aware of any voices, you may want to observe feelings or images instead.) Does one voice predominate, or do several voices vie for your attention? Do they criticize or encourage you? Shame or praise you? Or do they focus primarily on the other people in your life? Do any of the voices argue with one another?

What kind of emotional tone do these voices have? Are they loving and gentle or angry and impatient? Does one voice sound more like you than the others? Do any of them remind you of people in your life — past or present? How do these voices make you feel?

Allow ten minutes for this exercise initially. When you have the knack of it, you can stop from time to time during the day and pay attention to your inner dialogue. The important point is that you're not your thoughts — and you don't necessarily have to believe the messages they impart. (See the sidebar "You are not your thoughts or feelings" in this chapter.)

Discovering how turbulence clouds your mind and heart

Needless to say, when you're experiencing inner turbulence, you may find it difficult to connect with *being* when you sit down to meditate. Sometimes, of course, you may have moments when your mind just settles by itself and you can see all the way down to the bottom of the lake. (To use another nature metaphor, think of those overcast days when the cloud cover suddenly parts and the sun shines through with all its warmth and radiance.) These moments may be marked by feelings of inner peace and tranquility, upsurges of love and joy, or intimations of your oneness with life. But most of the time, you may feel like you're doing a breaststroke through muddy water.

The turbulence and confusion you encounter when you meditate doesn't suddenly materialize on cue. It's there all along, clouding your mind and heart and acting as a filter that obscures your clear seeing. You may experience it as an inner claustrophobia or density. In other words, you're so full of your own emotions and opinions that you have no room for the ideas and feelings of others or even for any new or unfamiliar ideas and feelings that may well up inside you. Or you may get so caught up in your drama that you're not even aware that you're filtering your experience.

Consider these two examples:

✔ Person A, a computer programmer, received plenty of love and support as a child. Now, as an adult, he thinks of himself as inherently competent and worthy, even though he's no Steve Jobs. As a result, he enjoys his career, experiences only minimal anxiety when he makes work-related decisions, sees others as inherently supportive, and exudes a palpable self-confidence that draws others to him and invites them to trust him.

✔ Person B, an independent entrepreneur, has several advanced degrees and has taken countless work-related training courses but believes deep down that he's inherently unworthy. No matter how hard he works, he can't seem to get ahead. Besides, he doesn't really enjoy his work because he's constantly anxious that he may fail, and he imagines that others are conspiring to undermine or discredit him.

In each case, the way each person views himself and interprets what's going on around him determines whether he's happy or stressed out.

As these examples indicate, it's the inner turbulence and confusion through which you filter and distort your experiences — not the experiences themselves — that cause most of your suffering and stress. The good news is that meditation can teach you how to calm the troubled waters of your mind and heart, turn some of your inner claustrophobia into inner spaciousness, and find your way past your filters (or avoid them altogether) so you can experience life more directly — and reduce your stress in the process.

Book VII

Meditation, Mindfulness, and Letting Go of Stress

You are not your thoughts or feelings

Find a quiet spot where you can sit for the next ten minutes. When you're comfortably settled, do the following:

1. **Take a few slow, deep breaths.**

2. **Turn your attention to your thoughts. (If you tend to be an emotional person, you can do the same exercise with your emotions.)**

Instead of getting caught up in your thoughts (or emotions) as you may usually do, watch them closely, the way an angler watches the tip of a rod or a tennis player watches a ball. If you find your attention wandering, come back to the task at hand.

At first, your mind may seem like wall-to-wall thoughts or emotions, and you may have difficulty determining where one thought leaves off and the next one begins. You may also find that certain thoughts or emotions keep recurring like popular tunes (for example, repetitive worries or favorite images or fantasies). If you're especially attentive, you may begin to notice that each thought or emotion has a beginning, a middle, and an end.

(continued)

(continued)

3. **At the end of the ten minutes, stop and reflect on your experience.**

   Did you experience some distance from your thoughts or emotions? Or did you keep losing yourself in the thinking or feeling process?

   The point of this exercise is not to see how well you can track your thinking or feeling; instead,

the point is to give you the experience of being the observer of your thoughts. Believe it or not, you're the thinker, *not* the thoughts themselves! As you begin to gain some perspective on your thoughts through the practice of meditation, you may find that your thoughts start losing the power they once had over you. You can have your thoughts, but they won't have you.

The Bad News: How Your Mind Stresses You Out

Here's a story: A woman in her mid-30s decided to ask for a raise. Even though she'd worked with the company as a graphic designer for years and was long overdue for a pay increase, she was overcome with self-doubt. Every day as she drove to work, she agonized and obsessed as conflicting voices and feelings battled it out inside her.

In particular, she kept rehearsing her upcoming conversation with her boss and reviewing all the things she'd done to make her worthy of more money. She ran through all the projects she'd completed as well as the successful ads and brochures she'd designed. Sometimes she emerged from these imaginary conversations feeling triumphant; other times she emerged crestfallen and defeated. As she listened to all this mind chatter, her feelings fluctuated wildly, from excited and confident to afraid and uncertain.

At times, she heard a barely audible voice (sounding suspiciously like her father's) arguing that given her overall ineptitude, she didn't deserve a raise and that she was lucky to have a job at all. In response, she felt ashamed and hopeless. Next, an angry, vindictive voice stepped in, arguing that her boss was an ungrateful autocrat and that she should barge into his office and put him in his place. Then a confident, affirmative voice reminded her how much she contributed at work and what a fine person she was overall. Finally, a voice that sounded a lot like her mother's counseled her to stay calm and unruffled and be thankful for whatever crumbs life sent her way.

After nearly a week of intense inner struggle and stress, during which she had difficulty sleeping and could barely function at work, the designer finally made an appointment with her boss. Filled with conflicting emotions, she entered his office. She was immediately offered a raise even larger than the one she had planned to request! As it turned out, all the images, emotions, and ideas her mind and body had churned out over the days leading up to the meeting had no connection with what ultimately happened.

Does any of this sound familiar? Like the woman in the story — indeed, like just about everyone — you may spend much of your time engrossed in the captivating but ultimately illusory scenarios fabricated in the original "fantasy factory" (the one that predates Disney and Pixar), the *neocortex.*

One moment you may be worrying about the future — how am I going to make enough money, orchestrate a great vacation, impress my lover, amuse my kids? — and subsequently lost in a reverie filled with hope and fear. The next moment, you may be obsessed with the past — why didn't I tell the truth, take that job, accept that proposal? — and you're overcome with regret and self-recrimination.

And like the woman in the story, you may have noticed, much to your chagrin, that you have remarkably little control over the worrying, fantasizing, and obsessing your mind generates. Instead of having thoughts and feelings, it may often seem that the thoughts and feelings are having you!

The reason these thoughts and feelings seem uncontrollable is that they spring from a deeper story or life script that may be largely unconscious. For example, you may hold the subliminal notion that nothing you do is quite good enough, so you push yourself anxiously to make up for your shortcomings. Or, quite the contrary, you may believe that you deserve more than you're getting, so you're unhappy with what you have. Perhaps you believe that you're inherently unattractive, so no matter how much you compensate, you feel embarrassed and uncomfortable around the opposite sex. Or maybe you see intimate relationships as inherently threatening, so you do all you can to avoid being vulnerable.

Your inner story or drama has a powerful momentum that carries you along, whether you're aware of it or not. Sometimes it may seem like a tragedy, complete with villains and victims. At other times, it may seem more like a comedy, a romance, a fantasy, or a boring documentary. The point is, you're the center around which this drama revolves, and you're often so enthralled by the scenery that you can't really see what's going on outside in the real world around you.

As a result, you may be constantly acting and reacting excessively and inappropriately, based not on the actual circumstances but on the distorted pictures inside your brain. (You've no doubt had moments when you suddenly woke up, as though from a dream, and realized that you had no idea what the person you were interacting with really meant or felt.) Besides, you risk missing entirely the beauty and immediacy of the present moment as it unfolds.

It's this inner drama, not the experiences themselves, that causes most of your suffering and stress. Not that life doesn't serve up shares of difficult times and painful situations for everyone, including the homeless in American cities and the starving children in Africa. But the mind often adds an extra layer of unnecessary suffering to the undeniable hardships of life by interpreting experience in negative or limited ways. (See the sidebar "Distinguishing suffering, pain, and stress" in this chapter.) The following sections highlight some of the major ways your mind stresses you out.

Preoccupation with past and future

Like most minds, yours may flit from past to future and back again, and it may only occasionally come to rest in the present. When you're preoccupied with what may happen next month or next year, you churn up a range of stressful emotions based on hope, fear, and anticipation that have nothing to do with what's happening right now. And when you're reliving the past — which after all has no existence except as thoughts and images inside your brain — you may bounce from regret to resentment to sadness and grief.

Hearts and minds

In this discussion about how the "mind" causes suffering and stress, the term "mind" is used generically to include emotions as well as thoughts because the two are inseparable. Certain Eastern languages, such as Chinese and Sanskrit, even use the same word to refer to both mind and heart, and many Eastern sages teach that the mind actually resides in the heart center.

When you have a thought about potentially charged situations — such as relationships, work, financial problems, or life transitions — you almost invariably have an emotional response (subliminal though it may be). In fact, the field of mind-body medicine has corroborated the view that the mind and body can't really be separated. Thoughts give rise to chemical changes in the blood that affect metabolism and immunity, and alterations in blood chemistry, through drugs or environmental toxins or stressors, can change how you think and feel.

Similarly, the stories that run your life consist of complex layers of emotions, beliefs, and physical contraction that can't easily be teased apart. Through the practice of meditation, you can begin to peel back these layers, infuse them with awareness, and gain insight into the patterns that hold them together.

By contrast, when you meditate, you practice bringing your mind back again and again to the present moment, where, as the Persian poet Rumi says, "the, only news is that there's no news at all." By returning to the simplicity of the here and now, you can take refuge from the stressful scenarios of your mind. (See the section "Returning to the present moment" later in this chapter.)

Resistance to the way things are

Most people struggle unhappily to get what they believe they need in order to be happy while at the same time ignoring or actively disliking what they already have. Now, don't misinterpret the message here; no one is suggesting that you just sit back passively and do nothing to improve your life. But the secret to improving your life is first to accept things just the way they are, which is precisely what the practice of meditation can teach. In particular, resistance to the way things are usually comes in one of two flavors: resistance to change and resistance to pain.

Resistance to change

Like it or not, constant change is unavoidable. If you try to resist the current of change by holding on to some image of how things are supposed to be, you're going to suffer because you can't possibly get life to hold still and conform. As the Greek philosopher Heraclitus used to say, "You can't step into the same river twice."

Through meditation, you can discover how to flow with the current of change by developing an open, flexible, accepting mind. In fact, meditation provides the perfect laboratory for studying change because you get to sit quietly and notice the thoughts and feelings and sensations coming and going. Or you can stiffen up and resist and make the process more painful. Did you ever notice how some people become more crotchety and depressed as they age, while others age gracefully and with a joyful twinkle in their eyes? The difference lies in their ability to adapt to the challenging changes life brings their way.

Resistance to pain

Like change, pain is inevitable. So, too, is pleasure. In fact, you can't have one without the other, though most people would love to have it some other way. When you tighten your belly and hold your breath against the onslaught of pain, be it emotional or physical, you actually intensify the pain. And when you affix a story to the pain — for example, "This shouldn't be happening to me" or "I must have done something to deserve this" — you just attach an extra layer of suffering on top of the pain, which causes your body to tighten and resist even more and only serves to perpetuate the pain rather than relieve it.

Book VII

Meditation, Mindfulness, and Letting Go of Stress

Through meditation, you can learn to breathe deeply, soften your belly, cut through your story, and relax around your pain. Often, the pain naturally lets go and releases — and even when it doesn't, it generally becomes much easier to bear.

A judging and comparing mind

The tendency of your mind to compare you to others (or to some impossible ideal) and to judge every little thing you do as imperfect or inadequate just keeps you anxious, frustrated, and upset. Generally, this tendency originates in your stories or life script, a deeply held cluster of often negative beliefs. (See the "Negative beliefs and life scripts" section earlier in this chapter.) After all, if you believe that you're lovable and inherently perfect just the way you are, your mind has nothing to compare you with.

When you practice meditation, you can develop the capacity to observe the judgments and comparisons of your mind without identifying with them or mistaking them for truth. (For more on this capacity, see the "Penetrating your experience with insight" section later in this chapter.)

Learned helplessness and pessimism

As numerous psychological studies suggest, your ability to deal with stressful situations largely depends on whether you believe you have the resources necessary to cope. That's right. The *belief* that you have what it takes is perhaps your greatest resource. If your story keeps telling you that you're inadequate, it's just making stressful situations more stressful.

Meditation can teach you coping skills like focusing and calming your mind; returning to the present moment; and cultivating positive emotions and mind-states that help you avoid negative, distracting thoughts and empower you to deal with difficult circumstances and people. (See the section "The Good News: How Meditation Relieves Suffering and Stress" later in this chapter.) Ultimately, you can discover how to see beyond your story and make direct contact with the true source of optimism and joy, the wellspring of pure *being* inside you.

Overwhelming emotions

Although you can't necessarily identify your story, you may be painfully aware of how powerful emotions like anger, fear, longing, grief, jealousy, and desire cloud your mind, torment your heart, and cause you to act in ways you later regret.

Initially, meditation doesn't eliminate these emotions, but it does teach you how to focus and calm your mind and prevent the emotions from distracting you. If you want, you can then use meditation to observe these emotions as they arise without avoiding or suppressing them. Over time, you can develop penetrating insight into the nature of these emotions and their connection to the underlying stories that keep generating them. Ultimately, you can investigate these stories and even dismantle them entirely. (For more on meditating with challenging emotions, see Book VII, Chapter 5.)

Distinguishing suffering, pain, and stress

Suffering, pain, and stress? Yikes! Who wants to burden their brains with such unappetizing topics? However, the clearer you are about suffering, pain, and stress, the more easily you can minimize their impact on your life. Consider the following helpful (and admittedly unofficial) distinctions:

✔ *Pain* consists of direct, visceral experiences with a minimum of conceptual overlays. Your best friend says something mean to you, and you feel a painful constriction in your heart. You hit your thumb with a hammer, and it aches and throbs. You get the flu, and your head feels like someone's squeezing it in a vice. Pain hurts, pure and simple.

✔ *Suffering* is what happens when your mind makes hay with your pain. For example, you decide that because she hurt your feelings, your best friend must secretly hate you, which means something must be terribly wrong with you. And the next thing you know, you're feeling depressed as well as hurt. Or you turn your headache into a sure warning sign of some serious illness, which just heaps a big dose of fear and hopelessness onto an already difficult

situation. Suffering, in other words, results from seeing situations through the distorting lens of the story your mind tells you.

✔ The *stress response* is a physiological mechanism for adapting to challenging physical or psychological circumstances. Certain physical stressors, such as extraordinary heat or cold, an extremely loud noise, or a violent attack, are stressful no matter how your mind interprets them. But the stressful effect of most stressors depends on the spin your mind adds to the situation. For example, driving to work in heavy traffic, sitting at your desk for eight hours handling paperwork and phone calls, and then driving home may be only mildly stressful on a purely physical level. But when you're afraid of arriving late, have a conflicted relationship with your boss, feel angry at several of your clients or coworkers, and are still mulling over the argument you had with your spouse or best friend yesterday, it's no wonder you crawl home at the end of the day completely exhausted. Just as your mind can transform pain into suffering, so it can parlay ordinary stressors into extraordinary stress.

Book VII

Meditation, Mindfulness, and Letting Go of Stress

Fixation of attention

The tendency of the thinking mind to obsess or fixate on certain thoughts and emotions causes the body to contract in response. Have you ever noticed how tense and anxious you can get when you mentally rehearse the same scenario again and again, even when it's an ostensibly positive one? By contrast, an alert, open, fluid mind — which you can develop through the regular practice of mindfulness meditation (see Book VII, Chapter 4) — allows you to flow from experience to experience without getting fixated or stuck. Ultimately, you can practice *receptive awareness* (see Book VII, Chapter 3), the spacious, skylike quality of mind that welcomes whatever arises.

Clinging to a separate self

The great meditative traditions teach that the root cause of suffering and stress, which gives rise to your stories, is the belief that you're inherently separate from others, from the rest of life, and from *being* itself. Because you feel separate and alone, you need to protect yourself and ensure your survival at all costs. But you have only limited power, and you're surrounded by forces beyond your control. As long as you keep struggling to defend your turf, you're going to keep suffering no matter how hard you try. Meditation offers you the opportunity to relax your guard, open your awareness, and ultimately catch a glimpse of who you really are, beyond your stories and the illusion of a separate, isolated self.

The Good News: How Meditation Relieves Suffering and Stress

Now for the good news! In case you find all the talk earlier in this chapter depressing, be reassured: Your story or drama may masquerade as who you really are, but it's not. Your essential being remains pure and unharmed, no matter how elaborate and compelling your story becomes. Besides, as stubborn and intractable as they may seem, your mind and heart are actually malleable. Through the regular practice of meditation, you can reduce your suffering and stress by stilling and ultimately dissipating the turbulence and confusion inside you. As one ancient Zen master put it, "If your mind isn't clouded by unnecessary things, this moment is the best moment of your life."

To begin with, you can develop the skill of *focusing and concentrating* your mind, which calms it and prevents it from becoming agitated. As your concentration deepens, thoughts and feelings that have been building up inside naturally bubble up and evaporate in a *spontaneous release*.

When you've developed strong concentration, you can expand your awareness to include thoughts, feelings, and the deeper patterns and stories that underlie them. Then, through the power of *penetrating insight,* you can explore the various layers of inner experience, get to know how they function, and ultimately use this understanding to dismantle the patterns that keep causing you stress.

Extending the mind-body 'round the clock

The mind-body connection doesn't have to stop when you roll up your mat and put it away. You can take your lessons — and the wisdom you have gathered through them — along for the ride as you cruise through your day. You're likely to find other ways that work for you, too. Here are some suggestions:

✔ **Concentrate on breathing:** Train yourself to be aware of your breathing in all situations. You may be surprised at how often you catch yourself holding your breath. Really. If you're in a conversation, debate, discussion, or even an argument with someone, take a moment to breathe before you respond. Breathing alone can help slow your pulse and blood pressure.

✔ **Look inside yourself:** Think about how and why you feel and react the way you do in certain situations. Let yourself feel all during the day, in everything that you do, by looking inward in short meditative moments.

✔ **Observe the world around you:** Observe both yourself and others in daily interactions, without judgment. Don't think, "Oh, what I just said was so stupid," or "How could she ever have worn those odd shoes?" Instead, simply observe things around you and how they affect you, then acknowledge that reaction or affect. You'll eventually find more calm and peace day-to-day.

✔ **Send healing energy to someone else:** Use the awakened mental powers you develop from mind-body exercise to "beam" positive energy to someone else. Imagining healing energy enveloping another person can make that person's day (and yours) better.

✔ **Take 5 (or 10, or 20 . . .):** Everybody can find at least five minutes in the day for him- or herself. Writing down your daily schedule to figure out where those extra minutes get lost may be helpful. You can even pencil in a time you intend to take a break, or set an alarm on your watch so you don't get so wrapped up that you forget.

✔ **Find 5:** Find a minute or two to do a quick balance pose, stretch, alignment drill, or standing meditation many times during the day. Look for times when you're just waiting for something. How about when you fill your car's gas tank? You can do a standing or breathing exercise in that moment. See how easy it is to find a couple of dangling minutes in your day?

Developing focus and concentration

So your mind chatters constantly, swirling you up and stressing you out, and you're wondering what you can do to quiet it down. Well, you can begin by practicing a meditation technique that emphasizes concentration, such as following or counting your breaths (see Book VII, Chapter 4) or reciting a mantra (see Book VII, Chapter 3). When you get the knack, you can keep shifting from your inner dialogue to the present moment, wherever you happen to be. And if you're so inclined, you can develop positive qualities that counteract some of the negative tendencies of your mind and heart.

Stabilizing your concentration

If you've ever tried to quiet your mind by preventing it from thinking, you know how hopeless that can be. (See the sidebar "Stopping your mind" in this chapter.) But the more you invest your mental energy in a single focus during meditation, the more one-pointed your mind becomes, and the more the distractions recede to the background. Eventually, you can develop the ability to stabilize your concentration on a single focus for minutes at a time, gently returning when your mind wanders off.

With increased one-pointedness comes an experience of inner harmony and stillness, as the sediment in the turbulent lake of your mind gradually settles, leaving the water clean and clear. This experience is generally accompanied by feelings of calm and relaxation and occasionally by other pleasurable feelings like love, joy, happiness, and bliss (which incidentally originate at the bottom of the lake in pure *being*).

At deeper levels of concentration, you may experience total absorption in the object — a state known as *samadhi.* When this power of focused concentration is directed like a laser beam to everyday activities, you can enter what psychologist Mihaly Csikszentmihalyi calls *flow* — a state of supreme enjoyment in which time stops, self-consciousness drops away, and you become one with the activity itself.

Returning to the present moment

When you've begun to develop your concentration, you can use it to keep shifting in everyday life away from your inner drama and back to the present moment. You may not eliminate the turbulence, but you can keep seeing beyond it. It's kind of like taking off your sunglasses and looking at things directly or like opening your eyes wide when you start falling asleep. The more you look past the drama, the more you see the freshness of *being* itself reflected in what you see. Returning to the present moment again and again forges a trail that allows you to do an end run around your drama and strengthens your direct connection with life.

Cultivating positive emotions and mind-states

You can use the concentration you develop in meditation to cultivate positive alternatives to agitation, fear, anger, depression, and the other powerful emotions that arise when you're involved in your story. (In fact, the practice of cultivation itself can develop your powers of concentration.) These positive mind-states include lovingkindness, compassion, equanimity, and joy.

Allowing spontaneous release

When you meditate regularly, you start to notice that thoughts and feelings that have accumulated inside you naturally dissipate like mist rising from the surface of a lake. You don't have to do anything special to make this happen. It simply occurs naturally as your concentration deepens and your mind settles down. You may sit to meditate feeling weighted down by worries or concerns and then get up half an hour later feeling somehow lighter, more spacious, and more worry-free. Who knows how this mysterious process happens? You may say that meditating is like lifting the lid on a boiling pot of soup: You create space for the water to evaporate and relieve the pressure that has been building up inside.

 To encourage this process of spontaneous release, you can practice meditation techniques that involve *receptive awareness* — open, spacious awareness that welcomes whatever arises. (You need to develop your concentration first.) When your mind is no longer fixated on a particular object — be it a thought, a memory, or an emotion — and is expansive and unattached like the sky, you're no longer investing energy in your drama. Instead, you're inviting whatever's churning inside you to unfold and let go.

Book VII

Meditation, Mindfulness, and Letting Go of Stress

Penetrating your experience with insight

The previous sections highlight concentration and awareness techniques that show you how to circumvent your drama, develop alternatives to your drama, and still your mind so that your drama doesn't disturb you. The problem with these techniques is that they leave your inner stories more or less intact, and when your concentration weakens or your lovingkindness wanes, the same old distracting thoughts and troubling emotions come back to stress you out!

Through the practice of penetrating insight, however, you can get to know your drama, gain an understanding of how it causes suffering, see beyond it, and eventually free yourself from it entirely.

Becoming aware of your inner experience

When you sit quietly for 10 or 15 minutes and notice your thoughts and feelings, you're making a radical shift in your relationship to your inner experience. (For more on observing thoughts and feelings, see Book VII, Chapter 5.) Instead of being swept away by the current, you become, for the moment, an observer on the shore, watching the river of your experience flow by. Though the difference may seem inconsequential and you may not feel that you're making any headway, you've actually begun to loosen your story's stranglehold on your life. Gradually, you begin to notice spaces in your mind's chatter, and what once seemed so serious and solid slowly becomes lighter and infused with fresh air. You may find yourself laughing at your tendency to worry and obsess, or perhaps you pause and notice what you're feeling before you react.

As you practice welcoming your experience just as it is, including your judgments and self-criticisms, you may also discover that your attitude toward yourself begins to change in subtle ways. Instead of impatience or contempt, you may begin to notice a certain self-acceptance creeping in as you become more familiar with the repetitive patterns of your mind. Hey, you may even develop a measure of compassion for yourself as you see how self-critical or distracted or frightened you can become.

Becoming aware of your story and how it confuses you

When you meditate regularly and observe your thoughts and feelings, you begin to notice recurring themes and story lines that keep playing in your mind. Perhaps you become aware of the tendency to obsess about all the times people misunderstood you or failed to give you the love you wanted. Maybe you see how you compare yourself to other people and judge yourself better or worse than them. Possibly you find yourself fantasizing about the ideal mate, even though you've been happily married for years. Or you may notice that you're constantly planning for the future while ignoring what's happening right here and now.

Whatever your particular patterns may be, you can observe how they keep arising to disturb you and pull you away from the reality at hand (which may be some simple task like following your breath or reciting your mantra). Gradually, you realize that your story is just that: a story your mind keeps spinning that separates you from others and causes you pain. As John Lennon put it, "Life is what's happening while you're busy making other plans." When you start seeing your story for what it is, you don't allow it to confuse you in the same way anymore.

Changing your story

As you may notice after you meditate for a while, just being aware of your story can begin changing it in subtle (or even not-so-subtle!) ways. When you develop a certain distance from your story — knowing at some level that it's just your story, not who you really *are* — you naturally become less reactive, people respond to you differently, and circumstances shift accordingly. Soon your life is just not the same old story anymore!

Of course, you may already be struggling to change your life by manipulating circumstances or reprogramming your mind with affirmations or positive thinking. But first you have to bring the power of penetrating insight to bear on your habitual patterns and stories; otherwise, healthier perspectives and patterns can't take root, and you just keep running in the same old grooves.

Seeing beyond your story to who you really are

Even though you may become aware of your story, gain some distance from it, and begin to alter it in certain fundamental ways, you may still identify with it until you can catch a glimpse of who you really are beyond your story.

Such glimpses can take a number of different forms. Perhaps you have unexpected moments of peace or tranquility, when your thoughts settle down — or even stop entirely — and a sweet silence permeates your mind. Or you may experience a flood of unconditional love that momentarily opens your heart wide and gives you a brief glimpse of the oneness beyond all apparent separation. Or maybe you have a sudden intuition of your inherent interconnectedness with all beings or a sense of being in the presence of something far vaster than yourself. Whatever the insight that lifts you beyond your story, it can irrevocably alter who you take yourself to be. Never again can you fully believe that you're merely the limited personality your mind insists you are.

Freeing yourself from your story

When you've caught a glimpse of who you really are, beyond your mind (and even your body), you can keep reconnecting with this deeper level of *being* in your meditations as well as in your everyday life. To resurrect the metaphor of the lake described earlier in the chapter, you can dive down to the bottom again and again because you know what it looks like and how to find it.

Even though your story may continue to play on the video screen of your brain, you can develop the capacity to disengage from it or even disidentify from it entirely. You even come to realize that the personality is a case of mistaken identity and that who you are is the vast expanse of *being* itself, in which your personal thoughts and feelings arise and pass away.

Such a profound realization may take years of meditation to achieve, yet it's always available to you no matter how long you've meditated — indeed, whether you've ever meditated at all! Many people report laughing uproariously when they finally see that their true natures were right there all along, as plain as the proverbial noses on their faces.

Book VII

Meditation, Mindfulness, and Letting Go of Stress

Stopping your mind

Many people believe that the point of meditation is to stop the mind. To get a visceral sense of the futility of such efforts, you can attempt to stop your mind and see what happens. Try the following exercise:

1. **Sit quietly and take a few slow, deep breaths.**

2. **For the next five minutes, try to stop thinking.**

   That's right. Do whatever you can to keep your mind from generating more thoughts. Try humming to yourself or concentrating on your big toe or recalling a beautiful day in nature. Or just try being as still as you possibly can. Do whatever you think will work for you.

3. **At the end of five minutes, reflect on your experience.**

   How successful were you? Could you actually stop thinking for an extended period of time? Did you find that the struggle to stop thinking just generated more thoughts? In case you hadn't noticed, this exercise reveals how stubborn and tenacious your thinking mind can be.

Contrary to popular belief, people who learn to integrate this realization and live their understanding in a moment-to-moment way don't become more detached and disengaged from life. Rather, because their stories and their senses of separation have lifted like a fog, they actually perceive situations and people with more immediacy and compassion, and they can act more appropriately according to the circumstances.

Chapter 2

Relaxed Like a Noodle: The Fine Art of Letting Go of Stress

*L*ife in general — not merely modern life — is inherently stressful. But not all stress is bad for you. The question is whether that stress is helping you or hurting you.

Psychologists distinguish between *distress* and *eustress* (good stress). Yoga can help you minimize distress and maximize good, life-enhancing stress. For example, a creative challenge that stimulates your imagination and fires your enthusiasm but doesn't cause you anxiety or lost sleep is a positive event. Even a joyous celebration is, strictly speaking, stressful, but the celebration isn't the kind of stress that harms you — at least not in modest doses. On the other hand, doing nothing and feeling bored to tears is a form of negative stress.

In this chapter, you discover how you can control negative stress not only through various yogic relaxation techniques but also by cultivating appropriate attitudes and habits.

The Nature of Stress

Your body has evolved to handle episodes of physical stress that arise and then subside. The fight-or-flight response you experience when you're in stressful situations helps you react to real threats in your physical environment. The alertness and physical energy you feel when your physical safety is threatened are truly life saving. These circumstances were the ones for which this capacity evolved.

Contrast this stress with the constant stress experienced in the course of modern life. The relentless demands — work, money woes, noise, pollution, a packed schedule, and so on — can put you in a chronic state of alertness that's extremely draining to your body's energies and resources. Instead of getting you to safety, the chronic stress that's part of today's lifestyles creates an imbalance in the body and the mind, causing you to tense your muscles and breathe in a rapid and shallow manner, perhaps with little relief. Under such chronic stress, your adrenal glands work overtime and your blood may become depleted of oxygen, thus starving your cells.

How can you deal with your stress response efficiently? Yoga suggests a three-pronged solution:

- ✔ Correct your stress-producing attitudes.
- ✔ Change habits that invite stress into your life.
- ✔ Release existing tension in the body on an ongoing basis.

Stress can occur without any obvious unpleasant stimulus. Even a birthday celebration can cause you stress, usually because of some hidden anxiety (like another year to mark off). Stress can be cumulative and can creep up on you so gradually that it's imperceptible — until its acute and adverse symptoms manifest.

Correcting wrong attitudes

Yoga's integrated approach works with both the body and the mind, offering potent antidotes to just the sort of attitudes that make you prone to stress, especially egotism, extreme competitiveness, perfectionism, and the sense of having to accomplish everything right now and by yourself. In all matters, yoga seeks to replace negative thoughts and attitudes with positive mental dispositions; it asks you to be kind to yourself. Yogic practice helps you understand that everything has its proper place and time.

If you, like so many stress sufferers, have a hard time asking for help, yoga can give you a real appreciation that everyone is interdependent. If it's your nature to distrust others, yoga puts you in touch with the part of your psyche that naturally trusts life itself. It shows you that you don't need to feel as if you're under attack, because your real life — your spiritual identity — can never be harmed or destroyed.

Wherever ego, I go

The ultimate source of stress is the ego, or what the yoga masters call the "I-maker" *(ahamkara)*, from *aham* ("I") and *kara* ("maker"). From the perspective of yoga, the ego is a mistaken notion in which people identify with their particular bodies instead of with the universe as a whole. Consequently, they experience fear of change and attachment to the body and the mind. This attachment, which is the survival instinct, gives rise to all those many emotions and intentions that make up the game of life. Keeping this artificial center — the ego — going is inherently stressful. Yoga masters all agree that relaxing the grip of the ego allows you to experience greater peace and happiness. Happy letting go!

Changing poor habits

People often desperately maintain a hectic schedule because they can't envision an alternative that includes time out. They fear what may happen if they slow down. But money and standard of living aren't everything; the *quality* of your life is far more important. Besides, if stress undercuts your health, you have to go into low gear anyway, and your climb back to health may prove costly. Yoga gives you a baseline of tranquility to deal with your fears and anxieties effectively — as long as you engage it at the mental level and not just the physical level.

Of course, you can take many practical steps to manage stress by reducing stressful situations: Don't wait until the last minute to start or finish projects, improve your communication with others, avoid unnecessary confrontations, and so on. Meditation, explained in Book VII, Chapters 3 through 5, is another way to reduce stress. Yoga recommends that you constantly remember your spiritual nature, which is beyond the realm of change and is ever blissful and at peace. However, it also asks you to care for others and the world you live in, all while appreciating that you can't step into the same river twice. These principles are explained in the next sections.

Embracing balance

Everything in the universe follows an ebb-and-flow pattern that you can count on. Seasons change, and newborn babies grow and eventually become elderly adults. Yogic wisdom recommends that you adopt the same natural patterns in your personal life. Notice and appreciate the cyclical change of the seasons, the myriad ways that you and your environment change and evolve. You may spend much of your time being serious, but you need to play, too. In fact, you need to make time to *just be,* with no expectations and

Book VII

Meditation, Mindfulness, and Letting Go of Stress

no guilt. Taking time to just be is good for your physical and mental health. Work and rest, tension and relaxation belong together as balanced pairs.

Letting go

Your inner wisdom tells you that your body and mind are subject to change and that nothing in your environment permanently stays the same. Therefore, there's no point in anxiously clinging to anything.

Yoga shows you how to cultivate the *relaxation response* throughout the day by letting go of your hold on things. Herbert Benson, MD, coined this phrase and was among the first to point out the hidden epidemic of hypertension (high blood pressure) as a result of stress. The yogic equivalent of the relaxation response is *vairagya,* which means, literally, "dispassion" or "nonattachment." We call it "letting go."

Feeling passionate about what you do (as opposed to having a lukewarm attitude) is good, but at the same time, you merely invite suffering when you become too attached to people, situations, expectations, and the outcome of your actions. Yoga recommends an attitude of inner detachment in all matters. This detachment doesn't spring from boredom, failure, fear, or apathy; it comes from inner wisdom. For example, if you're a mother, you love and take tender care of your children. But if you're also a yogini, you don't succumb to the stress-producing illusion that you *own* your children. Instead, you always remain aware of the fact that your sons and daughters have their own lives to live, which may turn out to be quite different from yours. You know that all you can do is guide them as best you can.

Releasing bodily tension

Yoga pursues tension release through all its many different techniques, including breathing exercises and postures, but especially relaxation techniques. The former are a form of *active* or *dynamic relaxation;* the latter are a form of *passive* or *receptive relaxation.*

Your daily Hatha Yoga routine, especially the relaxation exercises, can help you extend the feeling of peacefulness or calmness beyond the yoga session to the rest of the day. Pick some activities or situations that you repeat several times a day as reminders to consciously relax, such as when you go to the bathroom, wait at a traffic light, sit down, open or close a door, or look at your watch. Whenever you encounter these activities, exhale deeply and consciously relax, remembering the peaceful feeling evoked in your daily session.

Relaxation Techniques That Work

The Sanskrit word for relaxation is *shaithilya,* which is pronounced shy-theel-yah and means "loosening." It refers to the loosening of physical and mental tension and effort — all the knots that you tie when you don't go with the flow of life. These knots are like kinks in a hose that prevent the water from flowing freely. Keeping muscles in a constant alert state expends a great amount of your energy, which then is unavailable when you call upon your muscles to really function. Conscious relaxation trains your muscles to release their grip when you don't use them. This relaxation keeps the muscles responsive to the signals from your brain telling them to contract so that you can perform the countless tasks of a busy day.

Relaxation isn't quite the same as doing nothing. Often when you believe you're doing nothing, you're actually busy contracting muscles quite unconsciously. Relaxation is a conscious endeavor that lies somewhere between effort and noneffort. To truly relax, you have to understand and practice the skill.

Relaxation doesn't require any gadgets, but you may want to try the following:

- ✔ Practice in a quiet environment where you're unlikely to be disturbed by others or the telephone.

- ✔ Try placing a small pillow under your head and a large one under your knees for support and comfort in the *supine,* or lying, positions. Alternatively, use a folded blanket.

- ✔ Ensure that your body stays warm. If necessary, heat the room first or cover yourself with a blanket.

- ✔ Don't practice relaxation techniques on a full stomach; it can cause reflux.

Deep relaxation: The corpse posture

The simplest, yet most difficult, of all yoga postures is the corpse posture (*shavasana,* from *shava* and *asana,* pronounced shah-vah-sah-nah). This posture is the simplest because you don't have to use any part of your body at all, and it's the most difficult precisely because you're asked to do nothing whatsoever with your limbs. The corpse posture is an exercise in mind over matter. The only props you need are your body and mind.

If you're high-strung, asana practice helps make the corpse posture more easily accessible.

Here's how you do the corpse posture:

1. **Lie flat on your back, with your arms stretched out and relaxed by your sides, palms up (or whatever feels most comfortable).**

   Place a small pillow or folded blanket under your head, if you need one, and another large one under your knees for added comfort.

2. **Close your eyes.**

   Check out Figure 2-1 for a look at the corpse posture.

Figure 2-1:
The corpse is the most popular of all yoga postures.

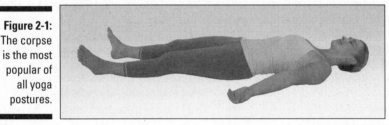

Photograph by Adam Latham

3. **Form a clear intention to relax.**

   Some people picture themselves lying in white sand on a sunny beach.

4. **Take a couple of deep breaths, lengthening exhalation.**

5. **Contract the muscles in your feet for a couple of seconds and then consciously relax them; do the same with the muscles in your calves, thighs, buttocks, abdomen, chest, back, hands, forearms, upper arms, shoulders, neck, and face.**

6. **Periodically scan all your muscles, from your feet to your face, to check that they're relaxed.**

   You can often detect subtle tension around the eyes and the scalp muscles. Also relax your mouth, jaw, and tongue.

7. **Focus on the growing bodily sensation of no tension, and let your breath be free.**

8. **At the end of the session, before opening your eyes, form the intention to keep the relaxed feeling for as long as possible.**

9. **Open your eyes, stretch, roll to one side, and get up slowly.**

Practice 10 to 30 minutes; the longer the duration, the better. But watch out; relaxing for too long can make you drowsy.

Ending relaxation peacefully

Allowing relaxation to end on its own is best; your body knows when it has benefited sufficiently and naturally brings you out of relaxation. However, if you have only a limited time for the exercise, set your mental clock to 15, 20, or however many minutes after closing your eyes, as part of your intention.

If you need to have a sound to remind you to return to ordinary waking consciousness, you can find any number of free or low-cost apps for your smartphone. You can set the timer for the length you like and be awakened by a pleasant sound of your choosing, like a bell or gong.

Staying awake during relaxation

The beautiful part of relaxation is that you're conscious throughout the experience and can control it to some extent. Through relaxation, you get more in touch with your own body, which benefits you throughout the day: You detect stress and tension in your body more readily and then take appropriate action.

If it looks like you're going to fall asleep while doing the corpse posture, try bringing your feet closer together. Also, periodically pay attention to your breathing, making sure it's even and unforced.

Afternoon delight

When your energies flag in the afternoon, try the following exercise as a great stress buster. You can practice it at home or in a quiet place at the office. Just make sure that you aren't interrupted. For this exercise, you need a sturdy chair, one or two blankets, and a towel or an eye pillow (small bags filled with light materials, usually plastic pellets, that not only block light but put slight pressure on the eyes). Allow 5 to 10 minutes.

1. **Lie on your back and put your feet on the chair, which faces you (see Figure 2-2).**

   Make sure your legs and back are comfortable. Keep your legs 15 to 18 inches apart. You can also put your legs and feet up on the edge of a bed. If none of the feet-up positions feels good, just lie on your back with your legs bent and feet placed on the floor. If the back of your head isn't flat on the floor, and if your neck and throat feel tense or your chin is pushed up toward the ceiling, raise your head slightly on a folded blanket or a firm, flat cushion so that you feel more comfortable.

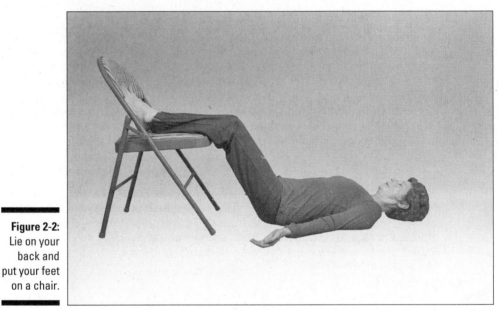

Figure 2-2:
Lie on your
back and
put your feet
on a chair.

Photograph by Adam Latham

2. **Cover your body from the neck down with one of the blankets.**

   Don't let your body cool down too quickly; it not only feels uncomfortable and interferes with your relaxation, but it also can cramp your muscles.

3. **Place the eye pillow or towel folded lengthwise over your eyes.**

4. **Rest for a few moments, and get used to the position.**

5. **Visualize a large balloon in your stomach: As you inhale through your nose, expand the imaginary balloon in all directions; as you exhale through your nose, release the air from the balloon.**

   Repeat this step several times until it becomes easy for you.

6. **Inhale freely, and begin to make your exhalation longer and longer.**

   Inhale freely, exhale forever.

7. **Repeat Step 6 at least 30 times.**

8. **When you finish the exercise, allow your breath to return to normal and rest for a minute or so, enjoying the relaxed feeling.**

   Don't rush getting up.

Magic triangles: Relaxing through visualization

The following relaxation technique utilizes your power of imagination. If you can picture images easily in your mind, you may find the exercise enjoyable and refreshing. For this exercise, you need a chair and a blanket (if necessary). Allow 5 minutes.

1. **Sit up tall in a chair, with your feet on the floor and comfortably apart, and your hands resting on top of your knees, as in Figure 2-3.**

   If your feet aren't comfortably touching the floor, fold the blanket and place it under your feet for support.

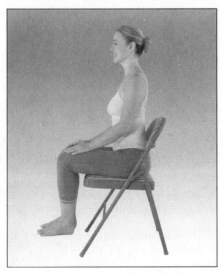

Figure 2-3:
Sit with your feet on the floor and your hands on your knees.

Photograph by Adam Latham

2. **Breathe through your nose, but allow your breath to move freely.**

3. **Close your eyes and focus your attention on the middle of your forehead, just above the level of your eyebrows.**

   Make sure you don't crinkle your forehead or squint your eyes.

4. **Visualize as vividly as possible a triangle connecting the forehead point and the palms of both hands.**

   Register (but don't think about) any sensations or colors that appear on your mental screen while you hold the triangle in your mind. Do this visualization for 8 to 10 breaths, and then dissolve the triangle.

5. **Visualize a triangle formed by your navel and the big toes of your feet; retain this image for 10 to 12 breaths.**

   If any part of the mental triangle is difficult to connect, keep focusing on that part until the triangle fully forms.

6. **Keeping your eyes closed, visualize again the first triangle formed between your forehead and your two palms, and then simultaneously visualize the second triangle (navel to toes).**

   This final step is more challenging. Picture both triangles together for 12 to 15 breaths, and then dissolve them.

Relaxation before sleep

If you want to enjoy deep sleep or you're experiencing insomnia (but you don't want to count sheep), the following exercise can help you. Many people don't make it to the end of this relaxation technique without falling asleep. For this exercise, you need the following props: a bed or other comfortable place to sleep, two pillows, and one or two blankets. Allow 5 to 10 minutes.

1. **Prepare yourself for sleep and get into bed, lying on your back under the blankets.**

   Your legs can be straight or bent at the knees, with your feet flat on the mattress.

2. **Place one pillow or a folded blanket under your head, and have the other one nearby.**

3. **With your eyes closed, begin to breathe through your nose, making your exhalation twice as long as your inhalation.**

   Keep your breathing smooth and effortless. Also, don't try to direct your breath to any part of your body. Let the breathing pattern be effortless, something you can keep up.

4. **Remain on your back for 8 breaths. Then roll onto your right side and place the second pillow between your knees.**

   Now use the same breathing ratio from Step 3 for 16 breaths.

5. **Finally, roll onto your left side, with the second pillow still between your knees, and use the breathing ratio for 32 breaths.**

Insomnia buster

This exercise is for people who suffer from insomnia but have an active imagination. Instead of watching your mind weave tale after tale when you can't sleep at night, why not recruit your imagination for the purpose of falling soundly asleep? Here's how.

If you're claustrophobic, this exercise may not necessarily work for you. But before giving up, you may first want to try evoking feelings of security and comfort, as when in a mother's womb or a favorite place in nature.

1. **Prepare yourself for sleep, and lie down comfortably in bed in any position.**

2. **With closed eyes, breathe evenly through your nose for a while.**

3. **Now visualize yourself snugly enfolded in a protective cocoon of purple.**

4. **While feeling safe in your purple environment, visualize a thin line of white light extending from the crown of your head to your solar plexus, just below your navel.**

This technique works even while traveling on a plane, with the jets roaring next to your ears. Just tell the flight attendant not to disturb you while you're sleeping.

Yoga Nidra: Catching Up on Your Sleep Quotient with Yogic Sleep

If your body-mind is slow to wind down to get its well-deserved rest, here's a potent technique to entice Mr. Sandman to visit you regularly. Yogic Sleep is a powerful relaxation technique that you can do when you gain some control over the relaxation response (discussed in the earlier section "Letting go"). When practiced successfully, this technique can be as restorative as sleep — except that you remain fully aware throughout.

To induce Yoga Nidra, you must listen to a set of instructions, similar to guided meditation. You can listen to a friend reading the instructions, but listening to a recording by someone else or by you yourself is more practical.

One feature of this practice is to focus in relatively quick succession on individual parts of the body. Mentally name each part, and then sense it as distinctly as possible.

In the beginning, you may find actually feeling certain body parts difficult. Don't let this setback dismay you; continue to rotate your awareness fairly swiftly. With practice, you can include even your inner organs and all kinds of mental states in this circuit.

Practicing Yoga Nidra before sleep is best because it's an excellent technique for inducing lucid dreaming and out-of-body experiences during sleep. *Lucid dreaming* refers to the kind of dream in which you're aware that you're dreaming. Great yoga masters remain aware even during deep sleep. Only the body and brain are fast asleep, whereas awareness is continuous.

Formulating your intention

Yoga Nidra serves as a potent tool for reprogramming your brain. If you do it correctly, it can accelerate your inner or spiritual growth. It allows you to cultivate good habits and attitudes. First, consider which specific habit or attitude you really want to replace with a more positive habit or attitude. This phase is called *formulating your intention*. Take your time to consider what you want to change about yourself.

Phrase your chosen intention in the following way: "I will become more [this or that]." This wording affirms your life's future trajectory by enlisting the unconscious mind. Worthy intentions may be to become more patient, more tolerant, or more loving. Also make your intention realistic and specific. "I will become enlightened" is specific but perhaps not very realistic, and "I will become a better person" is too vague. You want your intention to be something you can stick with until you realize it in your life, not one you have to abandon because it was too lofty or undefined.

When formulating your intention, try to evoke the corresponding feeling inside you so you know what it feels like to be loving, patient, forgiving, or whatever.

After you set an intention, you formally apply it during the actual Yoga Nidra exercise (described in the following section) by repeating it when prompted.

Performing Yoga Nidra

The following steps show you how to perform Yoga Nidra.

1. **Choose a clear intention (as described in the preceding section), and lie flat on your back, with your arms stretched out by your sides (or however feels most comfortable).**

   Place a pillow or folded blanket behind your neck for support, and use another pillow or folded blanket under your knees for added comfort. Refer to Figure 2-1 earlier in the chapter for an illustration.

2. **Close your eyes.**

3. **Repeat the clear intention you chose in Step 1 three times.**

4. **Take a couple of deep breaths, emphasizing exhalation.**

5. **Starting with your right side, rotate your awareness through all parts on that side of your body — limb by limb — in fairly quick succession.**

   Follow this progression: each finger, palm of the hand, back of the hand, hand as a whole, forearm, elbow, upper arm, shoulder joint, shoulder, neck, each section of the face (forehead, eyes, nose, chin, and so on), ear, scalp, throat, chest, side of the rib cage, shoulder blade, waist, stomach, lower abdomen, genitals, buttocks, whole spine, thigh, top and back of knee, shin, calf, ankle, top of foot, heel, sole, each toe.

6. **Be aware of your body as a whole.**

7. **Repeat the rotation in Step 5 on the left side, ending with the whole-body awareness described in Step 6.**

8. **Repeat Steps 5 through 7 one or more times until you achieve an adequate level of relaxation.**

9. **Continue to be aware of the whole body and the space surrounding it, feeling the stillness and peace.**

10. **Reaffirm your initial intention three times.**

11. **Mentally prepare to return to ordinary consciousness.**

12. **Gently move your fingers for a few moments, take a deep breath, and then open your eyes.**

No time limit applies to your Yoga Nidra performance unless you impose one. Expect to come out of Yogic Sleep naturally, whether you return after only 15 minutes or a whole hour. Or you may just fall asleep. If you have things to do afterward, make sure you set your phone or meditation app for a gentle wake-up call. Don't rush! Take your time to reintegrate with the ordinary world.

This practice is the most powerful yogic technique for personal change at the beginner level. Only the ecstatic state *(samadhi)* is more transformative. Several good recordings for practicing Yoga Nidra are available, but don't be surprised to discover that the instructions vary from recording to recording. Check out additional yoga resources at dummies.com.

Book VII

Meditation, Mindfulness, and Letting Go of Stress

Chapter 3

Getting Acquainted with Meditation

. . . .

In This Chapter

▶ Taking a close look at how life fails to live up to your expectations

▶ Assessing the high price of constant, rapid change

▶ Using meditation as a remedy for 21st-century ills like stress, anxiety, and alienation

▶ Cataloguing the many benefits of meditation

▶ Getting started with a quick taste of meditation

. . . .

The great thing about meditation is that it's actually quite simple. Just sit down, be quiet, turn your attention inward, and focus your awareness. That's all there is to it, really. Then why, you may be wondering, do people write so many books and articles about meditation? Why not just offer a few brief instructions and forget about all the verbiage?

If you're planning to take a long trip by car to some picturesque location, chances are you'll enjoy the trip more if you have a travel guide to point out the sights along the way. And you may feel more secure if you carry a troubleshooting manual to tell you what to do when you have problems with your car. Perhaps you'd like to take some side trips to scenic spots or even change your itinerary entirely and get there by a different route or a different vehicle!

In the same way, you can consider the practice of meditation to be a journey of sorts. This chapter provides an overview of your trip, offers some alternative routes to your destination, and explains the basic skills you need to know to get you there.

How Life Drives You — to Meditate

You know the old expression "If it ain't broke, don't fix it"? Well, the reality is that many people find that their lives are "broke" in some pretty significant ways.

Although you may be reluctant to admit it, at least publicly, life doesn't always live up to your expectations. As a result, you suffer — from stress, disappointment, fear, anger, outrage, hurt, or any of a number of other unpleasant emotions. Meditation teaches you how to relate to difficult circumstances and the tensions and emotions they evoke with balance, equanimity, and compassion. But before you delve into the positive solutions that meditation has to offer — and rest assured, there are plenty — take a whirlwind tour of the problems they're intended to solve.

The myth of the perfect life

Many people suffer because they compare their lives to some idealized image of how life is supposed to be. Cobbled together from childhood conditioning, media messages, and personal desires, this image lurks in the shadows and becomes the standard to which every success or failure, every circumstance or turn of events, is compared and judged. Take a moment to check out yours.

Perhaps you've spent your life struggling to build the American dream — two kids, house in the suburbs, brilliant career, what Zorba the Greek called the "full catastrophe." Only you're juggling two jobs to save the money for a down payment, the marriage is falling apart, and you feel guilty because you don't have enough time to spend with the kids. Or maybe you believe that ultimate happiness would come your way if you could only achieve the perfect figure (or physique). The problem is, diets don't work, you can't make yourself adhere to exercise regimens, and every time you look in the mirror, you feel like passing out. Or perhaps your idea of earthly nirvana is the perfect relationship. Unfortunately, you're watching the years pass by and you still haven't met Mr. or Ms. Right.

Whatever your version of the perfect life — perfect vacations, perfect sex, perfect health, even perfect peace of mind or total freedom from all tension and stress — you pay a high price for holding such high expectations. When life fails to live up to those expectations, as it inevitably does, you end up suffering and blaming yourself. If only you had made more money, spent more time at home, been a better lover, gone back to school, lost those extra pounds . . . the list is endless. No matter how you slice it, you just don't measure up.

The great meditative traditions have a more humane message to impart. They teach that the ideal earthly life is a myth. They remind you that far more powerful forces are at work in the universe than humans. You can envision and intend and strive and attempt to control all you want — and ultimately even achieve some modicum of success. But the truth is, in the long run, people have only the most limited control over the circumstances of their lives.

When things keep falling apart

Because it runs counter to everything you've ever been taught, you may have a difficult time accepting the basic spiritual truth that you have only limited control over the events in your life. After all, isn't the point of life to go out and "just do it," as the old Nike ads urged? Well, yes, you need to follow your dreams and live your truth; that's a crucial part of the equation.

But when life turns around and slaps you in the face, as it sometimes does, how do you respond? Or when it levels you completely and deprives you of everything you've gained, including your confidence and your hard-won self-esteem, where do you go for succor and support? How do you deal with the pain and confusion? What inner resources do you draw upon to guide you through this frightening and unknown terrain?

All things change and all things are impermanent

One day a woman came to see the Buddha (the great spiritual teacher who lived several thousand years ago in India) with her dead child in her arms. Grief-stricken, she had wandered from place to place, asking people for medicine to restore him to life. As a last resort, she asked the Buddha if he could help her. "Yes," he said, "but you must first bring me some mustard seed from a house in which there has never been a death."

Filled with hope, the woman went from door to door inquiring, but no one could help her. Every house she entered had witnessed its share of deaths. By the time she reached the end of the village, she had awakened to the realization that sickness and death are inevitable. After burying her son, she returned to the Buddha for spiritual instruction. "Only one law in the universe never changes," he explained, "that all things change and all things are impermanent." Hearing this, the woman became a disciple and eventually, it is said, attained enlightenment.

Life is a rich and perplexing interplay of light and dark, success and failure, youth and age, pleasure and pain — and, yes, life and death. Circumstances change constantly, apparently falling apart one moment, only to come together the next. The key to your peace of mind lies not in your circumstances, but in how you respond to them. As the Buddhists say, suffering is wanting what you don't have and not wanting what you do have, while happiness is precisely the opposite: enjoying what you have and not hungering for what you don't have. This concept doesn't mean that you must give up your values, dreams, and aspirations — only that you need to balance them with the ability to accept things as they are.

Meditation gives you an opportunity to cultivate acceptance by teaching you to reserve judgment and to open to each experience without trying to change or get rid of it. Then, when the going gets rough, you can use this quality to ease your ruffled feathers and maintain your peace of mind. (If you want to find out how to accept things the way they are, turn to Book VII, Chapters 4 and 5.)

Dealing with the postmodern predicament

It's news to no one that circumstances change constantly — certainly pundits and sages have purveyed this truth for ages. But at no time in history has change been as pervasive and relentless — or affected our lives so deeply — as during the past 10 or 15 years.

Sociologists call this period the *postmodern era,* when constant change is becoming a way of life and time-honored values and truths are being rapidly dismantled. How do you navigate your way through life when you no longer know what's true and you're not even sure how to find out? Do you search for it on the web or somehow glean it from the latest pronouncements of media soothsayers and corporate CEOs?

Such relentless change exacts a steep emotional and spiritual price, which people tend to deny in a collective attempt to accentuate the positive and deny the negative. Here are a few of the negative side effects of life in the postmodern age:

- ✔ **Anxiety and stress:** When the ground starts shifting beneath your feet, your first reaction as you attempt to regain your stability may be anxiety or fear. This gut-level response has been programmed into your genes by millions of years of living on the edge. These days, unfortunately, the tremors never stop, and small fears accumulate and congeal into ongoing tension and stress. Your body may feel perpetually braced against the next onslaught of difficulties and responsibilities — which makes it virtually impossible to relax and enjoy life fully (refer to Book VII, Chapter 1 for details on this phenomenon). By relaxing your body and reducing stress, meditation can provide a much-needed antidote.

✔ **Fragmentation:** Most Americans once lived, shopped, worked, raised their kids, and spent their leisure time in the same community. They encountered the same faces every day, worked the same job for a lifetime, stayed married to the same person, and watched their children raise their own children just down the block. Now they often shuttle their kids off to school or daycare and commute long distances to work, while checking their messages on the cellphone. On the way home, they may stop by the mall, and they may spend their evenings aimlessly surfing the web. They change jobs and partners more frequently than ever, and their grown children often move to another state — or another country! Although you may not be able to stay the tide of fragmentation, you can use meditation to connect you with a deeper wholeness that external circumstances can't disturb.

✔ **Alienation:** When your life appears to be made up of disconnected puzzle pieces that don't fit together, no wonder you wind up feeling completely stressed out. Never before, it seems, have human beings felt so alienated, not only from their work and their government but also from others, themselves, and their own essential being — and most people don't have the skills or the know-how to reconnect! By bridging the chasm that separates you from yourself, meditation can help to heal your alienation from others and the world at large.

✔ **Loneliness and isolation:** With people moving from place to place more frequently, and families fragmenting and scattering across the globe, you're less and less likely to have regular contact with the people you know and love — and even if you do, you may be too busy to relate in a mutually fulfilling way. Instead of sharing family dinners, mom, dad, and the kids call or text each other on the fly while hurrying from one activity or job to the next, rarely ending up in the same place at the same time. Of course, you may not be able to stem the forces that keep you apart. But you can use your meditation to turn every moment with your loved ones into "quality time."

✔ **Depression:** When people feel lonely, alienated, stressed out, and disconnected from a deeper source of meaning and purpose, it's no wonder that some end up feeling depressed. Millions of people take mood-altering chemicals each day to keep from feeling the pain of postmodern life. Meditation can connect you with your own inner source of contentment and joy that naturally dispels the clouds of depression.

✔ **Stress-related illness:** From tension headaches and acid indigestion to heart disease and cancer, the steady rise in stress-related illness reflects a collective inability to cope with the instability and fragmentation of the times — and fuels a billion-dollar healthcare industry that at times only masks the deeper problems of fear, stress, and disorientation. As numerous scientific studies have shown, the regular practice of meditation can actually reverse the onslaught of many stress-related ailments. (See the section "Surviving the 21st Century — with Meditation" later in this chapter.)

Book VII

Meditation, Mindfulness, and Letting Go of Stress

Four popular "solutions" that don't really work

Here's a quick look at a few popular approaches to handling stress and uncertainty that create more problems than they solve:

✔ **Addiction:** By distracting people from their pain, encouraging them to set aside their usual concerns and preoccupations, and altering brain chemistry, addictions mimic some of the benefits of meditation. Unfortunately, addictions also tend to fixate the mind on an addictive substance or activity — drugs, alcohol, sex, gambling, and so on — making it even more difficult for people to be open to the wonders of the moment or to connect with a deeper dimension of *being*. Besides, most addictions involve a self-destructive lifestyle that ultimately intensifies the problems the addict was attempting to escape.

✔ **Fundamentalism:** By advocating simple, one-dimensional answers to complex problems, offering a sense of meaning and belonging, and repudiating many of the apparent evils of postmodern life, fundamentalism — be it religious or political — provides a refuge from ambiguity and alienation. Alas, fundamentalists divide the world into black and white, good and bad, us and them, which only fuels the fires of alienation, conflict, and stress in the world at large.

✔ **Entertainment:** When you feel lonely or alienated, just turn on the tube, download a movie to your computer or smartphone, or head to your local multiplex. That will calm your anxiety or soothe your pain — or will it? In addition to providing entertainment, the media seemingly create community by connecting you with other people and the events around you. But you can't have a heart-to-heart conversation with a TV celebrity or hug your favorite movie star. Besides, the media (intentionally or not) manipulate your emotions, fill your mind with the ideas and images of the popular culture, and focus your attention outside yourself — rather than give you the opportunity to find out what you really think, feel, and know.

✔ **Consumerism:** This bogus solution to life's ills teaches that wanting and having more is the answer — more food, more possessions, more vacations, more of every perk that plastic can buy. As you may have noticed, however, the thrill fades fast, and you're quickly planning your next purchase — or struggling to figure out how to pay the credit-card bill that arrives like clockwork at the end of the month.

Surviving the 21st Century — with Meditation

Now for the good news! Meditation offers a time-honored antidote to fragmentation, alienation, isolation, stress — even stress-related illnesses and depression. Although it won't solve the external problems of your life, it does help you develop inner resilience, balance, and strength to roll with the punches and come up with creative solutions.

To get a sense of how meditation works, imagine for a moment that your body and mind are a complex computer. Instead of being programmed to experience inner peace, harmony, equanimity, and joy, you've been programmed to respond to life's inevitable ups and downs with stress, anxiety, and dissatisfaction. But you have the power to change your programming. By putting aside all other activities, sitting quietly, and attuning yourself to the present moment for a minimum of 10 or 15 minutes each day, you're developing a whole new set of habitual responses and programming yourself to experience more positive emotions and mind-states.

Of course, if you find it distasteful to think of yourself as a computer, you can picture life as an ocean, with the constant ups and downs you experience as the waves that churn and roil on the water's surface. When you meditate, you dive beneath the surface to a quiet place where the water is calmer and more consistent.

Whatever your favorite metaphor, the point is that meditation provides a way of transforming stress and suffering into equanimity and ease. In this section, you get to see how meditators have been reaping the remarkable benefits of meditation for millennia — and how you can, too!

The mind-body benefits of meditation

Book VII

Meditation, Mindfulness, and Letting Go of Stress

Although the earliest scientific studies of meditation date back to the 1930s and 1940s, research into the psychophysiological effects of meditation took off in the 1970s, fueled by a burgeoning interest in Transcendental Meditation (TM), Zen, and other Eastern meditation techniques. Since then, thousands of studies have been published, with an exponential increase in research in the past 10 to 15 years as brain-imaging technology has become increasingly sophisticated. Here is a brief synopsis of the most significant benefits of meditation:

Physiological benefits:

✔ Decreased heart rate

✔ Lower blood pressure

✔ Quicker recovery from stress

✔ Decrease in *beta* (brainwaves associated with thinking) and increase in *alpha, delta,* and *gamma* (brainwaves associated with deep relaxation and higher mental activity)

✔ Enhanced *synchronization* (that is, simultaneous operation) of the right and left hemispheres of the brain (which positively correlates with creativity)

✔ Fewer heart attacks and strokes

✔ Increased longevity

✔ Reduced cholesterol levels

✔ Decreased consumption of energy and need for oxygen

✔ Deeper, slower breathing

✔ Muscle relaxation

✔ Reduction in the intensity of pain

Psychological benefits:

✔ More happiness and peace of mind

✔ Greater enjoyment of the present moment

✔ Less emotional reactivity; fewer intense negative emotions and dramatic mood swings

✔ More loving, harmonious relationships

✔ Increased empathy

✔ Enhanced creativity and self-actualization

✔ Heightened perceptual clarity and sensitivity

✔ Reductions in both acute and chronic anxiety

✔ Complement to psychotherapy and other approaches in the treatment of addiction

Tuning in to your body

Like Mr. Duffy in James Joyce's novel *Ulysses,* most people "live a short distance" from their bodies. The following meditation, which has counterparts in yoga and Buddhism, helps reestablish contact with the body by drawing attention gently from one part to another. Because it cultivates awareness and also relaxes the muscles and internal organs, it makes a great preamble to more formal meditation practice. Allow at least 20 minutes to complete.

1. **Lie on your back on a comfortable surface — but not too comfortable, unless you plan to fall asleep.**

2. **Take a few moments to feel your body as a whole, including the places where it contacts the surface of the bed or floor.**

3. **Bring your attention to your toes.**

   Allow yourself to feel any and all sensations in this area. If you don't feel anything, just feel "not feeling anything." As you breathe, imagine that you're breathing into and out of your toes. (If this feels weird or uncomfortable, just breathe in your usual way.)

4. **When you're done with your toes, move on to your soles, heels, the tops of your feet, and your ankles in turn, feeling each part in the same way that you felt your toes.**

   Take your time. The point of this exercise is not to achieve anything, not even relaxation, but to be as fully present as possible wherever you are.

5. **Gradually move up your body, staying at least three or four breaths with each part.**

   Follow this approximate order: lower legs, knees, thighs, hips, pelvis, lower abdomen, lower back, solar plexus, upper back, chest, shoulders. Now focus on the fingers, hands, and arms on both sides; and then on the neck and throat, chin, jaw, face, back of the head, and top of the head.

   By the time you reach the top of your head, you may feel as though the boundaries between you and the rest of the world have become more fluid — or have melted away entirely. At the same time, you may feel silent and still — free of your usual restlessness or agitation.

6. **Rest there for a few moments; then gradually bring your attention back to your body as a whole.**

7. **Wiggle your toes, move your fingers, open your eyes, rock from side to side, and gently sit up.**

8. **Take a few moments to stretch and reacquaint yourself with the world around you before standing up and going about your day.**

Other great reasons to meditate

You don't have to join some cult or get baptized or bar mitzvahed to enjoy the benefits of meditation. And you don't have to check out of your everyday life and run off to a monastery in the Himalayas. You simply need to practice your meditation regularly without trying to get anywhere or achieve anything. Like interest in a money-market account, the benefits just accrue by themselves.

Awakening to the present moment

When you rush breathlessly from one moment to the next, anticipating another problem or hungering for another pleasure, you miss the beauty and immediacy of the present, which is constantly unfolding before your eyes.

Meditation teaches you to slow down and take each moment as it comes — the sounds of traffic, the smell of new clothes, the laughter of children, the worried look on an old woman's face, the coming and going of your breath. In fact, as the meditative traditions remind you, only the present moment exists anyway — the past is just a memory and the future a fantasy, projected on the movie screen of the mind right now.

Book VII

Meditation, Mindfulness, and Letting Go of Stress

Making friends with yourself

When you're constantly struggling to live up to images and expectations (your own or someone else's) or racing to reinvent yourself to survive in a competitive environment, you rarely have the opportunity or the motivation to get to know yourself just the way you are. Self-doubt and self-hatred may appear to fuel the fires of self-improvement, but they're painful — and besides, they contribute to other negative mind-states, such as fear, anger, depression, and alienation, and prevent you from living up to your full potential (refer to Book VII, Chapter 1).

When you meditate, you learn to welcome every experience and facet of your being without judgment or denial. In the process, you begin to treat yourself as you would a close friend, accepting (and even loving) the whole package, the apparent weaknesses and shortcomings, as well as the positive qualities and strengths.

Connecting more deeply with others

As you awaken to the present moment and open your heart and mind to your own experience, you naturally extend this quality of awareness and presence to your relationships with family and friends. If you're like everyone else, you tend to project your own desires and expectations onto the people close to you, which acts as a barrier to real communication. But when you start to accept others the way they are — a skill you can cultivate through the practice of meditation — you open up the channels for a deeper love and intimacy to flow between you.

Relaxing the body and calming the mind

As contemporary health researchers have discovered — and traditional texts agree — mind and body are inseparable, and an agitated mind inevitably produces a stressed-out body. As the mind settles, relaxes, and opens during meditation, so does the body — and the longer you meditate (measured both in minutes logged each day and in days and weeks of regular practice), the more this peace and relaxation ripples out to every area of your life, including your health.

Lightening up!

Perhaps you've noticed that nonstop thinking and worrying generate a kind of inner claustrophobia — fears feed on one another, problems get magnified exponentially, and the next thing you know, you're feeling overwhelmed and panicked. Meditation encourages an inner mental spaciousness in which difficulties and concerns no longer seem so threatening, and constructive solutions can naturally arise — as well as a certain detachment that allows for greater objectivity, perspective, and, yes, humor. That mysterious word *enlightenment* actually refers to the supreme "lightening up"!

Enjoying more happiness

Research reveals that the daily practice of meditation for just a few months actually makes people happier, as measured not only by their subjective reports but also by brain-mapping technology. In fact, meditation is apparently one of the only things that can permanently change your *emotional set point* — your basic level of relative happiness that scientists say stays the same throughout your life, no matter what you experience.

If you want lasting happiness, leading-edge science and spiritual wisdom have the same advice to offer: Forget about winning the lottery or landing the perfect job and begin meditating instead!

Experiencing focus and flow

When you're so fully involved in an activity that all sense of self-consciousness, separation, and distraction dissolves, you've entered what psychologist Mihaly Csikszentmihalyi calls a state of *flow*. For human beings, this total immersion constitutes the ultimate enjoyment — and provides the ultimate antidote to the fragmentation and alienation of postmodern life. No doubt you've experienced moments like these — creating a work of art, playing a sport, working in the garden, making love. Athletes call it "the zone." Through meditation, you can discover how to give the same focused attention to — and derive the same enjoyment from — every activity.

Feeling more centered, grounded, and balanced

To counter the escalating insecurity of life in rapidly changing times, meditation offers an inner groundedness and balance that external circumstances can't destroy. When you practice coming home again and again — to your body, your breath, your sensations, your feelings — you eventually grow to realize that you're always home, no matter where you go. And when you make friends with yourself — embracing the dark and the light, the weak and the strong — you get thrown off-center less and less frequently by the "slings and arrows" of life.

Enhancing your performance at work and at play

Studies have shown that basic meditation practice alone can enhance perceptual clarity, creativity, self-actualization, and many of the other factors that contribute to superior performance. In addition, specific meditations have been devised to enhance performance in a variety of activities, from sports to schoolwork.

Increasing appreciation, gratitude, and love

As you begin to open to your experience without judgment or aversion, your heart gradually opens as well — to yourself and others. You can practice specific meditations for cultivating appreciation, gratitude, and love. Or you may find, as so many meditators have before you have, that these qualities arise naturally when you can gaze at the world with fresh eyes, free from the usual projections and expectations.

Aligning with a deeper sense of purpose

When you practice making the shift from doing and thinking to *being* (see Book VII, Chapter 1), you discover how to align yourself with a deeper current of meaning and belonging. You may get in touch with personal feelings and aspirations that have long remained hidden from your conscious awareness. Or you may connect with a more universal source of purpose and direction — what some people call the *higher self* or *inner guidance.*

Awakening to a spiritual dimension of being

As your meditation gradually opens you to the subtlety and richness of each fleeting but irreplaceable moment, you may naturally begin to see through the veil of appearances to the sacred reality at the heart of things — and you eventually may come to realize (and this one could take lifetimes!) that the very same sacred reality is actually who you are in your own heart of hearts. This deep insight — what the sages and masters call "waking up from the illusion of separation" — cuts through and ultimately eliminates loneliness and alienation and opens you to the beauty of the human condition.

Developing and Directing Awareness: The Keys to Meditation

If, as the old saying goes, a journey of a thousand miles begins with a single step, then the journey of meditation begins with the cultivation of *awareness,* or *attention.* In fact, awareness is the mental muscle that carries you along and sustains you on your journey, not only at the start but also every step of the way. No matter which path or technique you choose, the secret of meditation lies in developing, focusing, and directing your awareness. (Incidentally, attention is just slightly focused awareness, and the two terms are often used more or less interchangeably. See the section "Becoming aware of your awareness.")

In meditation, you can use awareness in different ways. You can increase your powers of awareness by developing *concentration* on a particular object. Then, when you've stabilized your concentration, you can, through the practice of *receptive awareness,* expand your awareness to illuminate the full range of your experience. Next, you can concentrate even further in order to *cultivate* positive emotions and mind-states. Or you can use awareness to investigate your inner experience and *contemplate* the nature of existence itself.

These four practices — *concentration, receptive awareness, cultivation,* and *contemplation* — constitute the major uses of awareness throughout the world's great meditative traditions.

Building concentration

To do just about anything well, you need to focus your awareness. The most creative and productive people in every profession — for example, great athletes, performers, businessmen, scientists, artists, and writers — have the ability to block out distractions and completely immerse themselves in their work.

Some people have an innate ability to concentrate, but most of us need practice to develop it. Buddhists like to compare the mind to a monkey — constantly chattering and hopping about from branch to branch, topic to topic. Did you ever notice that most of the time, you have scant control over the whims and vacillations of your monkey mind, which may space out one moment and obsess the next? When you meditate, you calm your monkey mind by making it *one-pointed* rather than scattered and distracted.

REMEMBER

Many spiritual traditions teach their students concentration as the primary meditation practice. Just keep focusing your mind on the mantra or the symbol or the visualization, they advise, and eventually you will attain what is called *absorption,* or *samadhi.* (See the nearby sidebar "The art of the mantra" for more on mantras.)

In absorption, the sense of being a separate "me" disappears, and only the object of your attention remains. Followed to its natural conclusion, the practice of concentration can lead to an experience of union with the object of your meditation. If you're a sports enthusiast, this object could be your tennis racket or your golf club; if you're an aspiring mystic, the object could be God or *being* or the absolute. (For more on the spiritual benefits of concentration, see Book VII, Chapter 6.)

Even though you may not yet know how to meditate, you've no doubt had moments of total absorption, when the sense of separation disappears: gazing at a sunset, listening to music, creating a work of art, looking into the eyes of your beloved. When you're so completely involved in an activity, whether work or play, that time stops and self-consciousness drops away, you enter into what psychologist Mihaly Csikszentmihalyi calls *flow.* In fact, Csikszentmihalyi claims that activities that promote flow epitomize what most people mean by *enjoyment.* Flow can be extraordinarily refreshing, enlivening, and even deeply meaningful — and it is the inevitable result of unbroken concentration.

Book VII

Meditation, Mindfulness, and Letting Go of Stress

The art of the mantra

As Herbert Benson, MD, explains in his groundbreaking book *The Relaxation Response* (HarperTorch), the meditative repetition of a mantra tends to calm the mind and relax the body. But the earliest practitioners of mantra had more spiritual intentions, such as invoking the power of a particular deity, cultivating and strengthening positive qualities, or achieving union with divine reality.

Though the term *mantra* (meaning "mind protection") derives from the Sanskrit, the practice appears in one form or another in virtually every religion. Sufis repeat the phrase *La ila'ha, il'alahu* ("There is nothing but God"), Christians say the "Our Father" or the prayer of the heart ("Lord Jesus Christ have mercy on me"), Buddhists intone sacred invocations like *om mani padme hum* or *namu amida butsu*, and Hindus repeat one of the many praises or names of God.

Essentially, mantras are sounds infused with numinous or spiritual power by a teacher or a tradition. When you repeat a mantra — aloud, under your breath, or mentally (actually considered the most potent method) — you resonate with a particular spiritual frequency and with the power and blessings the sound has accumulated over the years.

The practice of mantra focuses and stabilizes the mind and protects it from unwanted distractions. For this reason, mantra recitation often accompanies more formal meditation practices. To experiment with a mantra, just choose a word or phrase with deep personal or spiritual meaning for you. (Traditionally, you would receive a particular mantra directly from your teacher.) Then sit quietly and repeat it again and again, allowing your mind to rest on the sound and the feeling it evokes. When your mind wanders, just come back to your mantra.

Opening to receptive awareness

The great sages of China say that all things comprise the constant interplay of *yin* and *yang* — the feminine and masculine forces of the universe. Well, if concentration is the yang of meditation (focused, powerful, penetrating), then *receptive awareness* is the yin (open, expansive, welcoming).

Where concentration disciplines, stabilizes, and grounds the mind, receptive awareness loosens and extends the mind's boundaries and creates more interior space, enabling you to familiarize yourself with the mind's contents. Where concentration blocks extra stimuli as distractions to the focus at hand, receptive awareness embraces and assimilates every experience that presents itself.

Most meditations involve the interplay of concentration and receptive awareness, although some more-advanced techniques teach the practice of receptive awareness alone. Just be open and aware and welcome whatever arises, these techniques encourage, and ultimately you will be "taken by truth."

Followed to its conclusion, receptive awareness guides you in shifting your identity from your thoughts, emotions, and the stories your mind tells you to your true identity, which is being itself.

Of course, if you don't know how to work with attention, these instructions are impossible to follow. That's why most traditions prescribe practicing concentration first. By quieting and grounding the mind just enough so it can open without being swept away by a deluge of irrelevant feelings and thoughts, concentration provides a solid foundation on which the practice of meditation can flourish.

Using contemplation for greater insight

Although concentration and receptive awareness provide enormous benefits, ultimately it's insight and understanding — of how the mind works, how you perpetuate your own suffering, how attached you are to the outcome of events, and how uncontrollable and fleeting these events are — that offer freedom from suffering. And in your everyday life, it's creative thinking — free from the usual limited, repetitive patterns of thought — that offers solutions to problems. So *contemplation* is the third key component that transforms meditation from a calming, relaxing exercise to a vehicle for freedom and creative expression.

After you've developed your concentration and expanded your awareness, you eventually find that you have access to a more penetrating insight into the nature of your experience. You can use this faculty to explore your inner terrain and gradually understand and undermine your mind's tendency to cause you suffering and stress (refer to Book VII, Chapter 1). If you're a spiritual seeker, you can use this faculty to inquire into the nature of the self or to reflect on the mystery of God and creation. And if you're a person with more practical concerns, you may ponder the next step in your career or relationship or contemplate some seemingly irresolvable problem in your life.

Cultivating positive, healing states of mind

Some meditations aim to open the heart and develop certain life-affirming qualities like compassion, lovingkindness, equanimity, joy, or forgiveness. On a more practical level, you can use meditation to cultivate a proactive, healthy immune system or to develop poise and precision in a particular sport. For example, you can visualize killer T cells attacking your cancer or imagine yourself executing a dive without a single mistake. These are the kinds of meditations this book calls *cultivation*.

Book VII

Meditation, Mindfulness, and Letting Go of Stress

Where contemplation aims to investigate, inquire, and ultimately see deeply into the nature of things, cultivation can help you transform your inner life by directing the concentration you develop to strengthen positive, healthy mind-states and withdraw energy from those that are more reactive and self-defeating.

Becoming aware of your awareness

Most of the time, you probably don't pay much attention to your awareness. Yet the truth is that it's crucial to everything you do. When you watch TV, study for an exam, cook a meal, drive your car, listen to music, or talk with a friend, you're being aware, or paying attention. Before you begin to meditate in a formal way, you may find it helpful to explore your own awareness:

1. **First, notice what it's like to be aware.**

   Are there times in your life when you're not aware of anything? Complete this thought: "I am aware of . . . ." Do this again and again and notice where your awareness takes you.

   Do you tend to be more aware of internal or external sensations? Do you pay more attention to thoughts and fantasies than to your moment-to-moment sensory experiences? Notice whether a preoccupation with mental activity diminishes your awareness of what's happening right here and now.

2. **Next, pay attention to whether your awareness tends to focus on a particular object or sensation or tends to be more expansive and inclusive.**

   You may find that your awareness resembles a spotlight that flows from object to object. Notice how your awareness flows without trying to change it.

   Does it shift quickly from one thing to another, or does it move more slowly, making contact with each object before moving on? Experiment with speeding up and slowing down the flow of awareness, and notice how that feels.

   You may discover that your awareness is drawn again and again to certain kinds of objects and events, but not to others. Where does your awareness repeatedly wander? Which experience does it seem to selectively avoid?

3. **Now experiment with gently directing your awareness from one focus to another.**

   When you pay attention to sounds, you may notice that you momentarily forget about your hands or the discomfort in your back or knees. Try to focus on one object of attention for as long as you can. How long can you remain undistracted before your mind skips to the next thing?

REMEMBER

Mindfulness: Meditation as a way of life

Mindfulness refers to ongoing attention to whatever arises moment to moment.

Mindfulness, which blends concentration and receptive awareness, is one of the simplest techniques for beginners to learn and also one of the most readily adaptable to the busy schedules most people face. Like many, you may be primarily concerned with living a more harmonious, loving, stress-free life, not lifting off into some disembodied spiritual realm divorced from the people and places you love.

In fact, the beauty, belonging, and love you seek are available right here and now — you only need to clear your mind and open your eyes, which is precisely what the practice of mindfulness is intended to teach! When you pay attention to your experience from moment to moment, you keep waking up from the daydreams and worries your mind fabricates and returning to the clarity, precision, and simplicity of the present, where life actually takes place.

The great thing about mindfulness is that you don't have to limit your practice to certain places and times — you can practice waking up and paying attention wherever you happen to be, at any time of the day or night.

MEDITATION

Eating a piece of fruit

For this in-the-moment exercise, imagine that you've just arrived from another planet and have never encountered an orange before. Now take a few minutes to experience a piece of fruit in a fresh new way:

1. **Place an orange on a plate and close your eyes.**

2. **Set aside all thoughts and preconceptions, open your eyes, and see the fruit as though for the first time.**

   Notice the shape, the size, the color, and the texture.

3. **As you begin to peel the orange, notice how it feels in your fingers.**

   Notice the contrast between the flesh and the peel and observe the weight of the fruit in your hand.

4. **Slowly raise a piece of the orange to your lips and pause a moment before eating.**

   Notice how it smells before you begin.

5. **Open your mouth, bite down, and feel the texture of its soft flesh and the first rush of juice into your mouth.**

6. **Continue to bite and chew the orange, remaining aware of the play of sensations from moment to moment.**

   Imagining that this may be the first and last orange you will ever eat, let each moment be fresh and new and complete in itself. Notice how this experience of eating an orange differs from your usual way of eating a piece of fruit.

Getting Started with Meditation: It's Easier Than You Think

Meditation is simply the practice of focusing your attention on a particular object — generally something simple, like a word or phrase, a candle flame or geometrical figure, or the coming and going of your breath. In everyday life, your mind is constantly processing a barrage of sensations, visual impressions, emotions, and thoughts. In general, when you meditate, you narrow your focus, limit the stimuli bombarding your nervous system — and calm your mind in the process.

For a quick taste of meditation, follow these instructions. (For more complete meditation instructions, see Book VII, Chapter 4.)

1. **Find a quiet place and sit comfortably with your back relatively straight.**

   If you tend to disappear into your favorite chair, find something a bit more supportive.

2. **Take a few deep breaths, close your eyes, and relax your body as much as you can.**

   If you don't know how to relax, you may want to check out Book VII, Chapter 2.

3. **Choose a word or phrase that has special personal or spiritual meaning for you.**

   Here are some examples: "There's only love," "Don't worry, be happy," "Trust in God."

4. **Begin to breathe through your nose, and as you breathe, repeat the word or phrase quietly to yourself.**

   You can whisper the word or phrase, *subvocalize* it (that is, move your tongue as though you're saying it, but don't say it aloud), or just repeat it in your mind. If you get distracted, come back to the repetition of the word or phrase. (If you have difficulty breathing through your nose, by all means breathe through your mouth instead.)

   As an alternative, you can rest your attention on your breath as it comes and goes through your nostrils, returning to your breathing when you get distracted.

5. **Keep the meditation going for five minutes or more and then slowly get up and go about your day.**

How did you feel during meditation? Did it seem weird to say the same thing or follow your breath over and over? Did you find it difficult to stay focused? Did you keep changing the phrase? If so, don't worry. With regular practice, you'll gradually get the knack.

Of course, you could easily spend many fruitful and enjoyable years mastering the subtleties and complexities of meditation. But the good news is, the basic practice is actually quite simple, and you don't have to be an expert to do it or to enjoy its extraordinary benefits.

Book VII

Meditation, Mindfulness, and Letting Go of Stress

Chapter 4

Mindfulness Meditation: Awareness of the Here and Now

*I*f you're looking for simple, concise meditation instructions, you've come to the right chapter. You can muse forever about meditation's benefits or the nature of the mind, but there's nothing quite like attempting to practice to show you how stubborn and wild the mind can actually be.

As previous chapters mention, the Buddhists like to compare the mind to a monkey that swings uncontrollably from branch to branch — from plan to memory, thought to emotion, sight to sound — without ever settling down in one place. You can't overpower it or subdue it or sit on it until it agrees to obey. Well, the same holds true for your mind. In fact, if you attempt to force your mind to calm down, you just swirl it up even more and end up going nowhere fast.

Instead, the practice of meditation involves gently returning your mind again and again to a simple focus of attention. In this chapter, you find out how to meditate on your breath — one of the most popular forms of meditation throughout the world's spiritual traditions. You also discover mindfulness techniques that balance relaxation and alertness, and extend your meditation to include welcoming the full range of present-moment experience.

 The mundane, repetitive, seemingly inconsequential activity of attending to your breath can eventually lead to all the glamorous benefits meditation promises to provide, including reduced stress; enhanced performance; increased appreciation and enjoyment of life; deeper connection with your essential being; and even advanced meditative states, such as unconditional love or transformative insights into the nature of existence.

Preparing Your Body for Meditation

Meditation works best when you can keep your body relatively motionless and your back relatively straight. Here's why:

- When you're constantly acting and reacting in response to thoughts and outside stimulation, you don't have a chance to get to know how your mind works. By sitting still, you have a mirror that shows you just how slippery and elusive your mind can be.

- Keeping still gives you a tremendous edge when you're working on developing your concentration. Imagine a heart surgeon or a concert pianist who can't quiet her body while plying her craft. The fewer physical distractions you have, the easier it becomes to follow your breath, practice your mantra, or whatever your meditation happens to be.

- By aligning the spine and opening the channels that run through the center of the body, upright sitting encourages an unimpeded circulation of energy, which, in turn, contributes to wakefulness on all levels — physical, mental, and spiritual. Besides, it's a lot easier to sit still for extended periods of time when your vertebrae are stacked like a pile of bricks, one on top of the other. Otherwise, over time, gravity has this irritating habit of pulling your body down toward the ground — and in the process, causing the aches and pains so typical of a body at war with the forces of nature. So the most comfortable way to sit in the long run is straight, which puts you in harmony with nature.

A word of caution, however: These sitting instructions aren't intended to turn your body into a stone. The point is to set your intention to sit still and notice what happens. The Buddha liked to use the metaphor of a stringed instrument like a sitar or guitar — if the strings are too loose, you can't play it, and if they're too tight, they'll break. If you're too rigid with yourself, you'll just end up miserable — but if you keep shifting your body this way and that, you'll never get your mind concentrated and quiet enough to reap the benefits of meditation.

Popular positions for the lower half of your body

Just as a tree needs to set down deep roots so it won't fall over as it grows, you need to find a comfortable position for the lower half of your body that you can sustain for 5, 10, or 15 minutes — or longer, if you want to obtain the maximum benefits from meditation. After several millennia of experimentation, the great meditators have come up with a handful of traditional postures that seem to work especially well. Different though they may appear from the outside, these postures have one thing in common: The pelvis tilts slightly forward, accentuating the natural curvature of the lower back.

The following poses, shown in Figure 4-1, are arranged more or less in order from the easiest to the hardest to do, though ease all depends on your particular body and degree of flexibility. Don't worry about which looks the coolest; just experiment until you find the one that works best for you.

- ✔ **Sitting in a chair:** The operative term is sitting, not slouching (see Figure 4-1a). The trick to meditating in a chair is positioning your buttocks somewhat higher than your knees, which tilts your pelvis forward and helps keep your back straight. Old-fashioned wooden kitchen chairs work better than the upholstered kind; experiment with a small cushion or foam wedge under your buttocks.

- ✔ **Kneeling (with or without a bench):** Kneeling (see Figure 4-1b) can be hard on your knees unless you have proper support. Try placing a cushion under your buttocks and between your feet — or use a specially designed *seiza bench,* preferably one with a soft cushion between you and the wood. Otherwise, your bottom and other tender parts may fall asleep.

- ✔ **Burmese position:** Used throughout Southeast Asia, the *Burmese position* (see Figure 4-1c) involves placing both calves and feet on the floor one in front of the other. Though less stable than the lotus series, it's much easier to negotiate, especially for beginners.

With all the cross-legged poses, first bend your leg at the knee, in line with your thigh, before rotating your thigh to the side. Otherwise, you risk injuring your knee, which is built to flex in only one direction, unlike the ball-and-socket joint of the hip, which can rotate through a full range of motion.

- ✔ **Quarter lotus:** This position is exactly like half lotus (see the following item on this list), except that your foot rests on the calf of your opposite leg rather than on the thigh (see Figure 4-1d).

- ✔ **Half lotus:** The half lotus is easier to execute than the famous full lotus (see the following item) and nearly as stable (see Figure 4-1e). With your buttocks on a cushion, place one foot on the opposite thigh and the other foot on the floor beneath the opposite thigh. Be sure that both knees touch the floor and your spine doesn't tilt to one side. To distribute the pressure on your back and legs, remember to alternate legs from sitting to sitting, if you can — in other words, left leg on the thigh and right on the floor, then left on the floor and right on the thigh.

- ✔ **Full lotus:** This position is considered the Everest of sitting positions (refer to Figure 4-1f). With your buttocks on a cushion, cross your left foot over your right thigh and your right foot over your left thigh. As with its more asymmetrical sibling, half lotus, it's best to alternate legs in order to distribute the pressure evenly. *Note:* Don't attempt the full lotus unless you happen to be particularly flexible — and even then by stretching first.

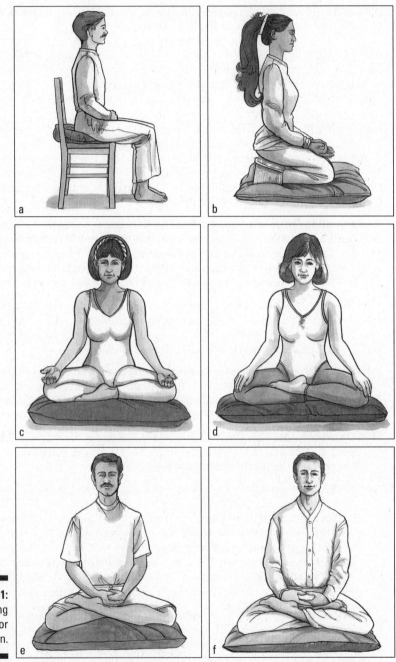

Figure 4-1:
Sitting
positions for
meditation.

Illustration by Pam Tanzey

Extending your spine

When you're settled into a comfortable sitting position, with your pelvis tilted slightly forward, you can turn your attention to straightening your back. Unfortunately, the natural curves of your spine are often exaggerated by the demands of computer workstations and other sedentary environments, and you gradually get into the habit of sitting hunched over, with your shoulders rounded, your upper back collapsed, and your neck and head craned forward like a turkey vulture.

You may not be able to reverse sitting habits like these in a few sessions of meditation, but you can experiment with *extending* your spine — a more accurate term than straightening — and slowly but surely softening those curves back to their natural, graceful arch. You may find yourself carrying these new sitting habits into your other activities so that in time, you're gently correcting your posture while driving your car or sitting at your desk, for example.

Try one or all three of the following images to help you discover what a straight or extended spine feels like. Don't bother to look in the mirror or compare yourself to some ideal you've picked up in books (even this one). The important thing is how your body feels from the inside. You want to feel centered, stable, grounded — and aligned with the force of gravity:

- ✔ **Suspending your head from a string:** Imagine that your entire body is suspended in the air from a string attached to the crown of your head. (The *crown* is the highest point on the top of your skull, toward the back.) As you feel the string pulling your head up into the air, notice how your spine naturally lengthens, your pelvis tilts forward, your chin tucks, and the back of your neck flattens slightly.

- ✔ **Stacking your vertebrae one on top of another:** Imagine your vertebrae as bricks that you're stacking one on top of the other, beginning with the first at the base of the spine. Feel your spine growing up toward the sky brick by brick, like a skyscraper.

- ✔ **Sitting like a mountain or tree:** Imagine your body as a mountain or tree with a broad base that extends deep into the earth and a trunk or peak that reaches toward the sky. Notice how stable, grounded, and self-sufficient you feel.

When you know what it feels like to sit upright with your spine extended, you can rock your body from side to side like a pendulum, first broadly and then in gradually decreasing arcs until you come to rest in the center. Next, you can tilt your pelvis forward slightly, accentuating the natural curvature of your lower back, and then lean forward and backward from the waist

Book VII

Meditation, Mindfulness, and Letting Go of Stress

(keeping your back straight) until you come to center. Finally, tuck your chin and draw your head back gently. Now you're ready to begin your meditation.

Turning Your Attention Inward

As the old saying goes, a journey of a thousand miles begins with a single step. In the case of meditation, this simple but essential step involves turning your mind away from its usual preoccupation with external events — or, just as often, with the story it tells you about external events — and toward your inner sensate experience.

If you're like most people, you're so caught up with what's happening around you — the looks in other people's eyes, the voices of family and coworkers, the latest news on the radio, the messages appearing on your computer screen — that you forget to pay attention to what's happening in your own mind, body, and heart. In fact, popular culture has been designed to seduce you into searching outside yourself for happiness and satisfaction. In such a confusing and compelling world, even the most rudimentary gesture of self-awareness can seem like a challenge of monumental proportions.

Just take a few minutes right now to turn your mind around and pay attention to what you're sensing and feeling. Notice how much resistance you have to shifting your awareness from your external focus to your simple sensate experience. Notice how busily your mind flits from thought to thought and image to image, weaving a story with you as the central character.

Because these habitual patterns are so deeply rooted, doing something as seemingly innocuous as returning your attention again and again to a basic internal focus, like your breath, can take tremendous courage and patience. This shift from outer to inner is precisely the simple but radical gesture that meditation requires. The shift has several related dimensions:

- ✔ **Content to process:** Instead of becoming engrossed in the meaning of what you're sensing, thinking, or feeling, you can shift your interest and attention to *how* experiencing occurs or to the mere fact of experience itself. For example, instead of getting lost in thinking or daydreaming, you can notice how your mind flits from thought to thought — or merely observe that you're thinking. Instead of becoming transfixed by your fear or what you imagine it means or is trying to tell you, you can notice how the waves of tension move through your belly — or simply note that you're feeling.

- ✔ **Outer to inner:** Initially, you need to balance your usual tendency to be so outer-directed by paying particular attention to inner experience. Eventually, you'll be able to bring the same quality of awareness to every experience, whether inner or outer.

✔ **Secondhand to direct:** Even more helpful than inner and outer is the distinction between secondhand experience and direct experience. *Secondhand experience* has been filtered and distorted by the mind and is often concerned with thoughts about the past or future, whereas *direct experience* is found only in the present and accessed through the senses. In addition to turning inward, meditation involves turning your attention away from the story your mind spins about your experience and toward the direct experience itself. (Refer to Book VII, Chapter 1 to find out more about this "story" your mind tells you.)

✔ **Doing to being:** You spend virtually all your waking hours rushing from one task, project, or activity to another. Do you remember what it's like to just *be,* the way you did when you were a baby or a little child, whiling away a summer afternoon just playing or lying in the grass? Meditation gives you the opportunity to make this crucial shift from doing to being.

Relaxing Your Body

As the field of mind-body medicine reiterates — and yogis and sages have been saying for millennia — your body, your mind, and your heart form one seamless and inseparable whole. When your thoughts keep leaping like the proverbial monkey from worry to worry, your body responds by tightening and tensing, especially in certain key places like the throat, the heart, the solar plexus, and the belly. When the discomfort gets intense enough, you register it as an emotion — fear, perhaps, or anger or sadness.

Because meditation connects you with your direct experience — and ultimately with a realm of pure *being* beyond the mind — it naturally relaxes your body while it focuses your mind. As a beginner, though, you may not experience this natural relaxation for days or even weeks. So practicing one of the techniques in the following list *before* you meditate can be helpful, especially if you tend to be noticeably tense. Of course, relaxing your body has its own wonderful benefits, but your body won't stay relaxed until you're able to work with your mind.

If you've never deliberately relaxed your body before, start with the meditation in the "Deep relaxation" sidebar nearby. Because the meditation takes at least 15 minutes to complete, you probably won't do it each time you meditate, but it does show you how to relax your body part by part. When you've practiced this exercise a few times, your body will remember what being deeply relaxed feels like, and you can then advance to one of the five-minute relaxations listed here. (By the way, deep relaxation is a great antidote for insomnia; just practice it in bed and then drift off to sleep!)

Deep relaxation

Here's a meditation you can do any time you have 15 or 20 minutes to spare and want to shed some of the tension you've accumulated in your busy life. It's also a great way to prepare for the other meditations in this book because it leaves you feeling relaxed, refreshed, and in touch with yourself.

1. **Find a comfortable place to lie down. Take off your shoes, loosen your belt and other tight clothing, and stretch out on your back with your arms resting at your sides, legs slightly apart.**

2. **Sense your body as a whole, including the places where it contacts the surface of the bed or floor.**

3. **Close your eyes and bring your awareness to your feet. Wiggle your toes, flex your feet, and then let go of all tension as much as you can, allowing your feet to melt into the floor.**

4. **Shift your awareness to your lower legs, thighs, and hips. Imagine them becoming heavy and relaxed and melting into the floor.**

   If the image of melting doesn't appeal to you, you can try dissolving, sinking, or disappearing.

5. **Bring your awareness to your lower abdomen. Imagine all tension draining away, your breath deepening, and your belly opening and softening.**

6. **Bring your awareness to your upper abdomen, chest, neck, and throat, feeling the areas opening and softening.**

7. **Bring your awareness to your shoulders, upper arms, lower arms, and hands. Imagine them becoming heavy and relaxed and melting into the floor.**

8. **Bring your awareness to your head and face. Feel the tension melting away from your face across your head and into the floor.**

9. **Scan your body from head to toe, searching for any remaining areas of tension or discomfort.**

   If you find any, just imagine them relaxing completely.

10. **Experience your body as one field of relaxation, without parts or edges.**

11. **Continue to rest in this way for five or ten minutes more; then very slowly begin to wiggle your fingers and toes, stretch your arms and legs, open your eyes, and gradually come up to a sitting position.**

Check in with yourself and notice how you feel. Do you feel more relaxed? Does your body feel lighter or more expanded? Does the world appear different in any way? Now gently get up and go about your day.

So here are five brief relaxation techniques:

- ✔ **Shower of relaxation:** Imagine taking a warm shower. As the water cascades across your body and down your legs, it carries with it all discomfort and distress, leaving you refreshed and invigorated.

↙ **Honey treatment:** Imagine a mound of warm honey perched on the crown of your head. As it melts, it runs down your face and head and neck, covering your shoulders and chest and arms, and gradually enveloping your whole body down to your toes. Feel the sensuous wave of warm liquid draining away all tension and stress and leaving you thoroughly relaxed and renewed.

↙ **Peaceful place:** Imagine a safe, protected, peaceful place — perhaps a forest, a meadow, or a sandy beach. Experience the place fully with all your senses. Notice how calm and relaxed you feel here; now allow that feeling to permeate every cell of your body.

↙ **Body scan:** Beginning with the crown of your head, scan your body from top to bottom. When you come to an area of tension or discomfort, gently allow it to open and soften; then move on.

↙ **Relaxation response:** Choose a word or brief phrase that has deep spiritual or personal significance for you. Now close your eyes and repeat this sound softly, again and again.

Developing Mindfulness

This chapter highlights an approach to meditation known as *mindfulness* — moment-to-moment awareness of your experience as it occurs. Mindfulness combines *concentration* (highly focused awareness) and a more receptive awareness that simply welcomes whatever arises. Because mindfulness grows like a house on a foundation of concentration, you need to strengthen and stabilize your concentration before you can proceed to the full practice of mindfulness. That's why the initial meditations provided here emphasize focusing on a particular object of concentration — your breath.

Ultimately, the goal of mindfulness meditation is to develop the capacity to be fully present for whatever is occurring right here and now. When you've stabilized your concentration by focusing on your breath, you can expand your awareness to include the full range of sensations, both inside and outside, and eventually just welcome whatever presents itself, including thoughts, memories, and emotions.

Though supremely simple, this advanced technique can take years of patient practice to master, but you may have glimpses of a more expanded awareness after only a few weeks of regular meditation.

Book VII

Meditation, Mindfulness, and Letting Go of Stress

TIP

Letting go of your expectations

When you invest in the stock market or work out at a gym, you expect results, and you keep checking the quotes or the scale to tell you how well you're doing. If you bring the same attitude to meditation, however, you're defeating the purpose, which is to let go of your thoughts altogether and just be present in the here and now. One of the great paradoxes of meditation is that you can't reap the benefits until you drop all your expectations and accept things the way they are. Then the benefits come back to you a thousandfold.

When you begin meditating, you're going to keep wondering whether you're doing it right. But don't worry; there's no wrong way to

meditate — except perhaps sitting and trying to measure how well you're doing! One day you may feel like you're on top of the world. You're full of energy, your mind is clear, and you can follow your breath with relative ease. "Wow, now I'm getting the hang of it," you think. The next day you're so overwhelmed by thoughts or emotions that you sit for 20 minutes without even noticing your breath. Welcome to the practice of meditation! The point isn't to do it right, but just to do it — again and again.

One Zen teacher used to compare meditation to walking in the fog on a warm summer day: Though you may not pay attention to what's happening, pretty soon you're soaking wet.

Focusing on your breath

Compared to posting on Facebook or catching a movie on HBO, watching your breath may seem like a boring way to spend your spare time. The fact is, the media have conditioned people to be stimulation junkies by flooding the senses with computerized images and synthesized sounds that change at laserlike speed. The head of an ad agency once bragged about how his latest TV spot bombarded the viewer with six images per second — far faster than the conscious mind can possibly register them.

By contrast, paying attention to the coming and going of your breath slows your mind to match the speed and rhythms of your body. Instead of six images per second, you breathe an average of 12 to 16 times per minute. And the sensations are far subtler than anything you'll see or hear on TV — more like the sights and sounds of nature, which is, after all, where you and your body came from.

Besides, the great thing about your breath as a focus of meditation is that it's always available, always changing, yet is always more or less the same. If your breath were totally different each time, it wouldn't provide the stability necessary for you to cultivate concentration; if it never changed in any way, you'd quickly fall asleep and never have an opportunity to develop the curiosity and alertness that are so essential to the practice of mindfulness.

The meaning of the breath

Traditional cultures identified the breath with the life force that animates all things. For example, the Latin word *spiritus* (the root of both *spirited* and *spiritual*), the Greek word *anima* (from which the word *animated* derives), the Hebrew word *ruach,* and the Sanskrit word *brahman* may sound quite different, but they have one thing in common: They all mean both *breath* and *spirit* or *soul.* When you follow your breath with awareness, you're not only harmonizing your body and mind, which gives you a sense of inner harmony and wholeness, but also exploring the living frontier where body, mind, and spirit meet — and attuning yourself to a spiritual dimension of being.

As a preliminary to the practice of following your breath, you may want to spend a few weeks or months just counting your breaths. It's a great way to build concentration, and it provides a preestablished structure that constantly reminds you when you're wandering off. If you were a neophyte Zen student, you might spend years counting your breaths before you graduated to a more challenging practice. But if you're feeling adventurous or already have some confidence in your concentration, by all means start with following your breath. Trust your intuition to tell you which method is right for you.

Book VII

Meditation, Mindfulness, and Letting Go of Stress

Counting your breaths

Begin by finding a comfortable sitting position that you can hold for 10 or 15 minutes (refer to the earlier section "Preparing Your Body for Meditation" for details). Then take a few deep breaths and exhale slowly. Without trying to control your breath in any way, allow it to find its own natural depth and rhythm. Always breathe through your nose unless you can't for some reason.

Now begin counting each inhalation and exhalation until you reach ten; then return to one. In other words, when you inhale, count "one," when you exhale, count "two," when you inhale again, count "three," and so on up to ten. If you lose track, return to one and start again.

To help you concentrate, you may find it useful to extend the number in your mind for the full duration of the inhalation or exhalation, instead of thinking the number quickly once and then dropping it. For example, allow "o-o-o-n-n-n-e" to last as long as the inhalation, "t-w-o-o-o-o" to last as long as the exhalation, and so on. You may also find it helpful to subvocalize the numbers, especially at first, saying "one" ever so softly to yourself as you inhale, "two" as you exhale, and so on.

As ridiculously easy as this exercise may seem at first-read, you may be surprised to discover that you never manage to reach ten without losing count — or go on autopilot and suddenly find yourself on breath 29! You don't have to stop your mind chatter in any way. But if you get distracted by your thoughts and lose track of your breath, come back to one and start again.

When you get the knack of counting each in-breath and out-breath — say, after a month or two of regular practice — you can shift to counting only the exhalations. If your mind starts wandering on the inhalations, though, just go back to the first method until you feel ready to move on again. Eventually, you may want to simplify the practice even further by simply noting "in" on the inhalation and "out" on the exhalation.

When you first begin paying deliberate attention to your breath, you may be surprised and somewhat frustrated to discover that your body tenses up and your breathing becomes stiff, labored, and unnatural. Don't worry: You're not doing it wrong. You just need to develop a lighter, gentler touch with your awareness so you're following but not controlling your breath. You may find it helpful to begin by exploring your breathing, without necessarily trying to track it from breath to breath. Notice what happens when you breathe: how your rib cage rises and falls, how your belly moves, how the air passes in and out of your nostrils. You may find that some breaths are longer and deeper, while others are shorter and shallower. Some may go all the way down into your belly, while others barely reach the upper part of your lungs before exiting again. Some may be rough or strong; others smooth or weak. Spend five or ten minutes exploring your breathing with the fresh curiosity of a child encountering a flower or a butterfly for the first time. What did you discover that you didn't know before? How does each new breath differ from the last? When you feel comfortable with your breath, you can begin the practice of counting or following your breaths.

Following your breaths

Begin by sitting and breathing exactly as you did for counting your breaths. When you feel settled, allow your attention to focus either on the sensation of your breath coming and going through your nostrils or on the rising and falling of your belly as you breathe. (Although you're welcome to alternate your focus from one session to the next, you're better off sticking with a single focus for the entire meditation — and eventually using the same focus each time you meditate.)

Give your full attention to the coming and going of your breath the way a mother tracks the movements of her young child: lovingly yet persistently, softly yet precisely, with relaxed yet focused awareness. When you realize that your mind has wandered off and you're engrossed in planning or thinking or daydreaming, gently but firmly bring it back to your breath.

At the end of your exhalation (and before you inhale again), there's often a gap or a pause when your breath is no longer perceptible. At this point, you can allow your attention to rest on a predetermined touchpoint, such as your navel or your hands, before returning to your breath when it resumes.

Thoughts and images will definitely continue to skitter and swirl through your mind as you meditate, but don't worry. Just patiently and persistently keep coming back to your breath. Gradually, you may even develop a fascination with all the little sensations of your belly and rib cage shifting and opening and changing shape as you breathe; or of your breath caressing the tip of your nose, tickling your nostrils, and cooling your nasal passages as it enters and leaves. You may also notice that your mind tends to quiet down or your thinking tends to change on either the exhalation or the inhalation. By attuning to a subtler level of experience while you meditate, you can open yourself to a subtler appreciation of each moment of life as it unfolds.

Expanding to sensations

As soon as you've developed a certain ease in following your breath, you can expand your awareness as you meditate to include the full range of sensations both inside and outside your body: feeling, smelling, hearing, seeing. Imagine that your awareness is like the zoom lens on a camera. Until now, you've been focused exclusively on your breath; now you can back away slightly to include the field of sensations that surrounds your breath.

If you find it difficult to expand your awareness all at once, you can begin by exploring a sensation when it calls attention to itself. For example, you're following your breath when a pain in your back cries out for your attention. Instead of staying focused on your breath as you would have done before, you can turn your attention to the pain and explore it fully until it no longer predominates in your field of experience. Then come back to your breath until you're once again called away.

You can also experiment with expanding your awareness to include one particular kind of sensation, such as bodily feelings or sounds. For example, you can spend an entire meditation just listening to the sounds around you, without focusing on any sounds in particular. In this way, you're able to balance the highly concentrated awareness required to follow your breath with the more receptive, all-inclusive awareness necessary to welcome a broad range of sensations. This blend of focus and receptivity lies at the heart of the practice of mindfulness.

As you get the knack of including sensations in your meditations, you can experiment with expanding your awareness to include the full sensate field

Book VII

Meditation, Mindfulness, and Letting Go of Stress

Just sitting

As an alternative to mindfulness meditation, you may want to experiment with the Zen practice known as *just sitting*, which usually involves two phases or steps: just breathing and just sitting.

When you're adept at following your breath, you can practice *becoming your breath* — merging yourself completely with the flow of the inhalation and exhalation, until you, as a separate observer, disappear and only your breath remains. Now you're no longer breathing; instead, your breath is breathing you. Like welcoming whatever arises, this practice, known as *just breathing,* is supremely simple but requires a quality of awareness that's both focused and relaxed.

The next step, *just sitting,* involves expanding to include the whole realm of sensate experience. But instead of being aware or mindful of your experience, you "disappear," and only your experience remains — seeing, smelling, hearing, sensing, thinking. As one Zen person put it, "When you sit, the walls of the meditation hall come down, and the whole world enters." Ultimately, this practice takes you to the same place as mindfulness; it's simply the Zen alternative.

(that is, hearing, seeing, smelling, touching, and tasting). Begin by following your breathing and then just open your lens wide, allowing sensations to arise and pass away in your awareness.

Welcoming whatever arises

When you become accustomed to including sensations in your meditation practice, you can open your awareness wide and welcome any and every experience — even thoughts and emotions — without judgment or resistance. Just like sensations, thoughts and feelings come and go in your awareness like clouds in the sky without pulling you off center. If you do lose your balance, by all means just return to open, nonjudgmental, present-moment awareness.

Just as the sky is never disturbed or constricted no matter how many clouds pile up, so this spacious, open awareness is undisturbed by the experiences that pass through. At first, you may find your attention drawn here and there like a flashlight, exploring one object and then another. But just keep coming back to this open, skylike awareness. (For more on welcoming whatever arises, see Book VII, Chapter 5.)

Chapter 5

Meditating with Challenging Emotions

*M*editation tends to make you calmer, more spacious, and more relaxed — at least most of the time. When you follow your breath, repeat a mantra, or practice some other basic technique every day, your mind begins to settle down naturally while thoughts and feelings spontaneously bubble up and release like the fizz in a bottle of soda. The process is so relaxing that the folks in Transcendental Meditation call it *unstressing*.

When you meditate regularly for a period of time, however, you may find that certain emotions or states of mind keep coming back to distract or disturb you. Instead of dispersing, the same sexual fantasies, sad or fearful thoughts, or painful memories may keep playing in your awareness. Instead of watching the mist rising from the lake, you've begun your descent into the muddy and sometimes turbulent waters of your inner experience.

At first, you may be surprised, dismayed, or even frightened by what you encounter, and you may conclude that you're doing something wrong. But have no fear! The truth is, your meditation has actually begun to deepen, and you're ready to expand your range of meditation techniques to help you navigate this new terrain.

At this point, you may find it helpful to extend your practice of mindfulness (covered in the preceding chapter) from your breathing and your bodily sensations to your thoughts and emotions. As you gently focus the light of your awareness on this dimension of your experience, you can begin to sort out what's actually going on inside you. In the process, you can get to know yourself better — even make friends with yourself. If you keep it up, you can eventually start to penetrate and even unravel some old habitual patterns of thinking, feeling, and behaving — patterns that have been causing you suffering and stress and keeping you stuck for a long, long time. (For more on how the mind causes suffering and stress, see Book VII, Chapter 1.)

Making Friends with Your Experience

If you're like most people, you tend to be exceptionally hard on yourself. In fact, you probably treat yourself in ways you wouldn't consider treating any of your loved ones or friends. When you make a mistake, you may call yourself names or heap harsh judgments and criticisms on yourself, including a laundry list of all the other mistakes you've made over the years. When you feel some tender or vulnerable emotion, you may dismiss it as weak or wimpy and attempt to push past it rather than give yourself time to feel it fully.

Most people hold some image of how they're supposed to act, think, and feel, and they're constantly struggling to get their experience and behavior to conform to it — and they blame themselves when they don't. In meditation, you have an opportunity to reverse this trend and explore your experience just the way it is without trying to judge it or change it. To replace the stress, conflict, and turbulence inside you with peace and harmony, you need to make friends with yourself, which means treating yourself with the same kindness, care, and curiosity that you would give to a close friend. You can begin by bringing a gentle, nonjudgmental awareness to your thoughts and feelings.

Embracing your thoughts and feelings

When you're familiar with following your breath and expanding your awareness to include sensations (refer to Book VII, Chapter 1), you can expand your awareness even further to include thoughts, images, memories, and feelings. As with sensations, begin by following your breath and then allow yourself to explore a thought or feeling when it becomes so strong that it draws your attention to it. When it no longer predominates in your field of awareness, gently return to your breath.

Of course, if you've been meditating for a while, you may have noticed that you're constantly being carried away by the torrent of thoughts and feelings that flood through your mind. One moment you're counting or following your breaths or practicing your mantra, the next moment you're mulling over a conversation you had yesterday or planning tomorrow's dinner. When this happens, you simply need to notice that you've wandered and immediately return to where you began.

Now, however, instead of viewing this dimension of your experience as a distraction, include it in your meditation with mindful awareness. When you find your attention wandering off into a thought or feeling, be aware of what you're experiencing until it loses its intensity; then gently return to your primary focus.

Naming your experience

As you expand your meditation to include thoughts and feelings, you may find it helpful to practice *naming,* or noting, your experience. Begin with mindful awareness of your breath, and then start silently naming the in-breath and out-breath. When you get really quiet and focused, you may even want to include subtleties such as "long breath," "short breath," "deep breath," "shallow breath," and so on.

Keep the naming simple and subdued, like a gentle, nonjudgmental voice in the back of your mind. As Buddhist meditation teacher Jack Kornfield says in his book *A Path with Heart* (Bantam), give "ninety-five percent of your energy to sensing each experience, and five percent to a soft name in the background."

When you become adept at naming your breath, you can extend the practice to any strong sensations, thoughts, or feelings that draw your attention away from your breath. For example, as you follow and name your breath, you may find your focus interrupted by a prominent emotion. Name this experience softly and repeatedly for as long as it persists — "sadness, sadness, sadness" or "anger, anger, anger" — then gently return your attention to your breath. Take the same approach with thoughts, images, and mind-states: "planning, planning," "worrying, worrying," or "seeing, seeing."

Use the simplest words you can find, and focus on one thing at a time. This practice helps you gain a little perspective or distance from your constantly changing inner experience, instead of becoming lost in the torrent.

By naming particular thoughts and emotions, you're also acknowledging that they exist. As mentioned earlier in this chapter, people often attempt to suppress or deny experiences they deem undesirable or unacceptable, such as anger, fear, judgment, or hurt. But the more you try to hide from your experience, the more it can end up governing your behavior, as Freud so wisely pointed out more than a century ago.

Naming allows you to shine the penetrating light of awareness into the recesses of your heart and mind and invite your thoughts and feelings to emerge from their hiding place into the light of day. You may not like what you encounter at first, but you can name your self-judgments and

Book VII

Meditation, Mindfulness, and Letting Go of Stress

self-criticisms as well. Ultimately, you may notice that you're not surprised anymore by what you discover about yourself. And the more you make friends with your own apparent shortcomings and frailties, the more you can open your heart to the imperfections of others as well.

Constant naming has disadvantages, however, because it separates you from your direct experience by placing words and concepts between your awareness and reality. So if you use this technique, do so lightly and judiciously as a first step in becoming acquainted with your inner life and making friends with yourself. Then gradually let go of the habit as you become more comfortable with being present for your experience just as it is.

Welcoming whatever arises

When you become accustomed to including sensations, thoughts, and feelings in your meditation, you can open your awareness gates wide and welcome whatever arises without judgment or resistance. Imagine that your mind is like the sky and that inner and outer experiences come and go like clouds.

At first, you may find your attention drawn here and there, exploring one object and then another. You don't have to control your attention in any way; just allow it to wander where it will, from thoughts to sensations to feelings and back again.

Eventually, you may have periods in your meditation when your mind feels spacious and expanded and doesn't seem to be disturbed by thoughts, feelings, or outside distractions. Whatever you experience, just keep opening your awareness and welcoming whatever comes.

A note of caution, however: This practice, though supremely simple, is actually quite advanced and requires well-developed powers of concentration to sustain. It's also difficult to teach — rather like riding a bicycle. First, you have to *discover* what it feels like to hold your balance, and then you just keep returning to the balance point whenever you start to fall off.

Meditating with Difficult Emotions

Many people believe they have a Pandora's box of ugly, disgusting emotions like rage, jealousy, hatred, and terror hidden inside them, and they're afraid that if they open it up, these demonic energies will overwhelm them and those they love. For another thing, they tend to think that these "negative" feelings are bottomless and irresolvable and that they're better off avoiding them no matter how painful it may be to hold them in.

Unfortunately, you pay a steep price indeed if you spend your life resisting and denying your feelings. Unacknowledged negative feelings can impede the flow of more positive feelings like love and joy. As a result, you may end up feeling lonely and unhappy because you lack close emotional contact with others, and you may be unable to give and receive love when you have an opportunity to do so.

In addition, negative feelings that build up inside you tend to cause stress and depression, suppress the immune system, and contribute to stress-related ailments like ulcers, cancer, and heart disease. They also hold valuable life energy that you may otherwise channel in constructive or creative ways. Besides, emotions that are persistently suppressed and denied have an annoying habit of bursting forth inappropriately when you least expect them, prompting you to do and say things you may later regret.

Of course, some people go to another extreme and seem to be so completely awash in powerful emotional reactions that they can't make simple decisions or carry on a rational conversation. But these people aren't really experiencing their emotions; they're indulging them and allowing them to run their lives.

Meditation offers you an alternative way of relating with your emotions. Instead of suppressing, indulging, or exploding, you can directly experience your emotions as they are — as an interplay of thoughts, images, and sensations. When you've become skillful at following your breath and expanding your awareness to include the flow of thoughts and feelings — which may take months or even years — you can focus your attention on particular emotions that you find challenging or problematic and develop *penetrating insight* into the nature of the experience.

Instead of being bottomless or endless, as some people fear, you may find that even the most powerful emotions come in waves that have a limited duration when you experience them fully. As one meditation teacher used to say, "What you resist persists" — and what you welcome has a tendency to let go and release. (See the sidebar "Facing your demons" later in this chapter.)

In the following sections, you find some guidelines for exploring a few of the most common emotions. Although feelings come in many shapes and sizes, they're all more or less variants or combinations of a few basic ones: anger, fear, sadness, joy, excitement, and desire. Just as an artist's rich palette of colors can ultimately be broken down into blue, red, and yellow, the difficult or challenging emotions like jealousy, guilt, boredom, and depression are combinations (or reactions) to four basic feelings: anger, fear, sadness, and desire. (If you find a certain feeling problematic, work on it as you would one of these four.)

Book VII

Meditation, Mindfulness, and Letting Go of Stress

Anger

Many people, especially women, have a taboo against getting angry because they weren't allowed to express their anger, even as children. So they expend enormous amounts of energy trying to skirt around the feeling. Other people seem as though they're perpetually seething with current anger and old resentments, although they may not realize it themselves.

When you meditate with your anger, you may begin by noticing where and how you experience it in your body. Where do you find yourself tensing and contracting? What happens to your breathing? Where do you notice a buildup of energy? How does it affect softer emotions? As you continue to be aware of your anger, do you notice it shifting or changing in any way? How long does it last? Does it have a beginning and an end?

Next, you can turn your attention to your mind. What kinds of thoughts and images accompany the angry feelings? Do you find yourself blaming other people and defending yourself? If you investigate further and peel back the initial layer of anger, what do you find underneath? Anger generally arises in response to one of two deeper emotions: hurt or fear. When you're hurt, you may lash out in anger against the one you believe hurt you. And when you're afraid, you may protect yourself with the sword and armor of anger rather than acknowledge your fear, even to yourself. Beneath the hurt and fear, anger generally masks an even deeper layer of attachment to having things be a certain way. When circumstances change or don't go according to plan, you feel hurt or afraid and then angry in response.

With anger, as with all emotions, set aside any judgment or resistance you may have and face the anger directly. You may find that it becomes more intense before it releases, but stay with it. Beneath the anger may lie deep wellsprings of power, which you may eventually discover how to evoke without getting angry.

Fear and anxiety

Many people are reluctant to admit they're afraid, even to themselves. Somehow, they believe that if they acknowledge their fear, they give it power to run their lives. In other words, deep down, they're afraid of their fear! Men, especially, often go to great lengths to hide their fears or anxieties behind a facade of confidence or anger or rationality. At the other extreme, of course, some people seem to be frightened of just about everything.

Facing your demons

The Tibetans tell a wonderful story about the great meditation master Milarepa, who lived about 900 years ago. Milarepa sought out remote caves high in the Himalayas where he practiced meditation. Once, he found himself in a cave inhabited by a company of demons that distracted him from his practice. (Demons apparently frequented caves in those days — looking for some action, no doubt!)

First, he tried to subdue them, but they wouldn't budge. Then he decided to honor them and extend friendliness and compassion to them, and half of them left. The rest he welcomed wholeheartedly and invited to return whenever

they wished. At this invitation, all but one particularly ferocious demon vanished like a rainbow. With no concern for his own body and with utmost love and compassion, Milarepa went up to the demon and placed his head in its mouth as an offering. The demon disappeared without a trace and never returned.

Consider the story of Milarepa the next time you're struggling with your own inner demons — emotions and states of mind you find challenging or unpleasant. Imagine what may happen if you welcomed them instead of trying to drive them away!

The truth is, if you're human — and not bionic or extraterrestrial — you're going to be afraid or anxious at least occasionally. In addition to the raw rush of adrenaline you feel when your physical survival seems to be at stake, you experience the fear that inevitably arises when you face the unknown or the uncertain in life, which can be quite often these days. Ultimately, you're afraid because you believe that you're a separate, isolated entity surrounded by forces beyond your control. The more the walls that separate you from others crumble through the practice of meditation, the more your fear and anxiety naturally diminish.

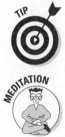

As with anger, you can use your meditation to explore and ultimately make friends with your fear. After all, it's just an emotion like other emotions, composed of physical sensations, thoughts, and beliefs. When working with fear, it's especially important to be kind and gentle with yourself.

Begin by asking the same questions you'd ask about anger: Where and how do you experience it in your body? Where do you find yourself tensing and contracting? What happens to your breathing? Or to your heart? Next, notice the thoughts and images that accompany the fear. Often fear arises from anticipating the future and imagining that you'll somehow be unable to cope. When you see these catastrophic expectations for what they are and return to the present moment — the sensations in your body, the coming and going of your breath — you may find that the fear shifts and begins to disperse. Then when it returns, you can simply call its name — "fear, fear, fear" — like an old, familiar friend.

Checking in with your inner child

When you're feeling agitated or upset, you may want to check in with the little child inside you, the part of you that feels things deeply. Here's a meditation to help reassure and nurture your inner child.

1. **Begin by noticing what you're feeling and where you're feeling it.**

2. **Take some time to breathe and relax into the feelings.**

3. **Imagine that there's a little boy or girl inside you having these feelings.**

   This child is the young, undeveloped part of you. You may have an image or just a gut sense or inner knowing.

4. **Ask yourself these questions: "How old is this child? What is this child's name? What kind of attention does this child want from me right now?"**

The child may want to be reassured or held, or he or she may just want to play.

5. **If possible, imagine giving the child what he or she wants.**

6. **Continue to commune with this child for as long as you like, giving and receiving words or physical contact as appropriate.**

7. **When you're done, notice how you feel.**

   You may be more relaxed or confident or at least less upset or afraid.

8. **Be sure to give your inner child a hug (if the child feels comfortable receiving one), tell the child that you love him or her, and reassure the child that you'll check in with him or her again from time to time — and please do!**

You may also want to amplify the sensations a little and allow yourself to shake or tremble, if you feel so inclined. You can even imagine the fear overwhelming you and doing its worst (knowing, of course, that you will survive). This approach is especially helpful if you're afraid of your fear, as so many people are. Facing your fear directly without trying to get rid of it or escape from it requires tremendous courage; yet these practices also have the capacity to bring you into the present moment and open your heart to your own vulnerability.

Sadness, grief, and depression

Most people find sadness easier to feel and express than anger or fear. Unfortunately, they don't give it the time and attention it deserves because they were told as children to stop crying before they were ready. Life inevitably presents you with a series of disappointments and losses; unexpressed sadness and grief can build up inside and ultimately lead to depression.

To make friends with your sadness, you need to hold it gently and lovingly and give it plenty of space to express itself. As with anger and fear, begin by exploring the sensations. Perhaps you notice a heaviness in your heart or a constriction in your diaphragm or a clogged sensation in your eyes and forehead, as though you're about to cry but can't. You may want to amplify these sensations and see what happens.

Then pay attention to the thoughts, images, and memories that fuel the sadness. Perhaps you keep reliving the loss of a loved one or the moment when a close friend said something unkind to you. If you're depressed, you may keep recycling the same negative, self-defeating beliefs and judgments, such as "I'm not good enough" or "I don't have what it takes to succeed."

As you open your awareness to include the full range of experiences associated with the sadness, you may shed some heartfelt tears. In the process, you may also feel yourself lightening up and your sadness lifting a little. Ultimately, as long as you're open to your own suffering and the suffering of others, you will experience a certain amount of tender sadness in your heart.

Unraveling Habitual Patterns with Awareness

As you explore your emotions (as described in the preceding section), you may gradually discover that they're not as overpowering or as endless as you feared. With mindful awareness, most emotions flow through your body and gradually release. For example, as you gently investigate your anger or fear, it may intensify at first, then break and disperse like a wave on the beach.

But certain persistent emotions and physical contractions, along with the thoughts and images that accompany and fuel them, seem to keep returning no matter how many times you notice and name them. These are the *stories* and habitual patterns that run deep in the body-mind like the roots from which recurring thoughts and feelings spring. (For more on these stories, see Book VII, Chapter 1.)

In your meditations, you may keep replaying a story from your past (including all the accompanying emotions and mind-states) in which you suffer some abuse or injustice. Perhaps you see yourself as a failure and fantasize obsessively about an imaginary future in which you're somehow happier and more successful. Or you may worry repeatedly about your job or relationship because you believe you can't trust people or because the world's not a safe place.

In his book *A Path with Heart,* Buddhist meditation teacher Jack Kornfield calls these habitual patterns *insistent visitors* and suggests that they keep returning in your meditation (and your life!) because they're stuck or unfinished in some way. When you give them the loving attention and deeper investigation they require, you may at first discover that they're more complex and deeply rooted than you had imagined. But with persistent exploration, they gradually unravel and reveal the hidden energy and wisdom they contain. In fact, the more you undo your patterns, the more you release the physical and energetic contractions that lie at their heart, and the freer, more spacious, more expansive — and, yes, healthier! — you become.

Here's a brief synopsis of the primary techniques for unraveling habitual patterns. Experiment with them on your own, and if you find them helpful, feel free to incorporate them into your meditation. If you get stuck or would like to delve deeper but don't know how, you may want to find yourself a meditation teacher or psychotherapist familiar with this approach.

- ✔ **Name your "tunes":** When a particular tune (habitual pattern) recurs, you can simply notice and name it without getting embroiled once again in the same painful pattern. This approach is another version of naming your experience.

- ✔ **Expand your awareness:** By welcoming the full range of thoughts, images, and feelings, you create an inner spaciousness in which the pattern can gradually unfold and release. Perhaps you keep feeling tense in your lower belly, and you don't know why. If you expand your awareness, you may discover that beneath the surface lies fear about the future, and under the fear lies a layer of hurt. When you include thoughts and ideas as well, you may find that, deep down, you believe you're inadequate. So you're afraid you can't cope, and you feel hurt when people criticize you because it just corroborates your own negative self-image.

- ✔ **Feel your feelings:** Patterns often persist until the underlying feelings are thoroughly felt. That's right, *felt* — not merely acknowledged or named! Many people keep their feelings at arm's length or confuse them with thoughts or ideas. Other people (as mentioned in the earlier section "Meditating with Difficult Emotions") get completely entangled in their feelings. As you expand your awareness, ask yourself, "What feelings haven't I felt yet?"

    Feeling your feelings doesn't make them bigger or worse, at least not in the long run. It actually allows them to move through and release!

- ✔ **Notice your resistance and attachment:** If a particular story or challenging emotion keeps replaying in your mind, explore your relationship to it. For example, ask, "How do I feel about this particular pattern or story? Do I have a vested interest in holding on to it? If so, what do

I get out of it? What am I afraid may happen if I let it go? Am I judging it as undesirable and struggling to get rid of it? If so, what don't I like about it?" When you can relax and gently open to accept the pattern with awareness, you may find that the pattern, which felt so tight and entrenched, relaxes as well.

✔ **Find the wisdom:** Sometimes recurring stories or patterns have wisdom to impart, and they won't stop nagging until you listen. If you keep having the same uncomfortable or difficult feeling during meditation and it doesn't shift or change with awareness, you may want to "give it a voice" and ask it to speak to you as though it were a close friend. Ask, "What are you trying to tell me? What do I need to hear?" You may discover that a tender, vulnerable part of yourself needs caring, nurturing attention. Other times, you may hear the voice of responsibility reminding you to tend to some important commitment.

✔ **Get to the heart of the matter:** Like the great Tibetan meditator Milarepa (see the sidebar "Facing your demons" earlier in this chapter), sometimes you need to stick your head into the demon's mouth before it disappears for good. In other words, you may need to explore the *energetic contraction* that lies at the heart of your pattern.

The term *energetic* here refers to the model of the human organism as a system of energetic pathways and centers that can get blocked or contracted. These blockages give rise to painful emotions and mind-states and may ultimately cause disease.

To explore the energetic contraction at the heart of your pattern, you can gently direct your awareness into the very center of the contraction and describe in detail what you find there. When you unearth the memory, feeling, or belief that holds the pattern together, you may find that the contraction releases, your awareness expands, and your meditation begins to flow more smoothly. (***Note:*** When you're dealing with exceptionally painful, deep-seated contractions, you may want to consult a qualified professional.)

✔ **Infuse the stuck place with being:** After you've meditated for a while and received some glimpses of your own inherent wholeness and completeness (your *being*), you may want to try the following shortcut. Set aside the thoughts and ideas that accompany your pattern and simply be aware of the physical and energetic contraction. Now shift your attention to your wholeness and completeness, which you may experience as a calm, relaxed energy in your body; a deeply loving feeling in your heart; a sense of expansiveness or space; or some other feeling unique to you. Imagine your wholeness and completeness gradually spreading, penetrating, and infusing the contraction with pure being. Continue this exercise as the contraction releases and dissolves into being.

Book VII

Meditation, Mindfulness, and Letting Go of Stress

Perhaps you're so full of negative thoughts and feelings that you find it virtually impossible to concentrate, even in meditation. The voices (or images) in your head keep spewing forth worries, regrets, judgments, and criticism with such volume and velocity that you can barely hear yourself think. If certain patterns persist — especially if they interfere with your capacity to do your work or maintain loving, satisfying relationships — you may consider psychotherapy.

Chapter 6

Cultivating Spirituality

*I*f you meditate regularly, you're going to have spiritual experiences — guaranteed. By following your breath or reciting a mantra or merely sitting quietly and listening with full attention to the sound of the wind through the trees, you're cutting through your usual preoccupations and attuning yourself to the present moment. That's where glimpses of the spiritual dimension of being generally occur — in the present. (In fact, being present with awareness is an inherently spiritual activity.) To paraphrase an old saying, spiritual experiences are accidents — but you make yourself accident-prone when you meditate. In this chapter, you find out how to use meditation to explore spirituality to your heart's content.

Now, this chapter doesn't give you detailed instructions on how to get enlightened or meet God directly — you may have to check out other books and teachers for that. But it does offer a brief glimpse of what the spiritual path has to offer so that you know which direction to take on your journey.

Dissolving or Expanding the Self: The Point of Spiritual Practice

The great spiritual traditions agree that the primary reason people suffer — and the primary problem they need to resolve — is the experience of being a separate, isolated individual, cut off from God or source or their own essential natures. When you meditate, you're bridging the apparent chasm that separates you and connecting with your breath, with your body and senses,

Mindfulness into meditation

To experience health and well-being, you must properly care for and feed the body, regulate your breath, exercise consciously and regularly, and care for the mind and your spirit. This is where meditation plays a practical key roll as part of your overall physical, emotional, mental, and personal health management.

Here are some effective tools and techniques to enhance your mindfulness and meditation practice. These tips come from San Francisco/Marin County yoga teacher Sherri Baptiste, born into a lineage of teachers at the forefront of yoga training in America and founder of Baptiste Power of Yoga:

1. **Find a quiet place.** Create a space in your home and set aside a daily time to just sit and practice meditation. The space should be warm and draft free, the phones should be turned off, and the lighting and music should be soft and unimposing.

2. **Determine how often and how long.** If you're a beginner, start with 3 to 5 minutes and let the time grow to 20 or more minutes as you become more adept. Practice a minimum of three times a week; the ideal is to practice daily. Meditation evolves over time, and when conditions are right, meditation will flow. Encourage yourself to be patient in the process and to practice without any expectations.

3. **Find a sitting technique that works best for you.** Book VII, Chapter 1 offers suggestions. Whichever sitting position you choose, remember that sitting straight is a key that heightens awareness and the quality of your breathing.

4. **Pay attention to your breath.** Breathe smoothly and evenly, using the lower, mid, and upper lungs without forcing. Establish a breath that is gentle and uninterrupted in quality and flow. You might say, "The breath rolls in like a wave and out like a wave" with a sense of expansion on the inhalation and relaxation on the exhalation.

5. **Cultivate the mind.** As you sit, notice your thoughts and then step back from those thoughts, watching them for a moment as they pass by. Then bring your awareness back to your breathing, using it as a tool, to calm the active mind and to direct the consciousness into new and deeper levels of awareness and insight.

6. **Go deeper.** At certain points as you guide yourself, use an inner dialog with words and phrases such as "Feel the stillness of your body"; "Relax more inside the throat"; "Notice the body breathing"; and "Listen to the breath with intimacy."

   Observe and notice any areas that may still be constricting, and then simply let them go, letting these areas completely release.

7. **Find space between your thoughts.** At this point, you let go of dialogue, leading yourself into the silence and space between the thoughts. Now sit here for the next few moments in stillness and silence. Remember, meditation goes beyond mindfulness techniques. It's a spontaneous flow and energetic quality. When all the conditions are just right, it will simply flow. The ideal here is to *be* in the moment as it unfolds.

8. **Bring yourself out of this practice slowly.** Use a soft tone of voice and then place your hands on your chest for three deep cleansing breathes. Open your eyes slowly. Encourage yourself to practice often.

with your heart, with the present moment, and ultimately with a greater reality. (It's this connection that promotes healing.)

You can believe in spirit, awaken to it, stay in touch with it, and become infused by it, but the ultimate aim of spiritual practice is to help you overcome all apparent separation and become one with spirit completely.

The approach of dissolving the self and the approach of expanding the self ultimately take you to the same place: the deep inner knowing that you and God or the ground of being are identical — "not two," as some teachers put it. Although most spiritual traditions tend to emphasize one approach over the other, they generally offer both as alternatives, depending on your inclinations.

Dissolving the self

What keeps you separate? Well, some traditions call it *ego* or *self;* others call it *personality, pride, self-image,* or *self-clinging.* Essentially, it's the beliefs and stories described in Book VII, Chapter 1: the inner turbulence and self-centered preoccupations and patterns that keep you from seeing things clearly. Of course, these preoccupations and patterns run deep and can take a lifetime (or lifetimes!) of dedicated practice to undo, but you can begin to unravel them using some of the meditative practices described in the preceding chapter. (At a deeper level of understanding, you're actually never separate from spirit even for an instant — you just think you are. But therein lies the riddle everyone needs to solve. As the great Indian sage Ramana Maharshi used to say, "The only thing that separates you from the Self is the belief that you're separate.") As you unravel these patterns, you gradually dissolve the limited self you thought yourself to be and realize your identity with the greater reality.

Book VII

Meditation,
Mindfulness,
and Letting
Go of Stress

This journey can take a long, long time (even lifetimes, if you believe in reincarnation), and it may be fraught with difficulties, fears, and uncertainties, as you'll discover if you read the biography of any great saint or sage. To navigate the journey at all, you need to develop a healthy measure of self-love and self-acceptance. You also need the guidance of an experienced teacher. For more on teachers, see the section "Finding a Teacher" at the end of this chapter.

Expanding the self

In addition to dissolving the self, you can also understand the spiritual journey as an expansion of identity from the narrow to the vast, until you're finally identified with the *luminous, eternal vastness* itself (also known as spirit or God). The ancient Indian sages used the model of the five bodies, which are subtler and subtler levels of identification beginning with the physical body and moving to identification with the ground of being or greater reality itself.

Here's a similar model (based on the five bodies and loosely adapted from the writings of philosopher Ken Wilber) that you may find helpful in understanding your own spiritual experiences and unfolding. Remember that each time you expand your identity to a new level, you incorporate the level that came before instead of leaving it behind:

- **Physical body:** Some people seem to think of nothing else but eating, drinking, working, sleeping, and sexing — they're largely identified with their physical needs and instincts.

- **Persona:** As you grow up and interact more with others, you develop a personality — a set of habits and tendencies and preferences — along with a self-image based largely on how others see you. Gradually, you begin to expand your identity to include this social persona, and you may become preoccupied with how you look or come across or the other accoutrements of a self-image, such as material possessions.

- **Mature ego:** If you spend enough time exploring your inner life and sorting through your deeper feelings, values, and visions, you may eventually develop a mature ego — a healthy, well-rounded sense of who you are, what you want, and how you can contribute to others.

- **Energy body:** Beyond the body-mind lies the *energy body* (the aura that surrounds the physical body), which expands and contracts depending on your mood, your energy level, and countless other factors. (Whether you notice it or not, you're constantly reacting to the energy bodies of the people you meet.)

The classic exercise for experiencing your energy body goes as follows: Rub your palms and fingers together vigorously for a few minutes, then hold them an inch or two apart and notice the energy field between them. Bring them closer together and farther apart, feeling the energy get denser and thinner and pulsate as your hands move. To explore this dimension further, check out the sidebar "Playing with your energy body" later in this chapter.

People who expand their identities to include their energy body realize that they're more than just their body-mind, which opens them to a spiritual dimension of being.

- **Transpersonal dimension:** This broad category encompasses the full range of nonordinary experiences, from clairvoyance and other forms of extrasensory perception (ESP) to rapture and bliss to visions of angels, gods and goddesses, and other otherworldly beings to direct communion

Playing with your energy body

Did you ever have the sense that you were bigger than your physical body? Or that the space you occupy expands and contracts depending on circumstances? Did you ever have the feeling that you had no boundaries and you went on forever? Well, you're experiencing the expansion and contraction of your energy body, the aura of energy that surrounds your physical body.

Here's a little exercise for playing with your energy body:

1. **Begin by sitting quietly; closing your eyes; and taking a few slow, deep breaths, relaxing a little on each exhalation.**

2. **Spend a few minutes imagining going for a walk in nature or spending time with someone you love.**

   Notice how big you feel.

   Then notice how your size (but not your waistline) changes when you imagine getting stuck in traffic or paying your bills or getting into an argument.

3. **Next, check out your energy body without imagining anything.**

   How far do you think it extends beyond your physical body? Six inches? Several feet?

Does it extend farther in front than behind? Farther above your body than below into the ground? Is it thicker than the air or thinner? Thicker in some places than in others?

4. **Pick a room where you feel comfortable, stand or sit near the center, and check out the boundaries of the room in every direction.**

5. **Fill the room with your energy — fill it with you!**

   Imagine it, sense it, visualize it, sing it — whatever helps you fill the space as much as you can.

6. **Draw your energy back in until it forms a sphere around you, about 2 or 3 feet away.**

   Notice how the energy becomes denser.

7. **Play with expanding and contracting your energy in this way several times; then relax and notice how you feel.**

By regularly experimenting with your energy body, you can acquire a direct understanding of the spiritual truth that you're more than your physical body. (This exercise is adapted from a series of exercises in the book *The Lover Within* by Julie Henderson [Station Hill Press].)

Book VII

Meditation, Mindfulness, and Letting Go of Stress

with your higher self — or even with a personal manifestation of God. When you expand your identity to include these subtler levels of being, you know without doubt that who you are is far vaster than you once believed, and you begin to access a deeper source of wisdom and compassion as well.

✔ **Glimpses of being:** When you experience *being* directly in all its innate perfection and completeness, you realize that you've never been separate from who you really are even for an instant.

✔ **Ground of being:** Only the great mystics and sages get this far. Now you're one with spirit or the ground of being without separation — in the words of the Indian scriptures, "You are That." Sure, you continue to eat, drink, sleep, and blow your nose, but you never forget even for an instant who you really are — and your being radiates wisdom and compassion to others.

The Path of Devotion: In Search of Union

If you believe in the existence of a personal God or have had experiences of a presence greater than yourself that inspired feelings of awe and reverence, you may be drawn to the path of devotion. It's the primary spiritual path in the Judeo-Christian tradition and Islam, and forms one of the main currents of Hinduism.

Although devotees may feel deeply connected to God and believe that a spark of divinity shines in their hearts, they often experience themselves to be painfully separate from God. As the anonymous author of the mystical Christian text *The Cloud of Unknowing* puts it, "The person who has a deep experience of himself existing far apart from God feels the most acute sorrow. Any other grief seems trivial in comparison." Through contemplation, mantra recitation (see the section "Mantra: Invoking the Divine in every moment" later in this chapter), chanting, selfless service, and other devotional practices, devotees seek to get closer to God by focusing all their love and attention on God — and ultimately, if they're mystically inclined, to merge with God completely in a state of ecstatic union.

The path of devotion has its own unique aspects or phases of development, which include the following:

✔ **Developing virtue:** In all the great devotional traditions, devotees are required to prepare themselves for union with God by living a life of purity and restraint.

✔ **Cultivating a higher octave of love:** The devotee may begin by feeling personal love for God or teacher, but eventually this love evolves into an unconditional, transpersonal love that knows no bounds and does not depend on the love object to evoke.

✔ **Overcoming duality:** Beginning with a painful sense of separation, the devotee gradually gets closer and closer and ultimately merges with God, until no trace of separation remains. As the Hindu sage Swami Vivekananda put it, "Love, the lover, and the beloved are one."

✔ **Transcending the personal God:** Ultimately, the devotee must transcend even God, if God is experienced as having a particular name or form. At this stage, the lover and the beloved dissolve into God as the absolute ground of being, the nameless, formless greater reality whose essence is love.

✔ **Everything is God:** The distinctions get pretty subtle at these higher levels, but here goes: When the devotee no longer needs to contemplate or meditate in order to experience oneness with God but sees God everywhere in every moment — waking or sleeping — he or she has reached the pinnacle of the devotional path. Now that the separate self and all self-centered striving have fallen away, every activity reflects a complete alignment with the divine purpose: "Not my will but Thy will be done."

To give you a flavor of the devotional path, here are two practices you may like to try. These have their counterparts in all the world's great spiritual traditions.

Mantra: Invoking the Divine in every moment

Throughout history, meditators and mystics in the great devotional traditions have recommended the constant recitation of a *mantra* (a sacred word or phrase usually transmitted directly from a teacher) to bring the devotee closer to the Divine. At first, you can practice repeating it aloud; then, when you become proficient, you can repeat it silently to yourself; and ultimately you can graduate to purely mental recitation (which is considered the most powerful).

Some practitioners of mantra also manipulate a rosary (or *mala* in Sanskrit) to help them keep track, ticking off one bead for each recitation. Or you can coordinate the sound with the coming and going of your breath.

Although you may begin by limiting your mantra recitation to a few minutes or hours of meditation each day, the traditional goal is constant practice. That is, you want to get to the point where you're repeating the sound or phrase nonstop in order to keep your attention focused on the Divine and away from habitual patterns of thought. Ultimately, your mind will become one-pointed, and you'll think always and only of God — which is the first step on the path to union.

Needless to say, you'll be lucky if you can remember your mantra for a few minutes at first. But if you've received a mantra from a teacher (or know a

Chanting and bowing

Besides meditation and contemplation, the devotional path usually involves active practices like chanting, singing, and bowing. As you may have noticed if you've ever sung along with a gospel choir or chanted Indian devotional hymns, you can lift your spirits, open your heart, and intensify your devotion by raising your voice in praise of the Divine. If you're devotionally inclined (or devotionally impaired!), try mixing your meditation with a little chanting or singing every now and then. Choose songs that have resonance or meaning for you.

Traditional wisdom suggests that chanting sacred words and phrases also has the power to open, stimulate, and harmonize your energy centers. In this way, chanting helps "tune up" your body and prepare it for meditation and other spiritual practices.

As for bowing: What better way to practice surrendering your self-centered preoccupa-tions and habitual patterns than by falling down on your knees on a regular basis? One famous Zen master wore a perpetual callus on his forehead from bowing repeatedly to soften his stubbornness.

Of course, bowing figures prominently in the Judeo-Christian tradition and Islam as well; like meditation, it's a universally recognized practice for overcoming separation and approaching the spiritual dimension of being.

But bowing doesn't mean giving up your autonomy to some outside power or force. When you bow — to God, Jesus, Buddha, or the picture of a teacher or saint — you're ultimately bowing to your own essential nature. Think of bowing as an expression of the essential oneness of inside and outside, the one bowed to and the one bowing. Or, as they say in India, "The divine in me bows to the divine in you."

mantra you find particularly meaningful or resonant) and you feel strong devotion, who can say how far you can go in your practice? (For inspiration on your path, you may want to read the spiritual classic *The Way of a Pilgrim*, the anonymous story of a devout Russian Orthodox peasant who chants the Jesus prayer day and night.)

The practice of the presence of God

Here's a time-honored practice that has counterparts in all the world's great spiritual traditions. When you catch a glimpse of the sacred, you can practice seeing it everywhere you look, in everyone and everything. One ancient Zen master used to say "Buddha! Buddha!" to every being he encountered. When the contemporary Tibetan teacher Kalu Rinpoche visited an aquarium in San Francisco, he went around tapping the glass to get the fishes' attention so he could bless them and wish them happiness and well-being.

The *practice* is just that simple: Remember to see the sacred or divine in every being and thing. You may believe that everything is God, or infused by God, or created by God, or has the spark of divinity inside. Whatever your belief, the practice reminds you to look not at the surface or at what you like, don't like, want, or need, but at the sacred, spiritual dimension that is perpetually present.

Of course, the practice may be simple, but it's certainly not easy. You may begin by doing it for ten minutes and see how it goes. If you enjoy it, you can naturally extend it as you feel inspired. (To help you remember, you may want to repeat a phrase like "This, too, is divine," not constantly like a mantra, but intermittently, as a reminder.)

The Path of Insight: Discovering Who You Are

If you find yourself seeking answers to core spiritual questions like "Who am I?" or "What is reality?" but don't have a particular interest in God or devotion, you may be drawn to the path of insight. Unlike devotion, which concentrates the mind on a representation of the Divine, the path of insight uses direct investigation and awareness of present experience to see beyond surface appearances to the deeper reality that underlies them. When you keep questioning and looking deeply into what is apparently real, you inevitably happen upon the ultimately real — the formless, indestructible essence of all appearances. (It's kind of like peeling the layers of an onion.)

Now, the point of this approach is not to deny the relative reality of ordinary people and things. Rather, the path of insight generally teaches that reality has two levels: the *relative* and the *absolute:*

- **On the relative level,** it's important to make a living, pay the bills, spend time with family or friends. If you pretend that the *relative* isn't real, you're going to have some problems. (Traffic court and bankruptcy spring immediately to mind!) As the Sufis say, "Trust in God, but make sure to tie your camel to the post."

- At the same time, though, there's **an absolute level** — a Divine presence or sacred dimension that underlies this world and gives it meaning. When you encounter this level, you see the deeper reality of things, just as the mystic sees God everywhere she looks. Whether directly or more gradually, the path of insight in its various incarnations leads you to an experience or knowing of this absolute level of reality. (In the East, they call this knowing *enlightenment* or *liberation.* In the West, they call it *gnosis* — the Latin word from which "knowing" derives.)

Book VII

Meditation, Mindfulness, and Letting Go of Stress

Discovering the sky of mind

Here's a brief meditation that you can do anytime you're outdoors to give you a taste of the vastness of your essential nature, which the Zen folks call, appropriately enough, "big mind."

1. **Preferably on a clear day, sit or lie down and look up at the sky.**

   Set aside your analytical mind for now and all you think you know about the sky.

2. **Take a few minutes to contemplate the vastness of the sky, which appears to stretch endlessly in every direction.**

3. **Gradually allow your awareness to expand to fill the sky — up and down, north and south, east and west.**

Let go of all sense of personal boundaries as you fill the sky with your awareness.

4. **Become the sky completely and rest in the experience for a few minutes.**

5. **Gradually return to your ordinary sense of yourself.**

   How do you feel? Has your awareness changed in any way?

After you get the knack of this exercise, you can do it for brief moments at any time of the day — for example, while walking your dog in the morning or gazing out your window on a break at work — to remind yourself who you are.

Most of the core practices highlighted in Book VII show you how to investigate your present experience so that you can eventually develop insight. To give you a glimpse of the absolute level, here are three exercises designed to cut through your usual way of perceiving things to reveal a deeper reality. Generally, they work best after you've been practicing some basic meditation technique like following your breath or reciting a mantra.

Expanding your boundaries

Picking up where the energy body meditation leaves off (see the sidebar "Playing with your energy body" earlier in this chapter), this technique shows you that you don't end with your skin — or with the farthest edges of the Milky Way, for that matter.

1. **Begin by sitting quietly, closing your eyes, and taking a few slow, deep breaths, relaxing a little on each exhalation.**

2. **Sense the solidity and density of your body as you usually perceive it.**

3. **As you inhale, imagine that your head is filling with a soft, clear mist; and as you exhale, imagine that all solidity and density drain from your head, leaving it pleasantly empty, spacious, and open to sensation and life-energy.**

   Don't worry; you won't disappear!

4. **Breathe the mist into your neck and throat, and breathe out any tension or density, leaving the area spacious and open.**

5. **Continue to apply this meditation to your chest, lungs, and heart; your arms and hands; your abdomen and internal organs; your pelvis, buttocks, and genitals; and your thighs, lower legs, and feet.**

6. **Feel your whole body completely empty, spacious, and open to the current of life energy.**

   Rest in this feeling for a few moments without thought or analysis. Enjoy the buzz!

7. **If certain areas still feel dense or solid, breathe into them until they're empty and open.**

   You may notice that the boundaries of your body are now diffuse — you're not sure where you leave off and the outside world begins.

8. **Expand the boundaries of your body and your awareness until you include the whole room and everything it contains.**

9. **Expand to include the whole building, then the whole block, the whole town or city, and the state.**

   Take a few minutes with each expansion.

10. **Expand even further to encompass the earth, then the solar system, the Milky Way, the universe, and beyond the farthest boundaries of the known universe.**

    Again, spend a few minutes at each level. You're vast beyond measure — you contain everything. Allow any thoughts, feelings, or sensations to arise within this vast expanse.

11. **After spending several minutes in the vastness, you can begin to pay attention to how you feel.**

    If you find it difficult to locate any feelings, that's fine — just enjoy the expansion for a few more minutes! Then check in with your body: Are you feeling more calm and relaxed than when you began? Has your breathing changed in any way?

12. **Gradually come back to your body before getting up and going about your day.**

    Notice whether your self-image or your experience of people and things has changed in any way.

You can practice the first part of this exercise (emptying and opening) by itself, if you like; it has the power to calm your mind and relax and harmonize your body. With regular practice, you'll be able to create a spacious, open, radiant feeling in your body with one sweep of your awareness.

Book VII

Meditation, Mindfulness, and Letting Go of Stress

Looking into the nature of mind

The Buddhists have devised some powerful techniques for exploring the mind and realizing its essential nature (which happens to be the greater reality mentioned earlier in this chapter). And you don't have to study with a Zen master to get a taste of this essential nature for yourself. Here's an exercise adapted from the Tibetan tradition:

1. **Begin by sitting quietly; closing your eyes; and taking a few slow, deep breaths, relaxing a little with each exhalation.**

2. **Meditate in your usual way for a few minutes to relax and focus your mind; then allow it to rest in its "natural state," as the Tibetans put it, without doing anything special.**

   If you can follow this exercise with your eyes open and gazing straight ahead at the space in front of you, great — that's how the Tibetans do it. But if you get distracted, you can close your eyes.

3. **Begin by noticing a particular thought as it arises and endures in your mind.**

   For example, you can take a memory, a plan, or a fantasy. Then ask yourself the following questions:

   • Does this thought have a particular shape or form? How big is it?

   • Does it have a particular color or colors?

   • Does it have a beginning, a middle, and an end?

   • Where is the thought located? Is it inside or outside your body?

   • From where did this thought arise? Where does it go when you're no longer thinking it? How long does it last when you continue to think it?

   • Does the thought have substance or is it just empty, open, and filled with space? Does it leave a trace in your mind, like footprints on the beach, or does it leave no trace, like writing on water?

4. **Turn your attention to your mind itself and ask the following questions.**

   Don't think about or analyze your mind or become preoccupied with its contents, such as thoughts or feelings. Instead, just look at your mind the way you would look at a bird or a tree. (Remember, the mind is what's important here, not the brain.) Take a few moments to respond to each question:

   • Does your mind itself have a shape or form? How big is it? Does it have a color or colors?

- Is your mind identical with your thoughts, or does it abide as the ground or space in which your thoughts arise and pass away?

- Where is your mind located? Is it inside or outside your body? Does it have a beginning or an end?

- Does your mind have substance like the earth or is it empty and spacious like the sky? Is it blank and dark, or is it bright and clear?

5. Allow your mind to rest for a few minutes in its "natural state."

Notice how the inquiry has affected you. Has your relationship to thoughts changed? Has your sense of identity shifted in some way? Do you feel calmer or more spacious? Take note of the changes; then gradually get up and go about your day.

Asking "Who am I?"

For as long as they've had the capacity to reflect on their experience, human beings have asked, "Who am I?" Zen masters, Sufi sheikhs, Indian sages, Jewish rabbis, and teachers of virtually every other spiritual persuasion have used this question to help their disciples see beyond their accustomed identities to a deeper realization of their essential nature.

When you first ask this question, you may come up with the usual answers: "I'm a woman," "I'm a father," "I'm an attorney," "I'm a runner." As you probe further, you may get more-spiritual answers, such as "I'm love incarnate" or "I'm a child of God." But if you just set these aside and continue to inquire, you'll eventually have a direct intuition of a more fundamental identity that has nothing to do with who you think you are.

Practice the following exercise with a partner, if possible. (One person begins by questioning; the other by answering.) If you don't have a partner handy, you can do it alone facing a mirror:

1. **Sit comfortably facing your partner, gazing at one another in a relaxed and natural way.**

2. **Allow the questioner to begin by asking, "Who are you?" Then the other person responds by saying whatever comes to mind.**

3. **After a pause, the questioner asks again, "Who are you?" and the other person again responds.**

   Of course, if you're doing it alone, you get to play both roles.

Book VII

Meditation, Mindfulness, and Letting Go of Stress

4. **Continue in this way for 15 minutes; then switch places for an equal amount of time.**

   If you're the questioner, don't critique or judge the answers in any way. Just listen, pause, and ask again.

   If you're the respondent, gently look for an answer; then respond. If you can't find one and have nothing to say for a moment or two, just sit with the silence and the not-knowing. You may become flustered or confused, start to laugh or cry, or have moments of deep stillness.

   Accept whatever arises, relax into the process, and keep going. Even a brief glimpse of who you really are can completely transform your life.

5. **When you're done, sit for a few minutes with your experience before getting up and going about your day.**

Finding a Teacher

A meditation instructor — someone who teaches you techniques, offers good advice on how to implement them, and helps you troubleshoot or fine-tune — can help you refine your practice and deal with basic questions that arise along the way. But if you want to deepen your practice and use it as a means to spiritual ends (as described in this chapter), you want to find a spiritual mentor or master.

Your spiritual teacher may coach and support you through the transformational process and even accelerate it by confronting the ways in which you resist or hold back. Some teachers act more like *spiritual friends,* treating you with the camaraderie and equality you expect from a peer, while also sharing their wealth of understanding. Others act more like *traditional gurus,* transmitting their understanding directly to you while actively pushing against your stuck places. (Of course, many teachers lie somewhere between these two extremes and combine a little of both styles.)

Whatever their approach, however, all good teachers help create and sustain, through their relationship with you, a sacred vessel or space in which the difficult, wondrous, and ultimately liberating process of spiritual transformation can take place inside you. They also possess these qualities (not all teachers will have every one of these characteristics, of course, but the more, the better):

- ✔ They're humble, ordinary, and down-to-earth, not arrogant or inflated. In Zen monasteries, the head monk cleans the toilets.

- ✔ They're honest, straightforward, and clear, not evasive or defensive. As people gain spiritual maturity, they become increasingly free of psychological baggage.

✔ They encourage independent thinking and open inquiry in their students rather than blind obedience to a particular dogma or ideology.

✔ They're primarily concerned with the spiritual development of their students, not with fame, power, influence, or the size of their organization.

✔ They practice what they preach instead of considering themselves exempt from the moral and ethical guidelines that others must follow.

✔ They embody the highest spiritual qualities, such as kindness, patience, equanimity, joy, peace, love, and compassion.

The process of finding a teacher can be as mysterious as the spiritual journey itself. For some people, it's a lot like finding a lover or a mate — it involves a complex mixture of luck, availability, and chemistry. For others, it's simply a matter of following the counsel of a friend or showing up at the right place at the right time. Ultimately, you need to trust your intuition, your own inner knowing, when choosing a teacher — it's the only reliable equipment you have for navigating in this flawed phenomenal universe.

Be open but not gullible, skeptical but not cynical. Feel free to ask questions, expect good answers, and take your time. According to the Dalai Lama, Tibetan students may spend years checking out teachers to make sure they embody the teachings they espouse. Just as you wouldn't rush into a marriage, you shouldn't rush into anything as intimate and deep as a relationship with a spiritual teacher.

Book VII

Meditation, Mindfulness, and Letting Go of Stress

Index

548 Yoga All-in-One For Dummies

About the Authors

Larry Payne, PhD, is an internationally prominent yoga teacher, author, workshop leader, and pioneer in the field of yoga therapy since 1980. Larry is the founding president of the International Association of Yoga Therapists and cofounder of the yoga curriculum at the UCLA School of Medicine. He was the first yoga teacher at the World Economic forum, was named "One of America's most respected yoga teachers" by the *Los Angeles Times,* and was selected as a yoga expert by Dr. Mehmet Oz, *Reader's Digest*, Web-MD, Rodale Press, and the *Yoga Journal.* In Los Angeles, Larry is the founding director of the Yoga Therapy Rx and Prime of Life Yoga programs at Loyola Marymount University. Larry is the coauthor of five books and is featured in the DVD series *Yoga Therapy Rx* and *Prime of Yoga.* Most recently he is coauthor "Yoga Therapy & Integrative Medicine" His website is www.samata.com.

Georg Feuerstein, PhD (1947–2012), studied and practiced yoga since his early teens and was a practitioner of Buddhist yoga. Internationally respected for his contribution to yoga research and the history of consciousness, he has been featured in many national magazines both in the United States and abroad. He authored more than 40 books, including *The Yoga Tradition*, *The Shambhala Encyclopedia of Yoga*, and *Yoga Morality*, which have been translated into eight languages. After his retirement in 2004, he designed and tutored several distance-learning courses on yoga philosophy for Traditional Yoga Studies, a Canadian company founded and directed by his wife, Brenda (see www.traditionalyogastudies.com).

Sherri Baptiste, an inspirational teacher at the forefront of yoga training in the United States, is the daughter of two of America's yoga-health-fitness pioneers — Magaña and Walt Baptiste — who established yoga on the West Coast in the mid-50s. Sherri has been teaching since her teens and is the founder of Baptiste Power of Yoga, a nationally recognized method of yoga, and Yoga with Weights. Sherri offers comprehensive training programs, including online learning and certification courses designed with mainstream appeal. These programs are registered and recognized by Yoga Alliance. A TV and radio personality, Sherri also teaches yoga classes throughout the United States and hosts retreats around the world. She is also a presenter for IDEA World Fitness, Western Athletics, Equinox, Gold's Gym, Body Mind Spirit, and ECA, and offers retreats at Montage Spas, Rancho La Puerta, Cal-A-Vie-Spa, Kripalu, Omega, International Yoga Therapy Conferences, Green Gulch and Tassajara Zen Centers, Esalan Institute, Noetic Institute, and Feathered Pipe Ranch. Her websites are www.powerofyoga.com and www.yogawithweights.com.

Doug Swenson is an internationally known yoga teacher and health educator. Doug began studying Yoga in 1964 with Dr. Ernest Wood and has been practicing and teaching Yoga ever since. Doug has studied under many great teachers, including Dr. Ernest Wood, Ramanand Patel, and K. Pattabhi Jois (guru of Ashtanga Yoga), from which Power Yoga was born. Doug is a master yoga practitioner and teacher dedicating his life to a holistic approach of yoga, learning from several different systems, and combining them with his interest in nutrition, concern for the environment, and warm, humorous approach to life to create his own unique and powerful system of yoga practice. Doug teaches yoga workshops and teacher-training courses across the U.S. and in other countries and is the author of three books on yoga and another book on diet and nutrition, plus many videos and DVDs. Contact Doug at dougswen002@yahoo.com or www.dougswenson.net.

Stephan Bodian is an internationally known author, psychotherapist, and teacher of mindfulness and spiritual awakening. As the founder and director of the School for Awakening, he leads regular retreats, workshops, and intensives and offers spiritual counseling and mentoring, by phone and Skype, to people throughout the world. His popular guidebook *Meditation For Dummies* (Wiley) has sold nearly a quarter of a million copies, and his digital program *Mindfulness Meditation (with Mental Workout)* has been praised in the *New York Times* and the *Wall Street Journal*. His most recent book, *Beyond Mindfulness* (available on Amazon.com), critiques the practice of mindfulness and offers a more direct approach to lasting happiness and peace. Stephan trained for many years as a Buddhist monk and edited the magazine *Yoga Journal* for a decade. His other books include *Buddhism For Dummies* (Wiley) and *Wake Up Now* (McGraw-Hill). For more information, visit www.stephanbodian.org.

Therese Iknoian, an internationally published and award-winning author and speaker, spent a decade as a newspaper reporter before launching a freelance career specializing in sports and fitness writing and instruction and earned her master's degree in exercise physiology. She, along with her husband, also operated a decade a successful news business for the outdoor and fitness industries for more than a decade. Today, Therese takes her adventurous spirit around the world, writing for their website, HI Travel Tales (www.HITravelTales.com) and working as a German-to-English translator (www.ThereseTranslates.com). She is a nationally ranked race walker and an ultra-runner. She has authored numerous books, including *Tai Chi For Dummies* (Wiley), *Mind-Body Fitness For Dummies* (Wiley), *Walking Fast* (Human Kinetics), and two editions of *Fitness Walking* (Human Kinetics). She was a contributing expert-author to *Precision Heart Rate Monitoring and Men's Fitness Magazine's Complete Guide to Health and Well-Being*, a contributing editor for the now-defunct Walking magazine, and the Ask the Coach columnist for eight years for *Trail Runner* magazine. She has been published in a wide range of popular magazines, including *Backpacker, Men's Health, Fitness, Health*, and *Women's Day,* and has written a self-syndicated fitness/sports newspaper column. She remains an American College of Sports Medicine-certified Health Fitness Specialist and a USA Track & Field Level II-certified endurance coach.

LaReine Chabut is a distinguished lifestyle and fitness expert, best-selling author, model, and mom. On *Focus on Feeling Better*, her weekly web series for MSN, LaReine took a well-rounded approach to healthy living as she helped everyday people deal with lifestyle issues and weight loss. LaReine's fitness books — *Lose That Baby Fat!*, *Exercise Balls For Dummies*,

Golf-All-in-One For Dummies (with Gary McCord), *Stretching For Dummies, Core Strength For Dummies, Dieting For Dummies*, and *Weight Training For Dummies*, among others — have sold over half a million copies. LaReine is the Director of Women's Health and Wellness for the International Sports Sciences Association. She is also the lead instructor of *The Firm*, a series of popular workout videos that have sold over three million copies worldwide. As a model, LaReine has appeared on the covers of *Shape, Health, New Body*, and *Runner's World*, and represents sports giant Nike. In addition, she has appeared on *Chelsea Lately* on E!, *Dr. Phil*, CNN, ABC, FOX News, *Extra, Access Hollywood*, and *Good Day LA*. To find out more about LaReine, go to www.LaReineChabut.com.

Deborah Myers, MS, CNS, is a lifetime practitioner of yoga, longtime student and writing associate of Larry Payne, PhD, and trained yoga teacher. Deborah brings yoga to her workplace and professional conferences in her field. In addition to her passion for yoga, Deborah is dedicated to improving the health and well-being of families. She is Chief of Nutrition and Breastfeeding Services at South LA Health Projects, a local agency of the USDA Special Supplemental Nutrition Program for Women, Infants, and Children (WIC).

Publisher's Acknowledgments

Acquisitions Editor: Tracy Boggier

Project Editor: Tracy L. Barr

Copy Editor: Megan Knoll

Technical Editor: Lisa Daugherty

Art Coordinator: Alicia B. South

Project Coordinator: Erin Zeltner

Illustrator: Pam Tanzey

Photographers: Bonnie Kamin, Adam Latham, Raul Marroquin

Cover Image: ©iStock.com/esolla